Rural Community
Mental Health Practice

Rural Community Mental Health Practice

by

John S. Wodarski, Ph.D.
Director, Research Center
School of Social Work
University of Georgia

University Park Press
Baltimore

UNIVERSITY PARK PRESS
International Publishers in Science, Medicine, and Education
300 North Charles Street
Baltimore, Maryland 21201

Typeset by Brushwood Graphics

Manufactured in the United States of America by Edwards Brothers

Library of Congress Cataloging in Publication Data

Wodarski, John S.
  Rural community mental health practice.

  Includes index.
  1. Rural mental health services. 2. Community mental health services. 3. Psychiatric social work—Study and teaching. I. Title. [DNLM: 1. Community mental health services. 2. Rural health. WA 305 W838r]
  RA790.5.W56   1983   363.2'0425   82–17464
  ISBN 0–8391–1785–X

Contents

v

Preface

This text represents the culmination of a five-year research project funded by the National Institute of Mental Health, Social Work Training Branch for the purpose of training graduate social work students for practice in rural community mental health. The project represents the intensifying interest in the practice of social work in rural areas. The country is witnessing a shift in population from urban to smaller towns and rural environments. Because people pack their troubles along with their belongings, community mental health services will certainly be necessary wherever the population moves. In recognition of this social change, my colleagues are expressing more interest in the area of rural social work. To date, seven Annual Institutes on Social Work in Rural Areas have taken place. Attendance and the number of papers presented have increased each year. At the Annual Program Meeting of the Council on Social Work Education the initial findings of our training program were presented. The turnout for our presentation and the lively discussion during and after gave evidence to the groundswell of interest in rural community mental health practice.

With the growing move toward smaller and more localized services comes a generated need for the identification of unique context attributes and specification of treatment rationale for rural practice. This text reviews initially requisite competencies for social workers practicing in rural community mental health. The conceptual competencies center on defining rural community mental health; labeling theory: heterogeneous versus homogeneous client groupings; de-institutionalization: assessment of individual attributes, community attributes, preparation of the community, preparation of individual, educating the individual and community, and maintaining placement; implementation of change strategy: where, by whom, why, how long, and on what level; and prevention. Seven general skills necessary for effective practice are reviewed: skills involved in relationship formation, interviewing skills, ability to define the target of change, competence in the assessment of the level on which the change strategy should be delivered, skill in choosing the appropriate change agent, skill in determining where treatment should be provided, and ability to specify the requisites for the evaluation of community treatment programs. Finally, means available to assess the competencies are elucidated: in-course training evaluation, practice observations, interviews, attitude testing, and follow-up procedures. The text concludes with a mention of the initial assessment of the program's effectiveness based on results of its implementation with the 18 Master's-level trainees.

There are many people who contributed to the successful execution of this training program. Specifically, I would like to thank Dr. Milt Whitman and Dr. Neilson Smith at the National Institute of Mental Health for their initial interest and subsequent conceptual and financial support throughout the duration of the program. Special appreciation goes to David Boyles, Ross Burggraf, and Ron Bates, who served as invaluable field instructors, and to the many agencies that provided our field work placements: Georgia Highlands Center, Canton, Georgia; Pineland Mental Health and Mental Retardation Services, Statesboro, Georgia; Alpine Center, Gainesville, Georgia; and Walton Area Mental Health Center, Monroe, Georgia. Next, recognition is given to the following students for their diligent work on this project in terms of executing requisite literature reviews for specific chapters of the text: Denise Dedman, Chapters 2 and 8; Linda Dimmock, Chapters 7 and 8; Alice Ford, general background information; June Leigh Green, Chapter 6; Ken McLeod, Chapter 1; Grace Riley, Chapter 5; Ron Sweet, Chapter 4; Vicky Young, Chapter 3; and Lisa Hawkins, Chapter 2. I would like to thank specifically one particular faculty member, Jeff Giordano, who helped me conceptualize and elucidate the competencies that were necessary for rural community mental health practice and who facilitated practicum placements of the students. Appreciation is expressed also to Dr. Steve Schinke who provided an invaluable analysis of the text and subsequently helped shape the final product.

To all who will in the future consider rural practice, I wish to emphasize the advantages of such a choice. Cedar and Salasin (*Research Directions for Rural Mental Health*. The MITRE Corp., McLean, Va., 1979) report that the positive aspects of rural area practice are often neglected and the negative ones emphasized. They see the high regard for professionals in a rural community as only one of many positive assets. Others include minimal pollution and traffic congestion, integration of family life, possibilities for unique career development and usually better housing opportunities. Students who will work in rural areas will experience these positive aspects of rural practice and be justly rewarded for their efforts.

I dedicate this book to my daughter Chrissie, whose early years were spent in an urban area but whose life, I am pleased to see, is greatly enriched through our move to a more small-town environment.

Rural Community
Mental Health Practice

Chapter 1

Rural Community Mental Health Practice

An Introduction

The last decade has witnessed a substantial change in the provision of services to major client groups as well as an increased interest in the provision of services to rural areas (Johnson, 1980; Walsh, 1981). Due to population shifts, in many respects rural practice could be considered a new frontier for the profession. Changing, too, is the tendency to remove individuals from their communities and to place them in institutions. Increasing emphasis now is on maintaining individuals in their communities through the provision of appropriate community-based residence care centers, family maintenance services, community support, outreach services, and so forth. This change in the provision of services promises a bright future for social workers practicing in rural community mental health. Not only does research evidence support the community health movement, that is, more normal and behavioral change and its maintenance can occur if clients are provided services in their daily interactional contexts, but additional supports are derived from improved economic and ethical aspects (Feldman, Caplinger, and Wodarski, 1983; Feldman, Wodarski, and Flax, 1973, 1975). Thus, it appears likely that the movement will continue to receive major emphasis in the years to come.

If social workers' involvement in rural community mental health is to continue to expand, practitioners must demonstrate specific competencies in this area. This text elucidates the rationale for conceptual, practice, and research competencies social workers must possess in order to claim a legitimate role in the practice of rural community mental health. It reviews the testing of a Master's level training program in rural community mental health funded for a 5-year period through the National Institute of Mental Health, Social Work Education Branch. The evolvement of the program through feedback from agencies and data provided by testing the adequacy of training through the competency-based model of education is elucidated. Implications are discussed for the education of social workers who will be prepared to practice in rural areas.

OVERVIEW OF PROGRAM

Rural trainees are enrolled in the Master's program at the University of Georgia School of Social Work. The present MSW program entails 18 months of training consisting of six quarters of class, laboratory, and fieldwork. Two quarters of course work precede three quarters of field instruction. Two 3-hour practice theory seminars are required during practicum. The final quarter of course work includes research, an advanced elective, and a required course in the student's specialty.

Students involved in the rural mental health project receive three specialized courses in mental health policy, treatment methods, and current issues in practice; one individual study course in rural mental health; and three practicum courses (4 days per week) in a rural mental health agency, totaling 50 hours of specialized course work.

Four practicum sites in rural Georgia were carefully selected. Students are placed in two different rural areas of the state, the mountains and the farmlands. Both areas consistently show rural characteristics. In the majority of situations students are placed in teams of two in each of the settings. Each site represents some variation in rural setting attributes. Perhaps this is best illustrated by the different work patterns that were adopted by the students, all of whom were located in satellites of community mental health centers. Students in the most rural areas worked several different counties using largely local, makeshift facilities, less frequently using the home satellite for client contact and traveling substantially to provide services. Students in a less rural setting often worked evenings and therefore developed specialized programs for evenings. Students in a third setting, a rural area between Atlanta and the home office located in a sizeable college community, had the most traditional work situation. At each setting MSW supervision was provided.

Every educational program, whether it occurs through undergraduate, graduate, or continuing education, should equip practitioners with the best empirically based rationale that exists for practice requisites (Wodarski, 1979a, 1981). Literature reviews have led to the isolation of five components that provide the rationale for the conceptualization of requisite practice competencies. These are: defining rural community mental health practice, covered in this chapter; labeling theory; procedures for deinstitutionalization; implementation of change strategy— where, by whom, why, how long, and on what level; and prevention. Additionally, a cluster of necessary practice skills have been identified and operationalized.

DEFINING RURAL COMMUNITY MENTAL HEALTH

Review of the literature reveals little agreement among mental health professionals as to the definitions of mental health and mental illness. Likewise, there is also difficulty in defining the parameters of community mental health. Bloom, in 1973 and 1977, suggested that community mental health refers to all activities under-

taken in the community in the name of mental health. He suggests nine characteristics of community mental health: 1) emphasis on practice in the community as
opposed to practice in institutional settings, for example, sending clients to
institutions for services as a last means of delivering services; 2) emphasis on total
defined population rather than on individual patients considered singularly, for
example, potential child abusers; 3) emphasis on preventive services as dis-
tinguished from therapeutic services, for example, stress reduction for hypertension (1, 2, and 3 stress application of public health concepts to the field of
psychotherapy); 4) emphasis on indirect services, for example, consultation,
education, and so forth are executed by the MSW trained practitioner, whereas the
bachelor's-level social worker provides direct service; 5) emphasis on innovative
clinical strategies, such as brief psychotherapy and crisis intervention. In social
work practice the task-centered model and other short-term treatment models are
appropriate. 6) Emphasis on the rational planning process in decision-making
regarding mental health programs; that is, assessing needs and planning requisite
intervention based on data and empirical theoretical rationale; 7) innovative use of
new sources of manpower, for example, "paraprofessional" or "indigenous
mental health worker," or the use of the natural helping networks that exist in rural
areas, such as the church and extended family; 8) commitment to community
control, for example, staff should join with the community or its representatives to
identify needs and purpose and to establish and evaluate programs; 9) view of the
community as having certain counterproductive stress-inducing properties, rather
than assuming psychopathology is exclusively an individual problem, for example, high unemployment, inadequate health facilities, and lack of appropriate
educational services are community variables.

Experience with undergraduates and the 20 previous graduate trainees in
community mental health at the University of Georgia is in accord with the
literature which indicates that community mental health workers must be prepared
to deal with the following practice tasks: needs assessment surveys; alcoholism
and drug abuse programs; mental health consultation by and for diverse groups;
varied types of crisis intervention programs; selection, training, and evaluation of
nontraditional helping agents, informal help-giving processes, natural care givers,
and community support networks; early detection and intervention; education and
prevention; and alternate service delivery models for inner city and rural individuals (Cowen, 1978). Thus, to ensure the quality of the services provided,
practitioners must be trained in such a manner to offer the foregoing services in a
competent manner (Berg, Cohen, and Reid, 1978; Feldman, 1978). A major step
toward meeting this objective would be to develop and evaluate methods of
training social workers for practice in rural community mental health. A first step
in attaining the first competency is to understand the parameters of rural practice.

Parameters of Rural Practice

Training procedures are geared toward helping students understand the culture of
rural settings, that is, distinctive living patterns. Characteristics elaborated on are

the isolation of clients and workers from other professionals, lack of transportation to secure the limited services available, the declining employment base resulting in limited incomes, how the established power structure will affect the worker's integration in the community, and the lack of formal education of clients. Personal attributes of rural individuals are emphasized to help students see how the emphasis on self-reliance and fatalism will affect the acceptance of services and what community networks, such as the church, farmer's cooperative, and formal and informal power structures can be used to facilitate the acceptance of services (Ginsberg, 1971). How such personal attributes influence who should be the primary providers of services is also reviewed. For example, in many instances the general practitioner (GP) is the professional the family deals with first, and through being a part of the culture, he or she can help the family accept services (Lerner and Blackwell, 1975; Weber, 1976).

Students also are helped to see how practice in rural community mental health will affect their professional activities in terms of lack of support due to the limited number of professional contacts in rural settings, how they will be called on to be a jack-of-all-trades, that is, in coordination and provision of services in terms of a micro-macro intervention continuum, how they must enlist the support of community leaders to gain the necessary community support for their programs, and how the social system is a major influence in who is labeled to receive services (Fenby, 1978; Horejsi and Deaton, 1977).

The program described here equips students to perform the following requisite roles for practice: the identification of primary health providers, both professional and paraprofessional; the provision of service through networks such as the church that will facilitate the worker's acceptance; development and coordination of services, that is, how to initially present mental health services to rural communities so as to maximize their acceptance; how to make use of indigenous caretakers and various professionals already residing in the community; and how to coordinate their services with existing indigenous caretaking networks in such a way that the former can improve the efficacy of the latter in dealing with the rural community's mental health needs (Katz, 1978; Kelley et al., 1977; Naftulin, Donnelly, and O'Halloran, 1974; Shupe, 1974). Minority content centers on black individuals because they constitute the primary minority group in the southeast. Special attention is paid to factors leading to hypertension; support networks available in black communities, that is, churches, families, and kinship groups; particular interpersonal difficulties associated with rural isolation of the aged black population; and so forth.

Characteristics of Rural Communities

The major characteristic of rural communities, as might be expected, is the higher incidence of poverty over their urban counterparts (Coppedge and Davis, 1977). Limitations in income inevitably affect one's ability to satisfy one's needs. In this case, lack of income may prohibit clients from gaining access to needed social services, such as mental health and welfare programs. Even when services are available, one's financial circumstances, in many instances, make them inaccessible. For example, a potential client of service agencies may be unable to secure help because the client cannot afford the transportation to the agency.

Money has been poured into rural communities through such programs as the Rural Development Act of 1972 for the purpose of increasing rural development and reducing unemployment. Programs designed to reduce unemployment and underemployment, however, have failed when they were not designed with an evaluation component to assess their effectiveness. Likewise, assessment data are necessary to alter the program when necessary to meet the needs of rural communities (Karsten, 1975; Wodarski, 1979b).

Personal satisfaction and happiness are adversely affected by poverty, and the public, in general, have a negative outlook on the poor, particularly those receiving government aid (Yokelson, 1975). This being the case, it is easier to understand the plight of rural community residents. They are locked into a situation which demands that they receive additional services but at the same time threatens their self-esteem and their standing in the community. To provide effective services, social work practitioners must be aware of this dilemma.

The rural community characteristically holds traditional views regarding sex roles (Cormican, 1979; Glenn and Hill, 1977). In rural areas the husband generally remains the head of the household. He is recognized as the one who maintains the family financially. In family matters that require an authority figure to make a decision, he, in the majority of instances, fills this role while the wife primarily maintains the role of homemaker. She rarely has a job outside of the home. Her role is to support the family by taking care of household responsibilities, tending to the children, and providing emotional support. She is submissive to her husband's position of authority. Now, however, with inflation affecting the rural communities, it has become necessary for women to work, thus creating another set of problems.

Another common characteristic of rural communities is that of rugged individualism and pride within the community (Cormican, 1979; Goudy and Wepprecht, 1977). This encompasses the notion of self-sufficiency. Rural community dwellers often hold individual accomplishment and hard work to be virtues. Although these may sound like attributes worthy of praise, they often entail the fatalistic attitude that they have no control over shaping their lives and destinies (Cormican, 1979). In other words, they feel that no matter what they do they have little control over the situations life thrusts upon them.

Rural communities are often suspicious of outsiders (Cormican, 1979). Newcomers are often scrutinized carefully to see if they will conform to the norms of the community, if they represent a threat to the status quo, and what value they are to rural ways of life. Those who conform are gradually accepted into the community. Those who do not are set apart and remain relatively isolated from the community.

A critical aspect of rural practice is that of understanding the power structure of a particular community (Cormican, 1979). In the majority of instances there is an informal network of control within the rural community that performs many of the same functions of its more formalized urban counterpart. How these networks are composed varies from one community to the next, but law enforcement personnel, church leaders, local businessmen, and farmers are typical components. If the professional intends to practice within the rural community, he or she must be aware of and work within this network to be most effective. Ignoring the network can lead to the isolation of service providers and to subsequent lack of support by community leaders, thus jeopardizing the provision of necessary service to clients.

Rural communities tend to hold conservative religious and political viewpoints (Glenn and Hill, 1977). Again, outsiders are often judged by whether or not they conform to or reject this viewpoint. Liberals who threaten or are seen as potential threats to the conservative foundations of the community are essentially set apart from the community and rendered ineffective. In many instances the community will take note whether or not one is affiliated with a religious group, supports local athletic teams, and attends community functions, and will use this as a measure of one's conservative or liberal biases.

In rural communities residents tend to know each other better than in urban areas (Goudy and Wepprecht, 1977). For this reason it is not easy to go unnoticed when one enters the rural setting. In such a situation, personal matters, which might otherwise go unnoticed, may become common knowledge within the community. Those who prefer leading more private lives than this may, unintentionally, leave the impression that they have something to hide and thus will not be integrated.

Finally, in rural communities physical isolation of the residents in the outermost areas of the community is a significant factor (Cormican, 1979). This isolation is often compounded by the lack of transportation and poverty, and at times may be total as a result of adverse weather conditions. The more isolated the people the more likely they are to exhibit "traditional" rural characteristics.

INTEGRATING THE WORKER INTO THE RURAL COMMUNITY

Community Attitudes and Expectations

Residents of small communities base their acceptance of each other on the basis of the person rather than the occupation (Wedel, 1969). Mental health professionals also will most likely be accepted or rejected on these same merits. Gaps in professional competence can be forgiven (or even welcomed) if the staff members are the kind of people whom you can "get along with." Thus, the new worker must be advised not to come on too strong during the initial integration period. That is, he or she must be careful not to use big words, to dress "differently," or to use professional titles inappropriately. Huessy (1972a) adds that clients do not relate to agencies, they relate to the people in the agencies. With this in mind, mental health practitioners should concentrate on the first requisite in building services in rural areas, that is, to produce effective workers and subsequently to build programs and facilities. This general interactional pattern and attitude has been referred to in the literature as the "Good Joe" complex (Buxton, 1973).

The implications of the practice context for the social work practitioner new to the rural area have been discussed by Buxton (1973), among others. In most cases, the mental health workers are visibly different from the "locals." They look, dress, and act differently and are rarely initially accepted as Good Joes. They are often not only viewed as outsiders, but also as a symbol of mass society and, as such, are not readily welcomed into the community and must work at being accepted. The tendency is for new rural mental health workers to respond to this coldness on the part of the community with a tendency to be behaviorally defensive and to maintain a professional distance which, at times, will have a negative bearing on the community's acceptance of the services and programs (Fenby, 1978).

Fenby (1978) points out two other significant facets of life in rural areas that can confound the new rural practitioner. The first of these is the existence of the grapevine, or gossip, circuit of communication. One of the encouraging features of this type of communication system is that any positive information passed along the grapevine about the professionals or the services will greatly enhance the early acceptance and utilization of the services by the general population. On the other hand, negative reports regarding the services or the behavior of the mental health professionals coursing through the grapevine may well seriously jeopardize the very existence of the program. This ties into the second facet of rural life, the visibility of both the worker and the client. As has been noted, the worker is usually visibly different and, in a small community in which everyone knows everyone else on a first name basis, the worker is under careful and constant scrutiny. Peculiarities, eccentricities, and objectionable or unacceptable behavior will readily become known throughout the community and will undoubtedly lead to rejection of both the worker and of the services he or she has to offer. Thus, the new worker must be careful not to exhibit behaviors that permit such a labeling process to occur.

New rural social work professionals must acknowledge and accept their vulnerability and cope with the pressures that accompany visibility. This is prerequisite to the professional's being able to help the clients accept and deal with their own unique problems of visibility. As mentioned by Gertz, Meider, and Pluckhan (1975), clients feel that the whole town sees them when they walk into the mental health center. It may well be that when they go to the center the event is transmitted through the grapevine with their appointment becoming generally known throughout the community, or it may simply be an expression of the client's feelings of vulnerability. In either case, the issue is a valid concern that must be addressed by the professional within the treatment context. Workers who are caught up in their own concerns of visibility will certainly be less able and willing to deal with the client's similar concerns and, consequently, will be less able to provide open, honest, and effective services to reduce these concerns.

New social workers in rural areas assume that nothing is happening in rural areas because there are no large groups of people or buildings. They erroneously posit that life in the rural community is simple (Buxton, 1973). These assumptions will undoubtedly lead new workers into a quagmire that will render them totally ineffective in the delivery of services to rural communities and areas. It is the responsibility of the professional to recognize and acknowledge the unique patterns in rural areas and to abide, to a degree, by the rules of the community. Gertz, Meider, and Pluckhan (1975) state that the professional must demonstrate an acceptance of the conservative rural ethic and integration into the small-town cultural patterns. There is a need to understand the community's "self-image," or the view of the community held by the inhabitants, combined with a recognition of the dynamic interplay of community forces (Klein, 1965). This includes issues such as a sensitivity to local concerns and etiquette along with a tuning in to the shared attitudes, feelings, values, and opinions of the residents in a community or area (Buxton, 1973; Cardoza, Ackerly, and Leighton, 1975). Even after the social worker has successfully dealt with these issues in the area or community, the task of establishing and delivering the services will be hampered by a general resistance to innovation and change found in many rural areas (Bachrach, 1977). This resistance may prove frustrating but it should not be an insurmountable obstacle to the development of effective services and programs in the community, provided the services can be identified as addressing a community-acknowledged need and are supported by the power structure.

Attitudes and expectations in rural areas have precipitated a debate or disagreement in the literature regarding semantics or terminology. Rands (1960) feels that there is likely benefit in avoiding the term *mental hospital* and similar terms due to the stigma or negative connotations attached to these terms. For the area in which he was involved, he proposed that the facilities be referred to as regional psychiatric centers. There was objection to the name change because people felt it would be better to put new meaning into the old term rather than attempting to avoid the stigmatization issues simply by changing a name.

Tranel (1970) also discusses a disagreement surrounding terminology in one small town during a discussion of the sign to put on the door of the mental health center. The mental health professional wanted to use the name *counseling center,* whereas the board, on the other hand, wanted the traditional name *mental health center* as it described the functions of the center as was consistent with their expectations. Again, this reflects a resistance to innovation and change as well as an example of the type of attitudes and expectations that exist in many rural areas. It cannot be stressed strongly enough that the social work professional unaccustomed to rural areas must progress carefully and be ever mindful of the pulse of the community and area. To do otherwise will prove to be both frustrating and unsuccessful in delivering of services in these areas.

Community Support and Involvement

Buxton (1973) states that social workers must work with the community to help the community solve its problems instead of trying to force change that is "good" for the community but that is contradictory to community desires. Additionally, as has been discussed, there must be recognition on the part of the professional that he or she is an outsider trying to gain support from insiders in the community (Kiesler, 1969). Overt violations of local norms frequently lead to painful confrontations and, due to the visibility issue, the rural professional has nowhere to go once he or she has violated the norms of the community (Ginsberg, 1969). Once this phenomenon occurs, the change agent's ability to provide requisite services is substantially compromised. Although these issues have been discussed in other sections of this chapter, it is believed that they are of sufficient import to justify their use in this discussion of community support and involvement.

As the building contractor acknowledges the importance of a firm, carefully constructed foundation before building a home in which he or she would be willing to live, so must the mental health professional be concerned with the type of community foundation on which he or she will build a program for service delivery. With a firm foundation, the program will also grow firmly and solidly in the community. One consideration involved in building this foundation is starting from where the community or area "is at." As has been discussed by Ramage (1971), these areas lack necessary medical, paramedical, rehabilitative, and other services, and facilities and initial efforts will have to be directed at mobilizing available community resources to meet these needs. Even greater effort will have to be made to educate and stimulate community leaders and to motivate political officials to enact social legislation to bring these support services to these areas. Along with this, the professional should have an awareness of formal and informal lines of communication and should take advantage of the local systems of communication to keep the community informed (Buxton, 1973; Jeffrey and Reeve, 1978). These community communication issues will be discussed later in more detail.

Utilization of local resources is crucial to the building of a foundation and to the success of a program as has been discussed by Buxton (1973) and Huessy (1972 a, b). Buxton states that local resources should be tapped as well as universities or other resources outside of the community. He feels the utilization of volunteers and advisory groups are a vital link to community attitudes and support. Huessy elaborates that one should look around the area to find out what skills are available in the population and should take advantage of those persons with such skills. He posits that it is advisable to use local talent to gear programs to the local personality rather than trying to force an area to adapt to a new system or design. Huessy points out that one way of accomplishing this is to find out who people turn to presently for mental health services in the community. It has been his experience that, in many cases, it is a former nurse or a current general medical practitioner. The use of local talent for programming of services will also positively affect the community acceptance of the services, providing the individuals have a position of esteem or positive regard in the view of the residents of the community or area.

Power Structure

The professional's understanding of community groups and power structure is prerequisite for effective practice. The nature of community groups and their characteristic interactional patterns vary from area to area and are radically different from those found in most urban areas (Klein, 1965). Likewise, there must be an awareness of the informal power structure in the community, an entity that is often ignored by many professionals who only contact the individuals in the formal power structure (Buxton, 1973). As is pointed out by Gurevitz and Heath (1969), the mental health professional in rural areas will have to contend with a variety of power alliances, traditions, sentiments, and control issues of the type to which he or she is totally unaccustomed. One way of approaching these issues is to develop partnerships with community groups to help alleviate suspicions about mental health programs and services (Gertz, Meider, and Pluckhan, 1975). In this manner, communication is enhanced and the opportunity for gaining community support and involvement is greatly improved.

It is essential that mental health practitioners in rural areas be aware that, in most cases, the total level of support in a community depends on the will of a few influential people in the community (Libo and Griffith, 1966). This is reiterated by Tranel (1970) who states that it is often easier to obtain wide community support for a program than it is to overcome the resistances and prejudices of a few key persons. This difficulty frequently is manifested in a situation in which the professional feels he or she has the general population in support of a program but still is confounded in efforts to get the program "rolling." The frustrated professional, upon closer examination, may find a group of businessmen, industrialists, large land owners, or other small but influential groups in opposition to the program and, consequently, subverting any efforts to establish the program in the community. If this is the situation, efforts will have to be directed toward engaging this power group to gain either their support or, in some cases, simply their permission to develop the program. This situation, as well as other factors, can contribute to what is described by Gurevitz and Heath (1969) as the differences between the "official" view of the community and that of the residents.

Rural politics plays a crucial role in the success or the demise of programs and ideas. As pointed out by Gertz, Meider, and Pluckhan (1975) in reference to rural programs, a knowledge of rural politics and power structures and the ability to develop informal patterns of communication with key community officials is essential to effective functioning. Ginsberg (1969) and Tranel (1970) add to this that rural government is less democratic than the urban counterpart. The decisions are usually made by a few for the majority, and this small elite usually expresses the inarticulate sentiments of the majority and rules over a numerically superior but powerless majority. Tranel also finds that governmental mechanisms are usually atrophied in rural communities and, consequently, are not employed in a meaningful way in the local decision-making process. The local government may or may not be comprised of the influential persons described previously, and it is the responsibility of the professional to determine where the "official" and the "real" power reside in the community.

Developing Community Support

A major means of educating and eliciting the support of the community, essential for acceptance of services, is through the use of a town meeting (Kiesler, 1969). The issues of community support and involvement and the use of a town meeting were elaborated on by Tranel (1970) in his discussion of the efforts to establish a successful community mental health program in one Wyoming community. The Chamber of Commerce was induced to appoint a steering committee, headed by a prominent businessman, to investigate a program and an effort was made to involve respected community leaders such as the newspaper editor, main street businessmen, the school superintendent, a physician, real estate dealers, and several other active community workers. This steering committee, in turn, sought to gain community support through the use of a town meeting and recruited about 75 people to function on various task forces. The town meeting can be an effective tool for eliciting community support and involvement but will prove still more effective if the professional can first gain the support of key, influential persons in the community and have those persons, rather than the mental health professional, organize and facilitate the town meeting.

At this time, it may prove beneficial to identify some of the individuals and groups that the mental health professional should contact for the development of cooperative working relationships, support, and involvement. The first group, the ministers in the community, have been discussed by numerous authors (Alexander, 1941; Cardoza, Ackerly and Leighton, 1975; Gurevitz and Heath, 1969; Libo and Griffith, 1966). Depending on the area, religion will play a greater or lesser role in the lives of the members of the community. In religious areas, acceptance of the mental health program by the religious leaders in a community will almost assure success in gaining the support of the community. In these areas, on the other hand, disapproval of the program by the influential ministers may result in the total inability of the professional to establish a program of services in that community or area. Also to be considered is the fact that most ministers are already involved in some degree of pastoral or mental health counseling and may or may not be receptive to abdicating this role to a new professional and mental health program. Although it is extremely doubtful that any professional would either desire or request total responsibility for a community's total mental health needs, some clergy may interpret the professional's entrance into the community as such. A far more frequent situation will arise in which the ministers want to voluntarily turn all their counseling responsibilites over to the new mental health professionals out of desire for the best possible treatment for their parishioners. In contacting them, the professional should encourage the ministers to continue their counseling roles while only referring especially difficult or problemmatic cases to the professionals. To accomplish this it may be helpful to offer the clergy in-service training to enhance their skills as counselors or other types of consultation, either on an individual basis or in groups. Ministers can provide important and complementary mental health services in the community if the effort is made by the professional to foster a sharing and cooperative working relationship.

A second constituency that should be contacted are the lawyers in the community (Huessy, 1972a). Lawyers may be disinterested initially in working with the mental health program, feeling that they have little need to get involved. It is the task of the professional to point out to the lawyers the many ways in which a cooperative working relationship can be mutually beneficial. In their practices, lawyers occasionally deal with issues such as guardianship for mental deficiency or incapacity cases, probate, involuntary commitment proceedings, and client competency hearings in regard to criminal cases. If the lawyers are aware that the mental health program includes diagnostic and consultation services, they may see the importance of their working with the professionals for the mutual benefit of their clients. The judiciary, likewise, is an important group to contact for the development of cooperative working relationships for many of the same reasons. Additionally, where the mental health program includes drug and alcohol treatment services, the judiciary should be made aware of both the capabilities and the limitations of these services to avoid misunderstandings and to enable appropriate disposition of cases from the bench.

Probation personnel also have been identified as a group to contact in the community (Libo and Griffith, 1966). In most areas, the probation officers play a major role in conducting the presentencing investigations and in making recommendations to the bench regarding the disposition of cases. If the mental health program is willing to accept mandated clients for drug, alcohol, or psychiatric treatment, these programmatic aspects should be cooperatively designed and mutually agreeable prior to any recommendations for treatment. With continued communication, both compliance and violation of mandated orders will be regularly reported for the most effective service delivery and fair disposition of these problemmatic cases to the satisfaction of all parties involved. In addition, if social and vocational rehabilitation services also are available through the mental health program, this information should be made known to the probation/parole personnel as it may prove to be of benefit and appropriate for the individuals under the supervision of the judicial system.

Another significant related group that should be contacted by the mental health professional is the law enforcement personnel (Gurevitz and Heath, 1969;

Libo and Griffith, 1966). The mental health program should be able to offer inservice training and consultation to assist them in dealing with psychiatric emergencies because, in most rural areas, they will be the initial respondent to community requests for aid. The professional might also consider having the staff available to respond to emergencies along with the law enforcement personnel to assist them in resolving domestic disputes and situations involving potentially suicidal or homicidal individuals. Because the situations are not rare in most rural areas, the offer of assistance will most likely be viewed positively by the law enforcement personnel and may serve to help avert a possible tragedy in the community. One substantial benefit to a good working relationship with law enforcement personnel is that, on those occasions when the professionals are confronted with a violent and/or assaultive client, the local constabulary will be more likely to respond readily to provide assistance in resolving the crisis. It is a well accepted fact that the presence of a uniformed officer will often calm the client and deter violence.

Health department officials, and specifically the public health nurses, are two related groups that also should be contacted (Libo and Griffith, 1966). In many rural areas, the health department can play a major role in the delivery of mental health services. The facilities of the health department can provide an economical and accessible site for traveling outpatient clinics and are currently used as such in many areas around the country. This type of relationship allows for the health department to have services readily available for the total health and well-being of its clients, not just physical health aspects. This local support also enhances the acceptability of mental health services in the community and legitimizes the professional's position in the eyes of the residents of the area. Public health nurses also can become important allies to the mental health professional in that they have more access to the community. They can act as a source of referrals and as legitimizing agents for mental health, and can provide monitoring activities and other information about a client's progress to the professional. In return, the professional will provide an avenue for referral and disposition of problemmatic mental health cases to relieve the nurses of this burden they often carry in rural areas. Likewise, the mental health professional can provide inservice training and consultation services for the public health nurses in an effort to make their jobs easier in dealing with certain clients. As has been discussed earlier, nurses often play a major role in the delivery of mental health services in areas that lack the services of mental health professionals. The new mental health professional should keep this in mind while developing a cooperative working relationship with nurses in the community so as not to inadvertently alienate them.

Nonpsychiatric physicians are another group that often have a major responsibility for the mental health needs and services in areas lacking professional services. They can continue to be important to the mental health professional as a program is being developed (Cardoza, Ackerly, and Leighton, 1975; Huessy, 1972a). Consultation and education services can be offered to the physicians by the mental health professional and consequently may prove to be of immense value with regard to early detection and prevention efforts in the community. The professional must be alert for any signs of resentment or negative attitudes toward the new mental health program and stress the cooperative nature of the relationship with the physicians. In most areas, however, the nonpsychiatric physicians will be more than willing to relinquish responsibilities for many of their counseling roles and will be quite cooperative with respect to medication monitoring and related aspects of the more traditional physician-oriented mental health services. Again, the cooperative relationship should be stressed, as opposed to a replacement approach, in the development of services in communities in which the physicians historically have played a consistent major role in the delivery of mental health services.

Welfare professionals also should be contacted for the development of a mutually beneficial cooperative working relationship. In many cases, welfare and mental health programs have a considerable number of clients in common and, therefore, a close working relationship is imperative for effective case coordination and management. The welfare workers, with in-service training and consultation, can become increasingly involved in prevention and early detection efforts within the community as well as in the referral of individuals and families when indicated. In addition, the mental health professional can offer child, adolescent, adult, and family counseling services to the clients of welfare personnel in an effort to remedy problems in cases involving neglect, abuse, or other family-oriented problems. With coordinated service delivery, the opportunity for beneficial impact on these types of family problems will be enhanced. Ongoing communication is one of the basic keys to the maintenance of a relationship oriented toward case coordination where mutual clients are involved (Wodarski and Feldman, 1974).

Family problems often can be identified and addressed through the development of a cooperative working relationship with school personnel. Often referrals that come from school personnel request treatment aimed toward extinguishing disruptive behavior as demonstrated by a student in the classroom. In-service training and consultation by the mental health professional may help school personnel to recognize types of behavior change that could be indicative of family problems at home as well as methods of initial intervention before referral to the professional. Through the proper working relationship, the professional can help teachers, principals, and others in the school system recognize that sudden manifestations of negative behavior are often linked to family problems and can best be effectively managed through family intervention. A good relationship with school personnel will also give the mental health professional an opportunity to engage in preventive practice with the student population through the use of presentations, group discussions, and other tenchiques specifically designed to engage children and adolescents for the purpose of promoting mental health. Specifics of such interventions will be elaborated in Chapter 5.

Civic community leaders have been identified and discussed previously, but their importance must be stressed once again in this discussion of groups and individuals who should be contacted for the development of cooperative working relationships (Eisdorfer, Altrocchi, and Young, 1968; Libo and Griffith, 1966). Support from this group can be critical in initial efforts to establish a mental health program; but it is also important on a continuous basis to encourage general community mental health, early detection and prevention, and appropriate use of treatment and services. Moreover, many service clubs will from time to time sponsor activities or fund-raising drives to financially support special mental health programs and services or in response to unique needs found in the community. In numerous instances, these service clubs have also assisted in individual cases to help clients with special needs purchase eyeglasses, hearing aids, and wheel chairs and to obtain limited traveler's-aid type of assistance. These clubs and organizations also provide the mental health professional an opportunity to make presentations about mental health and mental health services at their meetings, luncheons, and other events, thus providing a means of educating the community.

Private mental health practitioners in the community must not be neglected by the new mental health professional coming into the area (Libo and Griffith, 1966). The new professional occasionally may confront attitudes ranging from mild skepticism to open hostility on the part of the private practitioner; and it is the new worker who must take the responsibility for initiating contact with the private sector. The private practice community must be assured that the new program is not designed to compete with them, only to complement the service they are presently providing in the community. It may also be possible or desirable to engage these professionals in a mutual consultation relationship or to hire them as consultants to the new mental health program. An excellent means of soliciting support from the private sector is to ask them to serve as representatives on the advisory or executive board of the new program. This may help to dispel the suspicion and fear on the part of private practitioners with regard to their possible loss of livelihood with the advent of the new public mental health program. In most cases, the private practice community will be accepting and cooperative with the new program but, again, it is the responsibility of the new mental health professional to seek out the private practitioners in the community and to cultivate the cooperative working relationship. One cannot assume this cooperative relationship will automatically develop simply because both the private practitioners and the new program staff are involved in the delivery of mental health services in the community. With a paucity of mental health professionals in rural areas, the failure to take advantage of the presence of a valuable resource such as private practitioners would be a costly error on the part of the new mental health professional and would ultimately be a disservice to the community.

The preceding list of groups and individuals to be solicited by the mental health professional is far from exhaustive. It is, however, a sampling of the diverse types of groups in rural areas that have a potential impact on the development and operation of mental health programs. The identification of pertinent groups in each unique community should be accomplished during the initial assessment of the community or service area. The manner in which the professional approaches both the groups and the total community will have a decided effect on the overall effectiveness of the program and may in fact determine its very survival.

Public Education about Mental Health in Rural Communities

An initial task for the new mental health professional will be the attempt to dispel myths surrounding mental illness and to replace these myths with facts about mental health and community mental health treatment programs. For example, one myth commonly encountered in rural areas is that the mentally ill will not benefit from treatment on an outpatient basis in the home community. As pointed out by Bentz, Edgerton, and Kherlopian (1969), persons in the rural community often believe the mentally ill should be sent for treatment to the mental hospital or to the general hospital with a psychiatric unit. They apparently believe that these persons are sick and are best treated in hospital facilities by doctors.

The professional must be prepared to address this type of belief with patience and tolerance and be able to supply facts to counter the myths. This is particularly important when the major focus of mental health services is deinstitutionalization. Myths generally have firm basis in ignorance, false information, family values, and/or community tradition, and the community will likely part with their beliefs grudgingly, if at all. Likewise, educational level has been found to have a high correlation with one's ability to identify and perceive mental illness (Bentz, Edgerton and Kherlopian, 1969). As was discussed in an earlier section on differences between rural and urban areas, the rural area is significantly disadvantaged in both the general level of education of its residents and in the area of educational opportunity. With this in mind, it is not surprising that myths and misconceptions would be more prevalent in rural areas than in urban areas.

At the same time, the worker's educational level and his or her professional affiliations can create a communications gap rather than provide a tool for re-educating. Gertz, Meider, and Pluckhan (1975) emphasize that the mental health professional must take great care to translate terminology and jargon into language understandable to the local population. A failure to do so will promote suspicion, confusion, and, most likely, rejection of both the professional and the program of services. In contacting groups and individuals for the purpose of developing cooperative working relationships, the use of jargon and unfamiliar terminology will ultimately be viewed as insulting and intimidating. As a result, the professional is more likely to find resentment and hostility, rather than cooperation and support.

A major focus of educational programs should be on informing the population about available services. Rural residents frequently are not aware of even the meager mental health services that currently exist in the community (Edgerton and Bentz, 1969). This problem should be addressed in the growth and development stages of the mental health program but often is not given due consideration. Furthermore, Lee, Gianturco, and Eisdorfer (1974) state that real accessibility requires more than visibility or mere knowledge of the existence of a service. The lack of knowledge about what constitutes a mental health problem is a major barrier to obtaining services, primarily among the lower classes. Again, the absence of facts will often lead to the proliferation of myths and misconceptions about mental illness and mental health. It is the new mental health professional's responsibility to assess the overall impact of these characteristics in the community and to develop an educational program designed to address them accordingly.

Assessing Current Availability of Mental Health and Other Services

A first step in establishing a new center is to assess the nature of the existing human services system (Jeffrey and Reeve, 1978). The impact of a new center on the rural community is considerable as compared to the urban area. The new mental health professional must be attuned to not only the lack of professional mental health services and facilities as discussed by Libo and Griffith (1966), but he or she must have an awareness and consideration of the location in the community of various services, agencies, and institutions, such as social service agencies, schools, hospitals, and even main shopping areas (Klein, 1965). Considerations regarding availability of mental health and other services are discussed in Chapter 4. It is mentioned here, however, to reiterate the importance of assessing the availability of these in the initial phase of contact with the community.

Relationship to Other Service Providers

After the initial assessment of current services, an important consideration in the establishment of a service delivery system in rural areas is the development of the relationship with other professional personnel and agencies (Cardoza, Ackerly and Leighton, 1975; Clayton, 1977; Gurevitz and Heath, 1969; Huessy, 1972b; Ramage, 1971; Rands, 1960). Clayton (1977) points out the need for more coordination of services and programs due to the limited financial and manpower resources available in rural areas. To this end, Gurevitz and Heath (1969) suggest the creation of health systems composed of private practitioners, hospitals, and clinics, and using these systems to facilitate the creation of other systems whose mental health function is subsumed under their basic responsibilities, such as the schools, clergy, probation, and nonpsychiatric physicians.

Another approach involves the integration of services to help maximize the utilization of resources and manpower, avoid duplication of services, and assure maximum return on tax dollars (Ramage, 1971). This approach promotes a generalistic practice to reduce administrative costs and agency "hopping" by clients with the goal of providing more direct services. In reality, however, this type of service integration may not always be viewed as a reasonable alternative due to funding and administrative restrictions that supercede the authority and the desire to integrate on the part of the various programs and agencies in the community. But, whenever possible, the mental health facility should be amenable to coordinating other services under its roof, including offering office space to other agencies for their traveling representatives or contracting to provide services for other agencies (Huessy, 1972b).

The goal of the relationship with other service providers should be the centralization of responsibility and communication for the mental health care within the rural area or community (Gurevitz and Heath, 1969). The mental health professional will be more successful in meeting this goal through the use of a collaborative approach instead of taking an expert-teacher role (Cardoza, Ackerly, and Leighton, 1975). This approach is far less threatening and will enhance the type of cooperative working relationships discussed earlier. Again, the new professional, as an outsider, must approach the community agencies accordingly. Moreover, the new mental health professional cannot afford to become so intensively enmeshed in developing health systems, integrated services, coordinated services, and cooperative relationships that the services to clients suffer and their mental health needs become secondary in importance. The primary focus of the new program is mental health services and should not be abandoned in the zeal to gain acceptance in the community from other service providers—winning the battle while losing the war. The clients' needs must take priority, even at the risk of alienating, at times, some factions of the population within the community.

The problem of identification of the target population is important in developing relationships with other service providers in the community. There must be an awareness of the "skeletons" in rural areas so that the new mental health program does not inadvertently become embroiled in interagency conflicts and thus become identified as aligned with one agency or another (Jeffrey and Reeve, 1978). This type of situation would negatively affect the referrals to the mental health program, relationships with other programs and agencies, and, ultimately, the effectiveness of services to clients, especially where coordination of services is indicated as an appropriate response to client needs.

Although care and caution are necessary components of the new mental health professional's approach to other service providers in the community, the worker should not be hesitant or reluctant in developing relationships with these service providers. Their value as allies in the development of a new mental health program far outweighs the possible risks involved. It is important that the new professional contact local care-giving agencies to get a feel for the needs of the area (Gurevitz and Heath, 1969). One will find that an accurate appraisal of community needs is extremely helpful in approaching community agencies, especially those with fiscal responsibility (Eisdorfer, Altrocchi, and Young, 1968). A realistic assessment of community needs combined with logical and consistent plans for intervention will gain community support and acceptance far more readily than an idealistic theory purporting to solve the problems of the whole world while creating a mental health utopia, beginning with this community.

It should be noted that relationships between agencies are quite unsophisticated in rural areas and are oriented toward obtaining practical results

(Tranel, 1970). Often, there is a cynicism and apathy on the part of the community agency personnel who view the new mental health workers with skepticism when they refuse to accept the fact that some things cannot be changed. This knowledge should be used by the new professional to temper both vigor and aggressiveness to a degree while adjusting the approach so as to work within the present system to induce change in these professionals as well as in the community in general. These efforts can be assisted by the common feature of rural programs in that they are usually small, as compared to urban programs, and have a smaller staff. As Huessy (1972b) indicates, rural areas increase the feasibility of running programs without second-level management. He elaborates that the local representatives of any agency are few in number and are known to all other agency representatives, often on a first name basis. Due in part to this phenomenon, interagency cooperation is easier in rural areas. Through the use of these types of relationships, confidence in the new mental health professional's competence can be established with other service providers in the community. Once this competence has been established and the new professional has gained acceptance, the worker is better able to formulate plans and programs in a reality-oriented manner to address the mental health needs of the community and, possibly, to provide influence on some of the previously mentioned "things that cannot be changed." In some ways, the professional must first become a "Good Joe" in the eyes of the community service providers before they will give any credence to the worker's promulgations or observations on the state of the community or its needs.

Rural Community Mental Health Workers' Competencies

The practice foci of the community rural mental health social worker are arranged along a continuum. The initial competency entails knowledge of rural communities and how they function. Second, the bachelor's-level practitioner is conceptualized as the initial primary service worker. Thus, this individual should have an adequate knowledge of treatment and service modalities that can be employed in rural settings and must possess the ability to evaluate their effectiveness with clients. The competencies for the master's-level practitioner should possess advanced practice skills and knowledge. The additional functions that they should be able to perform are managerial, in terms of supervising BSW practitioners, executing administrative activities, such as funding programs and planning prevention at a macro-level. Finally, the practitioner should possess competence in research procedures that can be utilized to provide efficacious services to clients in rural areas.

SUMMARY

If social work's involvement in the area of rural community mental health is to continue to expand, practitioners must demonstrate specific competencies in this area of practice. This involves the elucidation of conceptual, research, and clinical competencies one must possess in order to claim a legitimate role in the practice of rural community mental health.

Despite the recent attention to competency-based education, there are not available well developed and evaluative training programs for social workers who practice in rural community mental health settings (Arkava and Brennen, 1975; Armitage and Clark, 1975; Duehn and Mayadas, 1977). The specification of competencies for training of social workers with delineation of pre-entrance and exit skills represents a critical, yet relatively unexplored area in facilitating the acquisition of practice skills needed by social workers in community mental health practice. Yet such specification will ensure that rural clients secure the services necessary to maintain themselves in their communities. The project described in this text involves the identification and evaluation of critical competencies. The goal has been to build a curriculum with specific learning and performance objectives relevant to rural mental health and, consequently, to develop in trainees competencies pertinent to rural practice. Chapter 2 reviews labeling theory and its implications for rural practice. Chapter 3 centers on deinstitutionalization and its significance for social work training and practice in rural areas. The implementation of change strategy: where, by whom, why, how long, and on what level is elucidated in Chapter 4. Chapter 5 covers prevention, a topic which is of increasing relevance in social work practice endeavors. Methods for preparing the rural practitioner to evaluate rural community mental health programs are elaborated in Chapter 6. Competencies for bachelor's- and master's-level workers are presented in Chapter 7. Practicum goals are detailed in Chapter 8. Chapter 9 elaborates outcome measures, both personal and behavioral, that were used to evaluate the programs. The final chapter covers issues in competency-based education with an elaboration of the implications for social work training.

REFERENCES

Alexander, F. D. 1941. Religion in a rural community of the south. Am. Sociol. Rev. 1:241–251.

Arkava, M. L., and Brennen, C. C., 1975. Toward a competency examination for the baccalaureate social work. J. Educ. Soc. Work 11:22–29.

Armitage, A., and Clark, F. W. 1975. Design issues in the performance based curriculum. J. Educ. Soc. Work 11:22–29.

Bachrach, L. L. 1977. Deinstitutionalization of mental health services in rural areas. Hosp. Community Psych., 28:669–672.

Bentz, W. K., Edgerton, J. W., and Kherlopian, M. 1969. Perceptions of mental illness among people in a rural area. Ment. Hyg. 53:459–465.

Berg, L. K., Cohen, S. Z., and Reid, W. J. 1978. Knowledge for social work roles in community mental health: Findings of empirical research. J. Educ. Soc. Work 14:16–23.

Bloom, B. L. 1973. Community Mental Health: A Historical and Critical Analysis. General Learning Press, Morristown, N.J.

Bloom, B. L. 1977. Community Mental Health: A General Introduction. Brooks/Cole, Monterey, Calif.

Buxton, E. B. 1973. Delivering social services in rural areas. Public Welfare 31:15–20.

Cardoza, V. G., Ackerly, W. C., and Leighton, A. H. 1975. Improving mental health through community action. Community Ment. Health J. 11:215–227.

Clayton, T. 1977. Issues in the delivery of rural mental health services. Hosp. Community Psych. 28:673–676.

Coppedge, R. C., and Davis, C. G. 1977. Rural Poverty and the Policy Crisis. Iowa State University Press, Ames.

Cormican, E. H. 1979. Characteristics of rural communities and their implications for social work. Arete 5:209–217.

Cowen, E. L. 1978. Some problems in community program evaluation research. J. Consult. Clin. Psychol. 46:792–805.

Duehn, W., and Mayadas, N. S. 1977. Entrance and exit requirements of professional social work education. J. Educ. Soc. Work 13:22–29.

Edgerton, J. W. and Bentz, W. K. 1969. Attitudes and opinions of rural people about mental illness and program services. Am. J. Public Health 59:470–477.

Eisdorfer, C., Altrocchi, J., and Young, R. F. 1968. Principles of community mental health in a rural setting: The Halifax county program. Community Ment. Health J. 4:211–220.

Feldman, R., Caplinger, T. E., and Wodarski, J. S. 1983. The St. Louis conundrum: Prosocial and antisocial boys together. Prentice-Hall, Inc., Englewood Cliffs, NJ.

Feldman, R., Wodarski, J. S., and Flax, N. 1973. Group integration and behavioral change: Pro-social and anti-social children at summer camp. Soc. Work, 5:26–37.

Feldman, R., Wodarski, J. S., and Flax, N. 1975. Anti-social children in a summer camp environment: A time sampling study. Community Ment. Health J. 1:10–18.

Feldman, S. 1978. Promises, promises or community mental health services and training: Ships that pass in the night. Community Ment. Health J. 14:83–91.

Fenby, B. L. 1978. Social work in a rural setting. Soc. Work J. 23:162–163.

Gertz, B., Meider, J., and Pluckhan, M. L. 1975. A survey of rural community mental health needs and resources. Hosp. Community Psych. 26:816–819.

Ginsberg, L. H. 1969. Education for social work in rural settings. Soc. Work Educ. Rep. September:28–32, 60–61.

Ginsberg, L. H. 1971. Rural social work. Encycl. Soc. Work 2:1138–1144.

Glenn, N. D., and Hill, L. 1977. Rural-urban differences in attitudes and behavior in the United States. Ann. Am. Acad. Polit. Soc. Sci. 429:36–50.

Goudy, W. J. and Wepprecht, F. E. 1977. Local and regional programs developed from resident's evaluations. J. Community Dev. Soc. 8:44–52.

Gurevitz, H., and Heath, D. 1969. Programming in a new region. In H. R. Lamb, D. Heath, and J. F. Downing (eds.), Handbook of Community Mental Health Practice. Jossey-Bass, San Francisco.

Horejsi, C. L., and Deaton, R. L. 1977. The cracker-barrel classroom: Rural programming for continuing education. J. Educ. Soc. Work 13:37–43.

Huessy, H. R. 1972a. Rural models. In H. H. Barten and L. Bellak (eds.), Progress in Community Mental Health, Vol. 2. Grune & Stratton, New York.

Huessy, H. R. 1972b. Tactics and targets in the rural setting. In S. E. Golann and C. Eisdorfer (eds.), Handbook of Community Mental Health. Appleton-Century-Crofts, New York.

Jeffrey, M. J. and Reeve, R. E. 1978. Community mental health services in rural areas: Some practical issues. Community Ment. Health J. 14:54–62.

Johnson, H. W. (Ed.) 1980. Rural Human Services: A Book of Readings. F. E. Peacock Publishers, Inc., Itasca, Ill.

Karsten, P. 1975. The rural development insurance fund: Another evaluation free "antipoverty" program. In D. Yokelson (ed.), Aspects of Low Income in America, Vol. 2. pp. 593–597. Hudson Inst., Croton-on-Hudson.

Katz, A. J. 1978. Problems inherent in multi-service delivery units. J. Sociol. Soc. Welfare 5:664–661.

Kelley, V. R., Kelley, P. L., Gauron, E. F., and Rawlings, E. I. 1977. Training helpers in rural mental health delivery. Soc. Work 22:229–232.

Kiesler, F. 1969. More than psychiatry: A rural program. In M. F. Shore and F. V. Mannino (eds.), Mental Health and the Community: Problems, Programs, and Strategies. Behavioral Publications, New York.

Klein, D. C. 1965. The community and mental health: An attempt at a conceptual framework. Community Ment. Health J. 1:301–308.

Lee, S. H., Gianturco, D. T., and Eisdorfer, C. 1974. Community mental health accessibility: A survey of the rural poor. Arch. Gen. Psych. 31:335–339.

Lerner, R., and Blackwell, B. 1975. The GP as a psychiatric community resource. Community Ment. Health J. 11:3–9.

Libo, L. M., and Griffith, C. R. 1966. Developing mental health programs in areas lacking professional facilities: The community consultant approach in New Mexico. Community Ment. Health J. 2:163–169.

Naftulin, D. H., Donnelly, F. A., and O'Halloran, D. B. 1974. Mental health courses as a facilitator for change in a rural community. Community Ment. Health J. 10:359–365.

Ramage, J. W. 1971. A basic philosophy in developing a rural mental health program. Public Welfare Fall:475–477.

Rands, S. 1960. Community psychiatric services in a rural area. Can. J. Public Health 51:404–410.

Shupe, A. D. 1974. Development of mental health services among existing community institutions in rural areas: The case of the Japanese Kumiai. Community Ment. Health J. 10:351–358.

Tranel, N. 1970. Rural program development. In H. Grunebaum (ed.), The Practice of Community Mental Health. Little, Brown & Co., Boston.

Walsh, M. E. Rural social work practice: Clinical Quality. Soc. Casework 62:458–464.

Weber, G. K. 1976. Preparing social workers for practice in rural social systems. J. Educ. Soc. Work 12:108–115.

Wedel, H. L. 1969. Characteristics of community mental health center operations in small communities. Community Ment. Health J. 5:437–444.

Wodarski, J. S. 1979a. Critical issues in social work education. J. Educ. Soc. Work 15:5–13.

Wodarski, J. S. 1979b. Requisites for the establishment, implementation, and evaluation of social work treatment programs. J. Sociol. Soc. Welfare 6:339–361.

Wodarski, J. S. 1981. Role of Research in Clinical Practice. University Park Press, Baltimore.

Wodarski, J. S., and Feldman R. 1974. Practical aspects of field research. Clin. Soc. Work J. 2:182–193.

Yokelson, D. (ed.) 1975. Public Attitudes Toward Poverty and the Characteristics of the Poor and Near-Poor, Vol. 3. Hudson Inst., Croton-on-Hudson.

Chapter 2

Labeling Theory

Implications for Rural Practice

INTRODUCTION

Rural communities were formed originally around kinship lines, religious affiliation, or race, and were later strengthened by the development of government, schools, industry, and trade. Rural communities generally are characterized, therefore, by stable social structures and high cohesiveness (Conklin, 1980). The social folkways and norms in rural areas are well defined and strictly enforced. Individuals who deviate from these norms are easily recognizable and often are outcast or at least considered "different." If the deviance continues, the individuals are labeled as having a personal deficiency that causes their behavior and they thus become prime candidates for interventions to alter the deficiency.

Distinctive characteristics of rural communities include religion as a significant social value and conservative political philosophies. Religion and churches play significant roles in the lives of rural society members. In rural communities people know more about each other, watch one another's church attendance, and use church facilities for social gatherings and community meetings (Ginsberg, 1977). Such activities facilitate high cohesiveness and provide the mechanism necessary for the identification and subsequent labeling of deviant behavior. Due to the lack of mental health professionals located in rural areas, ministers often serve as counselors for community residents and are often primary identifiers and labelers of deviant behavior.

In rural areas the media play an insignificant role in relaying news. Most news is passed orally and reaches the media only after everyone already knows it. "Gossip may be an all consuming pastime, which has a significant impact on the community life" (Ginsberg, 1977; p. 1233). The fact that many residents engage in gossip presents a real problem in engaging clients because they fear someone will find out they are receiving services and the stigma associated with mental illness will be ascribed to them. As a result of their visibility, rural residents are more likely than their urban counterparts to refuse to avail themselves of mental health services.

The professional worker is likewise affected by the exposure characteristic of the rural community. In the words of Shore and Mannino (1969),

> Rural areas offer no hiding places. The personal and family detachment and relative anonymity so often cherished and readily maintained by mental health professionals in metropolitan areas are neither possible nor desirable . . . very quickly we (rural social workers) learned how to handle repeated situations in which people we had seen in the office one day were introduced to us and our wives and our children in social or business settings the next day.

This chapter reviews the implications of labeling theory for the rural community mental health social worker in terms of who receives services and subsequent consequences of the labeling process. Implications of labeling theory for women and Blacks are stressed.

DETERMINANTS OF LABELING

Homogeneous versus Heterogeneous Grouping

The existing literature provides evidence of the pronounced tendency in our society for the helping professions to group clients together in the same context for treatment purposes, namely, to place the mentally ill in mental hospitals, criminals in prisons, mentally handicapped in schools for the retarded, and so forth. This process, in many instances, is reinforced through legal sanctions. Two reasons probably account for this segregation of exceptional individuals from interactions with so-called "normal" individuals. They are based on economic and theoretical factors that are interrelated in many instances. For economic reasons, helping institutions tend to treat individuals in the same context simply because it is easier, more efficient, and less costly to deliver services to sets of homogeneous clients. This is especially applicable to rural areas in which the agency catchment area is large. For theoretical reasons, it is believed that these types of groupings may lead to greater empathy among clients and increased understanding of common social problems, which in turn leads to their therapeutic improvement. In addition, if successfully treated, these clients provide adequate role models for others. Data are lacking to indicate that these therapeutic benefits actually accrue, however (Feldman, Caplinger, and Wodarski, 1983).

For example, homogenous client grouping is used extensively in the treatment of antisocial children even though data reveal little success with this procedure (Bailey, 1966; Bednar and Kaul, 1971; Feldman and Wodarski, 1975; Platt, 1969; Radzinowicz and Wolfgang, 1971; Warren, 1970; Wodarski and Pedi, 1977). Moreover, the following consequences have been observed to result from the grouping process:

1. As the antisocial child goes through the many institutional procedures to secure services, he or she becomes labeled and this results in stigmatization.
2. The antisocial child is not provided the opportunity to experience adequate role models because interaction with normal peers is discouraged and role models provided in segregated treatment settings may be more deviant than the ones provided in other settings. Thus, the likelihood of positive reinforcement from peers for prosocial behavior and generalization of such behavior is diminished. Moreover, the child may learn behaviors that are dysfunctional for interaction with his peers.
3. Homogeneous groupings prevent interactions between antisocial children and others with "regular" self concepts that may lead to the antisocial children developing self-concepts of deviancy.
4. The ability of antisocial children to learn prosocial behaviors is limited in segregated contexts, and even if prosocial behaviors are learned, the ability to generalize these behaviors to the open environment is minimal.

It is evident that these consequences can occur as well for other clients served by social workers, such as developmentally disabled populations (Begab and Richardson, 1975). Moreover, due to the nature of the rural environment, it is more likely that the consequences will occur for the rural client as compared to the urban client. Because of the closeness of social networks in rural practice contexts, individuals who exhibit deviant behaviors are labeled more readily, and the worker must be aware of the phenomenon in order to reduce its effects. In addition, the social system is the key variable that leads to individuals being labeled by significant others to secure services in rural areas as compared to urban areas in which self-referrals are more evident.

Practitioners must learn to determine what factors lead to the accurate perception of services offered and to the structuring and provision of service, and what processes operate to influence the services provided clients (Kazdin and Cole, 1981). When treatment takes place in the open community it is feasible to assume that more generalizability of behavior will occur. Thus, when possible, it is more desirable to locate treatment endeavors for clients within existing rural community agency systems rather than to remove them for treatment. Likewise, it is better to provide services to clients in systems in which they have the opportunity to interact with normal individuals. Satellite clinics are an example of bringing services closer to clients. Placing clinics near clients also facilitates the community's acceptance of the services, thus reducing the labeling effect. This alleviates many of the dysfunctional consequences discussed above and accomplishes one of the primary objectives of the community mental health movement, that is to provide services to clients in the least stigmatizing means possible (Feldman et al., 1972).

Within the training context of the project described herein, practitioners learn how traditional agencies, such as churches, schools, community centers, the

YMCA and YWCA, and day care centers, can be used to expedite implementation of rural community mental health services. Rural areas have a substantial advantage over urban areas in that support networks are stronger. That is, significant others are not as mobile as in urban networks (Collins and Pancoast, 1978). Students are instructed on how to use these resources. They learn to develop new and innovative resources based on their knowledge of the rural culture and the particular community characteristics. The use of such resources as church members, relatives, law enforcement officers, and so forth alleviates many of the dysfunctional aspects of providing traditional services through the homogeneous grouping of clients. Thus, a major contribution is the facilitation of the use of immense resources heretofore not utilized for the provision of community mental health services (Gottlieb and Schroter, 1978).

Social Reaction to Individual Differences

In order to understand how a person becomes a "client" the distinction must be made between individual differences in behavior and the social reaction to those individual differences (Denner and Price, 1973). The social reaction to a person's behavior determines whether the behavior will be seen as "normal" or "deviant." The social reaction also plays an important part in determining how much pressure and mechanisms the society will impose on the individual to alter his or her behavior. In one community a behavior may be considered "strange," whereas in another community exhibition of the same behavior may be considered acute psychotic symptomatology (Denner and Price, 1973). What causes this difference of perception in an identical behavior and, more importantly, what happens when an individual's behavior is labeled "deviant?"

> A partial list of factors which are important in determining the social reaction to individual differences might include community norms for the tolerance of various forms of behavior, the social and economic status of the person displaying the behavior, and the prevailing attitude toward and availability of mental health facilities (Denner and Price, 1973).

The preceding statement takes into account the importance of public reaction in the community in determining whether or not a person's behavior is considered "bizarre" and, to an extent, whether or not a person will be labeled as a "mental patient," "crazy," or "deviant." In communities low in social cohesion, if a person had been hospitalized and is exhibiting previously observed behavior which is not hurting himself or others, the behavior may be shrugged off as strange, but harmless. In another community with high social cohesion this person, exhibiting the same behavior, under the same circumstances, in many instances will be hospitalized (Denner and Price, 1973). It has been found to be the case that in many small, rural communities in which there are few mental health professionals, determination of need for hospitalization may be left to the discretion of the community power structure.

Visibility of the behavior is a crucial factor in determining the degree of labeling (Goffman, 1963). The size and social structure of the community can affect the visibility of the symptomatology, hence its definition and consequences (Denner and Price, 1973). In larger populations in which interpersonal relationships are based on a larger social network, the social visibility of a person lessens and symptoms will not be defined as quickly as in smaller, more intimate communities (Goffman, 1959).

LABELING AND STIGMATIZATION

Stigma refers to an "attitude which is deeply discrediting" (Goffman, 1963; p. 4). There are three types of stigma: abominations of the body, the various physical deformities; blemishes of individual character such as mental disorder, imprisonment, addiction, homosexuality, suicidal attempts, and endless others; and tribal stigma of race, religion, and nation, transmitted through lineage (Goffman, 1963). Stigma also connotes a lack of social acceptance by others. Those who do not deviate from society's expectations of them are known as "normals" whereas those who deviate from the norm are viewed as abnormal. For those with a stigma, normals tend to attach numerous additional stereotypes based on the original stigma. If a person has one imperfection in common with someone else, the individual is likely to find normals attributing other characteristics to him or her that are common to others with the same imperfection. For example, if a person meets a man with one arm who also happens to be irritable and deaf, they expect the next person they meet with one arm to exhibit similar traits. Consistency in perceptual process is a phenomenon of which rural practitioners have to be aware in assessing inaccurate labeling of clients (Gingerich, Feldman, and Wodarski, 1976a, b; Wodarski, 1977a).

Consequences of Stigmatization on Personality Traits

Many times stigmatized persons are defensive. This defensive response is often perceived as a direct expression of their defect, and consequently both defect and response are seen as a retribution for something he or she did. Hence, there is justification for the way one treats the stigmatized individual (Goffman, 1963). Although some pretend to accept those who are stigmatized, they may quite accurately be aware of the fact that no matter what they profess, they do not actually accept the individual. Not only do others not accept the person, but they are not willing to relate to the individual on equal grounds. The standards of society for the most part are obvious, and stigmatized individuals are painfully aware of the fact that they are "not fully equipped" or do not "fit in." These standards have made stigmatized persons intimately aware of what others see as their failing—inevitably causing them, if only for moments, to agree that they indeed fall short of what they ought to be (Goffman, 1963).

Because stigmatization usually is a basis for nonacceptance by others, the stigmatized individual often has feelings of self-hate. The individual cognitions center on "I am inferior. Therefore, people dislike me and I cannot be secure with them" (Perry, Gawel, and Gibbon, 1956; p. 145). Lacking interaction with others, either because they are not approached or because they are not secure enough in their self-image to approach others, self-isolates can become suspicious, hostile, depressed, anxious, withdrawn, and/or bewildered, thus enhancing the labeling of deviancy (Goffman, 1963).

Frequently, the stigmatized individual will be thrown into a relationship with others who possess the same stigma. Those relationships often foster a new sense of identity and new feelings of acceptance (Goffman, 1963). New relationships of this type are less likely to occur in rural communities, however, because there are fewer available programs in which people with like stigmas can meet and develop interpersonal relationships. Therefore, feelings of acceptance among those possessing a stigma are less prevalent and low self-esteem is more common to rural individuals with stigmas.

As mentioned previously, symptoms of deviancy are viewed as violations of social norms. The violation of the social norm is not in itself enough to be labeled as mentally ill. In many communities, people who exhibit bizarre behavior are ignored or, at most, labeled *"eccentric."* However, when the individual's behavior infringes upon community residents or becomes a public issue, the traditional stereotype of "crazy person" is adopted by those reacting to the individual, and many times by the individual himself (Lamb et al., 1971). When a person acquires the label *crazy* the stereotyped image may become a part of their self-concept and, in turn, may begin to guide their behavior.

When persons are labeled *deviant,* their behaviors induce anxiety, especially in the case of psychotic or other observable behavior. Consequently, deviant individuals are often singled out for care by professionals when their behavior is no longer ignorable.. People "exiled" to the care of professionals become separated from their peers and are partially or wholly excluded from normal community life. The "overriding" deviant behaviors of their lives are emphasized to the point that they become central (Lewis and Lewis, 1977).

When the stigma attached to the deviant role is strong, segregation is extreme, physically as well as socially divorcing the deviant from everyday community (Lamb et al., 1971). Public opinion of mental illness may have significant implications for persons who have been mental health patients (Lamy, 1973). There is a core element of historical values found in rural society. Those values are an emphasis on work (which many mental health patients are unable to perform), achievement, traditional moral orientations, group participation, and conformity (Park and Shapiro, 1976). Therefore, anything deviating, such as addiction or mental illness, from these norms or values would carry stigma (Williams, 1970). People who deviate from norms in rural areas are generally more visible and, thus, are more likely to hold a stigma.

The Result of Seeking Help

A major consequence endured by one who has experienced any labeling of deviancy is the stigma attached to receiving help (Goffman, 1959). The process of receiving help from a professional may alter others' reactions to the client (Denner and Price, 1973). The very act of seeking help, whether the person is diagnosed as mentally ill or not, may lead others to negatively react and/or attach a stigma.

In a study of community reaction to hypothetical individuals seeking help, when the helping source was a clergyman the community members' reactions were mild and little rejection was experienced. But, if the individual sought help from a psychiatrist or a mental hospital, the community reaction was much more severe and rejecting. Thus, even an attempt to seek help may elicit rejection by others (Denner and Price, 1973). There are different toleration levels for different behaviors, means to deal with them in rural areas, and natural helping networks are essential to reduce stigma.

In metropolitan areas, mental health seems to be gaining a sense of acceptance. In certain areas the elite in the community take pride in seeing a therapist. In rural areas, the traditional values hold on much more tightly. The only people who go to mental health centers are crazy people. The cultural isolation of rural communities, however, is under change (Hassinger, 1978). Perhaps with the influx of metropolitan cultural values and more trained professionals, attitudes about mental health in rural areas will become less negative.

The Effect of Stigmatization on the Realization of Potential

When people suffer a physical or mental *disability* or *impairment*, they are labeled in those terms and that label connotes dependence and limited worth (Lewis and Lewis, 1977). Those who carry stigmas suffer from a failure of their communities to recognize their potential to contribute to society. Mental health clients are seen as valueless people who are dependent upon the system for survival.

The perceived limitations imposed by society devalue the person, the most devastating effect of stigma. Victims are devalued to the point that their self-images are affected. One important aspect of reintegration of the deviant individual into the community is interaction with significant others in the community. Often, stigmatization limits or prohibits such interaction, further widening the gap between the devalued individual and the community, and thus decreasing that individual's sense of self-worth (Lewis and Lewis, 1977).

For example, upon release from the hospital and return to the community, ex-mental patients will find themselves stigmatized and rejected individuals. The stigma they carry will affect their interpersonal relations and, in many cases, results in job discrimination (Denner and Price, 1973). Even when able to get past the employer in the job interview, ex-mental patients are likely to be outcast by co-workers. This can lower their job satisfaction, decrease their self-esteem, and subsequently affect their performance, thus confirming the original assessments. Research shows that a mental hospital patient will be more employable and acceptable if he or she explains the hospitalization in terms of interpersonal problems than in terms of mental illness (Denner and Price, 1973). In short, stigmatization is the situation of the individual who is disqualified from the full acceptance of society, and who society feels is unable to contribute to the community because of inaccurate assessment of the person's potential. Moreover, primary group intimacy is denied the ex-mental patient. The high social cohesion characteristic of rural areas intensifies this process of exclusion.

Reaction of Others to Acquired Stigmas

Many times, as in cases in which individuals have contracted polio, affected persons are educated about the characteristic they have which is stigmatized, but they must be re-educated and must re-identify themselves when the illness strikes (Goffman, 1963). Persons the individuals were acquainted with *after* the onset of the unacceptable problem may see the individual as a faulted person, but still accept that person for who he or she is. Those who knew the individual before the onset of the problem, however, may still be attached to the conception of who they thought he or she was before being stigmatized. Because of this, they may be unable to treat the individual with formal tact or with the familiar full acceptance (Goffman, 1963). The fact that mental illness, once diagnosed, is seen as incurable by most people makes pre-stigma acquaintances unable to accept people receiving mental health services.

Familial Attitudes and Their Importance

One of the most significant abilities of a newborn child is that of expressing emotions, especially empathy. The baby is able to sense and respond to feelings of acceptance and rejection (Johnston, 1971). The child has physiological and psychosocial needs that must be met by the parents or other caretakers for optimal development.

The physiological needs are referred to as *primary needs,* for without any one of them the person will die. The primary needs are oxygen, food, shelter, and sleep. The major psychosocial or secondary needs are love, status and recognition, achievement, and identity (Johnston, 1971). These secondary needs, although not essential to life, play an important part in the formation of attitudes and values. The secondary needs are acquired through interacting with others. Thus, most of the socialization of the rural child occurs in the family (Lamb et al., 1971).

In child development, perhaps one of the most important concepts of growth is the development of identity. Through interaction with significant others, individuals define who they are, what they are, and what they can do (Johnston, 1971). A strong sense of identity is invaluable in defending oneself from stigmatization (Lewis and Lewis, 1977). The attitudes of the family that play a large role in forming the individual's attitudes are, for the most part, shaped by larger society. In rural areas, the community is a major force in forming family attitudes. One of the best therapeutic objectives a social worker can attain is helping mental health clients cope through increasing their positive self-concepts. The family can play an important role in assimilating the ex-mental patient into the community merely by accepting the person and subsequently reinforcing a sense of identity.

A great deal of time is required in changing attitudes, especially if the attitude is complex and has been held for a long period of time by a large number of people. Mental illness is one phenomenon that has had many different ascriptions and attitudes associated with it (Carroll, 1964). One way that attitudes are changed is through confrontation and presentation of different attitudes so that the original attitude is challenged and modified. In rural areas, attitudes are maintained more strongly due to a more stable social structure and also because of less influx of population with differing attitudes.

"The emotional basis of the attitude appears to be a mixture of fear and contempt, with fear predominating" (Carroll, 1964; p. 269). One theory about dealing with fear states that when people are fearful, they react with either "fight or flight." Both of these reactions are common in rural society for dealing with mental health. A major defense used in both reactions is denial. It is common for individuals and their families to deny that the member has mental illness. Many families are relieved when a family member is diagnosed mentally ill. When they know that person is sick they understand the exhibition of bizarre behavior and can excuse it (Park and Shapiro, 1976). However, many families regard the diagnosis as something of which to be ashamed. Being labeled as mentally ill can stigmatize the individual and separate him or her from family, friends, and community (Park and Shapiro, 1976). Thus, the practitioner's goals must be to re-establish these attachments.

It is becoming increasingly apparent that one of the major focuses of social work practitioners in rural areas must be the development of community acceptance of the client. The family's and the community's tolerance of the mental health client is one of the central factors in the determination of success at discharge (Park and Shapiro, 1976). There may be limitations in the person's ability to effectively communicate with people in his or her social environment due either to the client's lacking these skills or to the nature of the environment (Glasser and Glasser, 1970). Thus, when dealing with mental health or mental illness, there is a constant need for education. Part of the fear families feel and the misconceptions they hold are due to a lack of knowledge about mental health. By educating families of mental health clients, the mentally ill family member can gain a better sense of acceptance. Acceptance by the family is essential in treatment of the mentally ill. The prognosis of the patient is higher if the family is accepting of the person (Glasser and Glasser, 1970).

What Can Rural Mental Health Professionals Do to Reduce Stigma?

Part of the job of rural social workers is to decrease as much stigma as possible for the client. Labeling and stigmatization may be minimized somewhat by maintaining expectations that individuals live up to their potential, however high or low that may be (Lamb et al., 1971). The high-expectation approach emphasizes to clients that they do have strengths and in their own ways can contribute in a meaningful way to the communities in which they live. Thus, individuals are less likely to be stigmatized by themselves or by others (Hollingshead and Redlich, 1958).

In attempting to provide services in rural areas agencies should recognize indigenous helpers as a vital resource because of their knowledge of community attitudes and norms, their understanding of crises peculiar to their communities, and their willingness and ability to intervene. Such helpers can bridge the gap between existing services (Conklin, 1980).

In dealing with stigmatization in rural areas, the most important function of the worker is to reduce the misconceptions and fears about mental health. A continuous process of community education is essential for accurate assessment of behavior and subsequent referral. The reduction of misinformation can be dealt with in a variety of ways through community education and consultations with other service agencies. Interdisciplinary meetings, workshops, and other informative activities are helpful in building the reputation of the mental health centers, thus increasing referrals. With greater use, community fears about mental health are likely to decrease, resulting in the long run in less stigmatization for our clients.

LABELING THEORY AND MINORITIES

As mentioned earlier, distinctive attributes such as race and physical differences predispose the individual to labeling (Schneider, 1979). Any discussion of relevance of labeling theory for rural practice must necessarily review implications for minorities and women.

The literature has dealt primarily with the delivery of urban community mental health services to minorities with major focus on Blacks and Chicanos because they comprise the largest ethnic minority groups in the United States. The recent reinflux of people to rural areas, variously defined according to population density or distance from a metropolitan area of 40,000 population, or as any community with a specific lifestyle related to agribusiness or any community with less than 2,500 population, has brought to light the same kinds of flagrant discrimination in the delivery of mental health services to minorities in rural areas as exists in urban, that is, when and where rural area mental health services are offered. On this subject, Ginsberg (1969) is emphatic that rural people with problems are people who belong to groups with a high degree of cultural or linguistic visibility. Who fits both categories best? Rural Negroes, South Appalachian Whites, Mexican Americans, and American Indians.

According to Treiman, Street, and Shanks (1976), there is general agreement that Blacks constitute the largest ethnic minority in the United States and that they have been systematically discriminated against in every phase of life. In addition to racial inequality, Blacks that lived and live in rural areas are poor, very poor. Johnson (1967), in describing Negro life in the black belt (southern agricultural states), reports that their most distinguishing feature is poverty. He related this poverty not only to income but to education, housing, recreation, and any other indices of living conditions. The following figures are offered as "unequivocal evidence" by Korchin (1980) of continued racism: whereas 8.7% of all White families are officially designated as poor by the Census Bureau, 30% of all Black families, 34% of all Native American families, and 21% of all Spanish origin families are in that class.

Although Blacks are the largest ethnic minority in the United States, they are not the only victims of discriminatory practices. In 1971, almost nine million residents were identified as being of Spanish origin by the U.S. Bureau of the Census. They too suffer serious socioeconomic deprivation, and are accustomed to living in a culture of poverty.

Discrimination in Treatment

When one applies labeling theory to mental health services and to minorities (identified by the U.S. Government as Black, Hispanic, Asian, and Native Americans), there is ample support in the literature for the view that the comprehensive, culture-sensitive approach is almost nonexistent. Jackson (1976), for example, states that black individuals and their families are afforded different types of treatment than white individuals and their families whatever the mental health setting, be it inpatient or outpatient. Hollingshead and Redlick (1958) observed that because Blacks are less likely than whites to be offered psychotherapy, they are more likely to be offered custodial care and medication, and they have fewer good clinical services available to them (Berry and Davis, 1978; Couch et al., 1976; Gertz, Meider, and Pluckhan, 1975; Weber, 1976).

In addition, Padilla (1971) asserts that a minority member who seeks psychological or psychiatric assistance will most likely not see a psychologist or a psychiatrist and if he or she does, the treatment will be short-term, supportive psychotherapy or some form of physical treatment. Further support for this view is offered by Sue (1976) who conducted a 3-year study of client participation patterns in 17 community mental health centers in the Seattle area. He found that, as compared to whites, minority group clients were more likely to see paraprofessional staff members at intake and during therapy. In addition, as a single predictor of services received, ethnicity showed the greatest number of significant correlations. Cole and Pilisuk (1976) found similar occurrences in different communities in their study on quality of mental health services to Black, Chicano, and Asian clients. Likewise, two studies conducted in 1968 by Bloombaum, Yamamoto, and James and by Yamamoto, James, and Palley show that compared to Anglo controls, Spanish speaking, Spanish surname (SSSS) patients are referred for individual or group psychotherapy less often, receive less lengthy and intensive treatment, and are referred more often for ataractic medication.

Obstacles to Treatment

McGee and Clark (1976) express the view that the majority of the American population (whites) is not attuned enough to the cultural needs and experiences of blacks to be able to address their mental health needs. It would be reasonable to assume that this phenomenon would generalize to other ethnic minority groups in the United States, and there is sufficient literature support for this assumption. Bloombaum et al. (1968) indicate that a substantial number of psychotherapists involved in the delivery of mental health services to members of certain minority groups, that is, Caucasian, Negro, Mexican-American, and Oriental, exhibit similar negative prejudices found in the general population.

The literature supports the premise that the majority of the obstacles to minority utilization of mental health services are external. That is, these obstacles are often placed there and/or supported by the majority population who deliver mental health services to minorities. It has been indicated that many practitioners hold the view that White is superior and that "outsiders" have to conform to their (majority) view of cultural patterns of behavior. In his discussion of the low utilization rate of mental health services by Mexican-Americans in Texas, Jaco (1959) suggests that this is due mostly to their perception of any Anglo institutional structure as alien and hostile. Other minority group studies offer similar findings. Fugii (1976) found that frequent reasons for elderly Asian-Americans' failure to participate in public social and health service programs are racism, cultural differences, and general institutional alienation, whereas Korchin (1980) reports the significant variables involved in minorities' low utilization of services center on less access to resources, greater concern for stigma and shame, and language differences.

All data to date show that Spanish speaking, Spanish surname persons use mental health facilities far less than other population minorities. Fabrega (1970) indicates that definition of illness and lack of awareness of the need for treatment may be the underlying reasons. Johnson (1972), on the other hand, in an examination of mental health statistics on Mexican-American needs, found the absence of services in the barrios and the effects of discrimination major factors. Karno and Edgerton (1969) see the formidable language barrier, self-esteem-reducing nature of client-agency contacts for Mexican-Americans, past experiences, and paucity of mental health facilities in the Mexican-American community as being major contributors to underutilization of mental health services. Sensitivity to negativeness and lack of trust in service providers are reasons Paez (1975) gives for Chicanos waiting so long and bearing so much pain before seeking community mental health services.

WOMEN IN RURAL AREAS

Thirty year old mother
Autumn finds her pregnant once more
And the leaves like gold and copper
reminding her that she is poor
And her children often are hungry
And she hungers too, for knowledge
time and choices (Christian, 1977)

Rural women face the same problems as do their urban counterparts. They are discriminated against in the job market, their wages are less than those of equally qualified men, they may have difficulty obtaining credit or they may be discriminated against in inheritance laws. Women also face actual physical dangers of wife-beating and rape (Task Panel Reports, 1978). In short, sexual inequality has an effect on both the physical and psychological well-being of a substantial number of women.

Rural women are a special group of women. Throughout the nation, women tend to be "overrepresented among the mentally ill and underserved by the mental health system" (Task Panel Reports, 1978). Rural women have special and greater needs, however, resulting from the economic deprivation and high degree of sexual inequality prevalent in those areas (Task Panel Reports, 1978). The needs of this group are largely unmet and unexplored because ". . . rural women are rarely mentioned in rural research studies . . . and (they) are similarly overlooked in women's literature" (Moser and Johnson, 1973).

Rural and urban clients differ in the types of problems they present and in ways of responding to psychotherapeutic intervention (Fink, 1977; Millar, 1977). Techniques that may be effective in urban areas may be unsuccessful with rural clients (Nooe, 1977). Rural clients tend to be more concrete in thought, use more primitive defenses, and, generally, are less psychologically sophisticated than urban clients (Fink, 1977). Moreover, women have criticized current psychotherapy as promoting the sexist values of the society at large and it might be assumed that such therapy occurring in a rural context would increase the probability of promoting such values (Levine, Kamin, and Levine, 1974).

Use of interventions that conflict with the prevalent beliefs or traditions of the area may cause services to be rejected (Buxton, 1973). If traditional roles and relationships and political or religious structures are faced with change, rural inhabitants may feel threatened and resist not only the change but its provocateur. New therapeutic processes, especially ones that have political implications which alter many distressing factors to women—such as feminist therapy—may be difficult to introduce to rural areas because of their conservative nature. In the context of the traditional rural environment, the use of this new therapeutic technique raises several questions: What are some possible negative consequences of the use of feminist therapy in a rural area? What structures of the rural macrosystems would possibly limit the use of feminist therapy? Can feminist therapy keep its meaning if it is reduced to a nonpolitical tool? And, finally, are the values and techniques of feminist therapy applicable to rural women?

Conditions of Rural Women

The geographic factors and demographic composition of rural areas affect the lifestyle and attitudes of both the men and the women who have lived there. Rural clients tend to be isolated. Due to both the small population and the reluctance to associate with newcomers, their only associations frequently are with family and neighbors who have lived in the area most or all of their lives (Reul, 1974). Because fewer women than men work outside the home, this isolation of rural areas may have an even greater impact on women. This social detachment contributes to the tendency of rural people to be more reserved and to hold more traditional values than people in a more heterogeneous environment (Nooe, 1977; Reul, 1974). Outside help tends to be rejected and help is sought instead from traditional sources—preachers, teachers, doctors, and older family members (Bates, 1980; Nooe, 1977). Professional help is usually viewed as the last alternative and is used only when natural helping systems become overburdened or when they do not have the skills or ability to deal with the problem (Golan, 1980).

Utilization of natural helping systems is important in the rural community. Traditional area helpers are more readily accepted than outsiders. Because of the number of people who have mental health needs but will not go to the mental health center, "it is important to commit resources to an extensive development of consultations, agency staff training, citizen education, and prevention projects which will strengthen services to those clientele who are seeking help for their emotional and relationship problems somewhere else than at the mental health center" (Hollister, 1976, p. 64). By enhancing existing helping systems, the mental health center is responding to rural values (Task Panel Reports, p. 1165). Treatment personnel in rural mental health centers should take into account the rural people's suspicion of authority (Reul, 1974).

In rural areas the extended family is of great social importance. "The traditional rural family is patriarchal and has clear-cut divisions of tasks for men and women . . . Sex roles are taught in early childhood with an emphasis on what is proper behavior for boys or girls" (Reul, 1974). There may be little or no alternative offered to the roles of housewife and mother. Indeed, sexual equality is much further away for rural women than for urban.

Across the United States, for every 100 women admitted to treatment in community mental health centers, only 69 men are admitted (Cannon and Redlick, 1973). Excluding admissions to Veteran's Administration hospitals, women are the most frequent consumers of all mental health services, both public and private (Cannon and Redlick, 1973; Chesler, 1972). For women, seeking help for "nerves" or other mental illness, primarily depression, seems to be as culturally appropriate a role as seeking a husband and marriage (Chesler, 1972).

The most common diagnosis for women in outpatient treatment is depression. In the general population, more women than men experience depression. Married women whose children live at home have the highest incidence of depression (Task Panel Reports, 1978). The female response to loss or deprivation—be it tangible loss or losing power over their own lives—is depression instead of aggression (Chesler, 1972). Women have been taught to accept their positions and, lacking an overt method of creating conflict and raising their status, turn their frustration inward and become depressed (Chesler, 1972; Miller, 1971).

The rural life is not a pastoral, stress-free life. Economic hardship and lack of social services and other resources are common in rural areas. Much stress arises from the rural environment itself. Farm families, whose income is dependent on conditions suitable for the raising of produce or livestock, can be devastated by unfavorable weather or diseases (Reul, 1974). Shortages in fuel, fertilizer, pesticides, or types of feed can bring small farms to a complete standstill resulting in economic hardship, perhaps even the loss of the farm. Many rural areas are subject to frequent floods, most have little or no firefighting equipment (Reul, 1974). Combined, this means that rural people are still largely at the mercy of the elements. The stress of this uncertainty is an important consideration in assessing the mental health needs of both men and women in these areas.

Non-farm work in rural areas also tends to be stressful. In the Appalachian area, the two biggest non-farm employment sources are mining and textile or sewing factories (Reul, 1974). Both of these occupations are physically dangerous and involve unsafe and unpleasant working conditions. Mining employs relatively few women, where as textile workers are mainly women. Occupational stress is a significant problem for women working in these factories.

> Many women physically shake when they are on the job because of the tension caused by having to meet production quotas . . . Some women become so nervous at the end of a day's work that they can't eat, constantly drop things, talk incessantly, and lose their tempers easily . . . Factory workers often take drugs, smoke incessantly when they are not at work, and many die at an early age. The cause is simple; factory workers are overworked and underpaid in one of the most nerve-shattering jobs in the country (Kahn, 1972).

In addition to the working conditions, these jobs tend to be low paying, especially for the female workers. Rural men have much greater earning power than women: in 1974 there was a difference of almost $5,000—women earned $3,952 compared to $8,912 for men (Committee of Women's Issues, 1979). Another stress-producing element of factory work is the frequent lay-offs. A worker may be put on a "mandatory vacation" schedule of working for a week and then being off a week. Sometimes they are simply told that they are out of work but will be rehired whenever jobs are available again.

Implications for Practice

The isolation of rural inhabitants has led them to be more conservative in general than their urban counterparts. This conservatism might well lead both men and women in rural areas to reject certain therapies as being too different from their values. Rejection of the therapist or agency as well as the mode of therapy would be the most negative consequence of using inappropriate therapies in a rural area.

Rural areas uphold traditional social structures of extended families and male-dominated households. Sex role stereotypes are taught early in life and define strict rules of behavior. Such treatments as feminist therapy would oppose subjugation of women and would be seen as a threat to male domination of families. In addition, the process of consciousness-raising would cause women to view sex role stereotyping as a tool of oppression. Resistance to accepting traditional sex roles would also be quite threatening. Not only would rural men perceive these changes as dystonic, it is likely that rural women would, also. Both men and women reared in the same culture would view change as being difficult and might reject it without considering possible benefits. Rural women who might embrace the changes offered by feminist therapy would be the object of social pressure designed to maintain the status quo. Ostracism by friends, relatives, church members, and work associates, verbal criticism and abuse, and even the risk of physical abuse might be incurred by rural women who attempted to change traditional social structures. Given the likelihood of rejection of the mode of therapy, with potential for rejecting the clinician and agency, and the chance of women who became politically motivated risking censure by community and family, it seems that feminist therapy would have to be very limited initially in rural areas. In introducing a new mode of practice in a rural community it is best to move slowly in the beginning and lay the necessary groundwork (Chesler, 1972; Hopkins, 1980; Levine et al., 1974; Mander and Rush, 1974; O'Donnell et al., 1979; Task Force on Sex Bias and Sex Role Stereotyping, 1978; Thomas, 1977).

It is possible that tools of therapies, such as feminist therapy, would be suitable for use in rural areas. Certain values, for instance, reducing the authority of the traditional male or female therapist, would be very appropriate for dealing with rural female clients. Using groups to help women overcome their fear of seeking professional assistance would be complementary to the rural social mores. By using feminist therapy techniques to reduce the social distance between client and therapist, acceptance of the therapist as a helper in the rural community would increase. Another technique that, used out of its political context, would enhance therapy with rural women is consciousness-raising. By relating their experiences of daily living and seeing the areas of commonality, the sense of isolation would be diminished. Rather than direct the clients to use this experience to identify sex role stereotypes, the therapist would encourage the development of a feeling of community. Such changes as this would be of great help to rural women and, while leaving room for greater change in the future, are small enough not to threaten long standing social systems.

Most frequently, the therapist is not a local native but moves into the area from another urban or rural setting. As a newcomer, he or she is highly visible. Differences in the level of education, manner of speech, type of dress, and social attitudes may set the clinician apart from the local residents. Even so, exposure of the native to these differences increases the possibility for diversity in their own social attitudes. Especially in the case of a female therapist, role models that never existed before would be available to that rural area. To the clinician who is a feminist, small changes like this may seem insignificant; but, taken in the light of rural conservatism, all changes have a great impact on the community.

Conclusion

Much more must be learned about the conditions and needs of rural women. Because of the vast differences in lifestyle between women of various rural areas—the Great Plains states, Appalachian mountains, southern Black Belt, and many others—the needs of women in each area should be assessed. Economic factors, principal sources of employment, and geographic conditions should be evaluated. Information should be gathered regarding the incidence of female-headed households and spouse abuse. Such data would help determine if women in the area had special needs ranging from additional economic support to groups for single parents and battered wives. Women should be surveyed to ascertain what social problems they perceive as pressing in their area. In addition, information about their awareness of social services and willingness to seek help should be obtained.

Problems Peculiar to the Rural Clientele

A Michigan State University study indicated that because rural areas are not prime labor market areas and because they have dispersed populations, survey data collection is costly and many of the standard data are not computed for rural areas (1972). Yet, the data are continually used to assess rural as well as urban needs and this affects subsequent funding. This poses a problem in that delivery of mental health services in rural areas is often difficult because of the wide geographic area a mental health center must serve; and the geographic dilemma, in turn, demands heavy resources in travel budgets and maintaining satellite offices (Witt, 1977).

Agreement with Witt and an added dimension of concern are offered by Clayton (1977), who describes the geographic size of most rural community mental health center catchment areas as exceeding 5,000 square miles, with the average being approximately 17,000 square miles. This means that not only the expense Witt discussed must be addressed, but the door is open to unfavorable criticism and comparison of rural mental health workers to urban peers because less time is spent in treatment-related activities due to the heavy travel demands.

Programs unrealistically modeled after urban programs, poverty populations, high unemployment, and relatively few human service agencies all with generally inadequate resources are "external realities common to rural catchment areas" (Perlmutter, 1979). In discussing rural diversity, Cedar and Salasin (1979) indicate that rural populations differ from urban populations in many ways: average income, education, age, employment, and health status. Rural communities are more likely than urban communities to have inadequate services, housing, transportation, and an inadequate tax base. It cannot be concluded, however, from this general description of rural life that all rural areas require a set of mental health services, staffing, and rules and regulations different from urban areas, or that all rural areas can be treated conceptually and practically in the same way.

The composite picture of the rural American resident is presented by Witt (1977) in terms of percentages. For example, these residents equal "30 percent of the U.S. population, 40 percent of its poor, the homes of 55 percent of the Native Americans, 22 percent of the Blacks and 12 percent of our Spanish speaking citizens." Further delineation of the population composition is preferred by Cedar and Salasin (1979) who state "rural areas have a higher dependency ratio (the number of persons under 18 and over 65 years of age per 100 persons). The percentage of people living in poverty is higher for rural than urban areas: 9.8 percent urban compared to 16.2 percent rural/non-farm, and 17.9 percent rural farm."

Although there are rural poor everywhere, there are proportionately more poor among certain minority and ethnic groups, and they are more prevalent in certain regions of the country. For example, Weber (1976) reports that in 1969 more than half the total rural Black population were below poverty level. Migrant farm workers, Mexican-American farmers in the southwest, and Indians also comprised the poor population. Poor regions often coincide with location of this population as in Appalachia, the Ozarks, and farm and seacoast areas of the south.

Implications for Treatment

The outlook for treatment of the rural minorities is gloomy. Weber (1976) states that the physician-patient ratio in rural areas in 1969 equaled almost five times as many people per physician as the city. In addition, 4% of the practicing National Association of Social Work (NASW) members at the MSW and DSW levels were located in communities of 4,000 or less while almost 17% of these same NASW members were practicing in communities with 50,000 population or less.

Of those who practice in rural areas few are fully prepared for the intricacies of treatment for this population. Giordano and Giordano (1977) state that clinicians cannot deal with client issues unless their own prejudices are understood and until they are able to see themselves in relation to other groups. Especially critical areas of concern viewed by the Giordanos are emotional language, food differences, family symbolism, alienation, racism, and the variations of family roles. Wodarski (1977b) addressed the need to remove institutional racism from social work curricula by charging the professional social worker with developing the expertise and the opportunities to implement and support this change. He readily admits that although this is an enormous task, it is one of undebatable necessity. One prerequisite is to understand and be sensitive to the culture of different minority groups. Moreover, the social work student must understand and respect the "elements of custom, tradition, mores, folkways, norms and values" of the rural community. Implicit in this is a working knowledge and understanding of the formal and informal community systems and the desire to help consumers utilize available resources, even when resources are scarce (DeJong, 1975; Stanton, 1977).

SUMMARY

This chapter has reviewed the implications of labeling theory for social workers practicing in rural areas. Particular emphasis has been on the mentally ill, minorities and women. Labeling theory is particularly important to the practicing rural social worker in gaining an understanding of how clients secure services and how they are processed by the general community. Preliminary research seems to indicate that clients come to community centers because others, particularly individuals of stature in the community, believe that they need mental health care. More research is needed to indicate the significant variables involved in why and how communities process clients.

REFERENCES

Bailey, W. G. 1966. Correctional outcome: An evaluation of 100 reports. J. Crim. Law Criminol. Police Sci. 57: 153–160.

Bates, C. E. 1980. Developing a Comprehensive Community Helping System in a Rural Boom Town: A Potential for Informal Helping. Paper presented at the Council on Social Work Education Annual Program Meeting, March, Los Angeles.

Bednar, R. L., and Kaul, T. J. 1971. Empirical research in group psychotherapy. In A. E. Bergin and S. L. Garfield (eds.), Handbook of Psychotherapy and Behavior Change: An Empirical Analysis. Wiley, New York.

Begab, M. J. and Richardson, S. A. (eds.) 1975. The Mentally Retarded in Society: A Social Science Perspective. University Park Press, Baltimore.

Berry, B. and Davis, A. E. 1978. Community mental health ideology: A problematic model for rural areas. Am. J. Orthopsych. 48:673–679.

Bloombaum, M., Yamamoto, J., and James, O. 1968. Cultural stereotyping among psychotherapists. J. Counsel. Clin. Psychol. 32:99

Buxton, E. B. 1973. Delivering social services in rural areas. Public Welfare, 31:15–20.

Cannon, M., and Redlick, R. 1973. Differential utilization of psychiatric facilities by men and women, U.S. 1970. Statistical Note Number 81, NIMH.

Carroll, H. A. 1964. Mental Hygiene: The Dynamics of Adjustment, pp. 266–291. Prentice-Hall, Inc. Englewood Cliffs, N.J.

Cedar, T. and Salasin, J. 1979. Research Directions for Rural Mental Health. The MITRE Corp. Research and Development Resource Center for Rural Mental Health, July.

Chesler, P. 1972. Women and Madness. Doubleday, Garden City, N.Y.

Christian, M. 1977. "The rock will wear away". Face the Music. Olivia Records, Los Angeles.

Clayton, T. 1977. Issues in the delivery of rural mental health services. Hosp. Community Psych. 28:673–676.

Cole, J., and Pilisuk, M. 1976. Differences in the provision of mental health service by race. Am. J. Orthopsych. 46:510–525.

Collins, A. H., and Pancoast, D. L. 1978. Natural Helping Networks: A Strategy for Prevention. National Association of Social Workers, Washington, D.C.

Committee of Women's Issues. 1979. Womanpower. A newsletter of the National Association of Social Workers, September.

Conklin, C. 1980. Rural community care-givers. Soc. Work, November:495–596.

Couch, B., Dutton, E., Gurss, A., and Serpan, T. 1976. A specialist generalist model of social work practice for contemporary rural America. In R. K. Green and S. A. Webster (eds.), Social Work in Rural Practice. University of Tennessee, Knoxville.

DeJong, C. R. 1975. Field instruction for undergraduate social work education in rural areas. The Dynamics of Field Instruction: Learning Through Doing, pp. 20–30. Council on Social Work Education, New York.

Denner, B. and Price, R. H. 1973. The Making of a Mental Patient. Holt, Rinehart and Winston, Inc., New York.

Fabrega, H., Jr. 1970. Mexican Americans of Texas: Some social psychiatric features. In E. G. Brody (ed.), Behavior in New Environments: Adaptation of Migrant Populations pp. 249–273. Sage Publications, Beverly Hills.

Feldman, R. A., Caplinger, T. E., and Wodarski, J. S. 1983. The St. Louis Conundrum: Prosocial and Antisocial Boys Together. Prentice-Hall, Englewood Cliffs, N.J.

Feldman, R. A. and Wodarski, J. S. 1975. Contemporary Approaches to Group Treatment. Jossey-Bass Publishers, San Francisco.

Feldman, R. A., Wodarski, J. S., Flax, N., and Goodman, M. 1972. Treating delinquents in traditional agencies. Soc. Work 17:71–78.

Fink, R. L. 1977. The role of mental health programs in rural areas. In R. Green and S. Webster (eds.), Social Work in Rural Areas, pp. 328–340. Tennessee: University of Tennessee School of Social Work, Knoxville.

Fugii, S. 1976. Elderly Asian-Americans and use of public services. Soc. Casework 57:202–207.

Gertz, B., Meider, J., and Pluckhan, M. A. 1975. A survey of rural community mental health needs and resources. Hosp. Community Psych. 26:816–819.

Gingerich, W., Feldman, R. A., and Wodarski, J. S. 1976a. Accuracy in assessment: Does training help? Soc. Work 21:40–48.

Gingerich, W., Feldman, R. A., and Wodarski, J. S. 1976b. Accurate and inaccurate attributions of anti-social behavior: A labeling perspective. Sociol. Soc. Res. 61:204–222.

Ginsberg, L. H. 1969. Education for social work in rural settings. Soc. Work Educ. Rep. 17:28–61.

Ginsberg, L. H., 1977. Rural social work. Encycl. Soc. Work pp. 1231–1234.

Giordano, J., and Giordano, G. P. 1977. The Ethno-Cultural Factor in Mental Health: A Literature Review and Bibliography. Institute on Pluralism and Group Identity of the American Jewish Committee, New York.

Glasser, P. H. and Glasser, L. N. (eds.) 1970. Families in Crisis. Harper & Row, New York.

Goffman, E. 1959. The moral career of the mental patient. Psychiatry 22:123, 131.

Goffman, E. 1963. Stigma: Notes on the Management of Spoiled Identity. Prentice-Hall, Inc., Englewood Cliffs, N.J.

Golan, N. 1980. Intervention at times of transition: Sources and forms of help. Soc. Casework 61:259–266.

Gottlieb, G. N. and Schroter, C. 1978. Collaboration and resource exchange between professionals and natural support systems. Prof. Psychol. 9:622–641.

Hassinger, H. W. 1978. The Rural Component of American Society, pp. 147–151. The Interstate Printers and Publishers, Inc., Danville, Ill.

Hollingshead, A. B., and Redlich, R. C. 1958. Social Class and Mental Illness: A Community Study, pp. 180–186. Wiley & Sons, Inc.,

Hollister, W. 1976. Experiences in rural mental health. In L. Ginsberg (ed.), Social Work in Rural Communities, pp. 63–67. Council on Social Work Education, New York.

Hopkins, T. 1980. A conceptual framework for understanding the three "isms"—Racism, ageism, sexism. J. Educ. Soc. Work 16:63–70.

Jackson, A. M. 1976. Mental health center delivery systems and the Black client. J. Afro-Am. Issues 4:21–27.

Jaco, E. G. 1959. Mental health of the Spanish Americans in Texas. In M. K. Opler (ed.), Culture and Mental Health: Cross-Cultural Studies, pp. 467–485. The MacMillan Co., New York.

Johnson, C. S. 1967. Growing Up in the Black Belt: Negro Youth in the Rural South. Schocken Books, New York.

Johnson, H. S. 1972. Mental Health Needs of Mexican Americans. Prepared for the Regional Training Program to Serve the Bilingual/Bicultural Exceptional Child, Mental Educational Associates.

Johnston, M. K. 1971. Mental Health and Mental Illness. J. B. Lippincott & Co., Philadelphia.

Kahn, K. 1972. Hillbilly Women. Avon Books, New York.

Karno, M., and Edgerton, R. B. 1969. Perception of mental illness in a Mexican-American community. Arch. Gen. Psych. 20:233–238.

Kazdin, E., and Cole, P. 1981. Attitudes and labeling biases toward behavior modification: The effects of labels, content, and jargon. Behav. Ther. 12:56–68.

Korchin, S. J. 1980. Clinical psychology and minority problems. Am. Psychol. 35:262–269.

Lamb, R. H. and Associates. 1971. Rehabilitation in Community Mental Health. Jossey-Bass, Inc., New York.

Lamy, R. E. 1973. Social consequences of mental illness. In B. Denner and R. H. Price (eds.), The Making of a Mental Patient, p. 334. Holt, Rinehart, & Winston, Inc., New York.

Levine, S., Kamin, L., and Levine, E. 1974. Sexism and psychiatry. Am. J. Orthopsych. 44:327–336.

Lewis, J. A., and Lewis, M. D. 1977. Community Counseling: A Human Services Approach. John Wiley & Sons, New York.

McGee, D. P. and Clark, C. 1976. Critical elements of Black mental health. J. Afro-Am. Issues 4:21–27.

Mander, A., and Rush, A. 1974. Feminism as Therapy. Random House, New York.

Michigan State University. 1972. Labor Market Information in Rural Areas: Proceedings of a Conference. Center for Rural Manpower and Public Affairs.

Millar, K. 1977. Canadian rural social work. In R. Green and S. Webster (eds.), Social Work in Rural Areas, pp. 148–160. University of Tennessee School of Social Work, Knoxville.

Miller, J. 1971. Psychological consequences of sexual inequality. Am. J. Orthopsych. 41:767–775.

Moser, C., and Johnson, D. 1973. Rural Women Workers in the 20th Century: An Annotated Bibliography. Center for Rural Manpower and Public Affairs, Michigan State University, East Lansing.

Nooe, R. 1977. A clinical model for rural practice. In R. Green and S. Webster (eds.), Social Work in Rural Areas, pp. 347–399. University of Tennessee School of Social Work, Knoxville.

O'Donnell, M., Leoffler, V., Pollock, K., and Saunders, Z. 1979. Lesbian Health Matters. Santa Cruz Women's Health Center, Santa Cruz, Calif.

Padilla, E. R. 1971. The relationship between psychology and Chicanos: Failures and possibilities. In N. N. Wagner and M. J. Haug (eds.), Chicanos: Social and Psychological Perspectives, pp. 286–294. C. V. Mosby Co., St. Louis.

Paez, J. L. 1975. Minority cultures. Psych. Ann. 5:184–186.

Park, C. C. and Shapiro, L. N. 1976. You are Not Alone. Little, Brown, and Co., Boston.

Perlmutter, F. D. 1979. Consultation and education in rural community mental health centers. Community Mental Health J. 15:58–68.

Perry, H. S., Gawel, M. L. and Gibbon, M. (eds.), 1956. Clinical Studies in Psychiatry, p. 145. W. W. Norton & Co., New York.

Platt, A. 1969. The Child Savers: The Invention of Delinquency. University of Chicago Press, Chicago.

Radzinowicz, L. and Wolfgang, M. E. (eds.) 1971. The Criminal in Confinement. Basic Books, New York.

Reul, M. 1974. Territorial Boundaries of Rural Poverty. Center for Rural Manpower and Public Affairs and the Cooperative Extension Service, Michigan State University, East Lansing.

Schneider, D. J. 1979. Person perception. In C. A. Kiesler (ed.), Topics in Social Psychology Series. 2nd ed. Addison-Wesley, Reading, Mass.

Shore, M. F., and Mannino, F. V. 1969. Mental Health and the Community: Problems, Programs, and Strategies. Behavioral Publications, New York.

Stanton, O. L. W. 1977. Education for social work practice in rural and small communities. Doctoral dissertation, University of Michigan.

Sue, S. 1976. Client's demographic characteristics and therapeutic treatment: Differences that make a difference. J. Consult. Clin. Psychol. 44:864.

Task Force on Sex Bias and Sex Role Stereotyping in Psychotherapeutic Practice. 1978. Guidelines for therapy with women. Am. Psychol. 33:1122–1123.

Task Panel Reports. 1978. President's Commission on Mental Health. Vol. 3. U.S. Government Printing Office, Washington, D.C.

Thomas, S. 1977. Theory and practice in feminist therapy. Soc. Work 22:447–454.

Treiman, B. R., Street, P. B., and Shanks, P. 1976. Blacks and Alcohol: A Selected Annotated Bibliography. University of California, Berkeley.

Warren, M. O. 1970. Correctional treatment in community settings: A report of current research. Paper presented at 6th International Congress on Criminology, September, Madrid, Spain.

Weber, G. K. 1976. Preparing social workers for practice in rural social systems. J. Educ. Soc. Work 12:108–115.

Williams, R. M. 1970 American Society: A Sociological Interpretation, 3rd Ed., p. 456. Knopf, New York.

Witt, J. 1977. Meeting of mental health needs of rural communities beyond the cities. Ment. Hyg. 60:4–6.

Wodarski, J. S. 1977a. Anti-social children and labeling theory: A methodological critique. Corr. Psych. J. Soc. Ther. 23:122–128.

Wodarski, J. S. 1977b. Strategies for the alleviation of institutional racism in services offered by social work agencies. J. Soc. Welfare Spring:51–60.

Wodarski, J. S. and Pedi, S. J. 1977. The comparison of anti-social and pro-social children on multi-criterion measures at a community center: A three year study. Soc. Work 22:290–296.

Yamamoto, J., James, Q., and Palley, N. 1968. Cultural problems in psychiatric therapy. Arch. Gen. Psych. 19:45–49.

Chapter 3

Deinstitutionalization

Implications for Social Work Training and Practice in Rural Areas

INTRODUCTION

The implementation of deinstitutionalization programs in rural areas currently presents a perplexing and frustrating challenge to social workers and other mental health professionals. What individuals can be placed in the rural community? What resocialization processes are necessary? What community characteristics can be matched with individuals' attributes to facilitate placement and to enhance their functioning? What support systems are available to facilitate placement? These are all questions to be resolved prior to the placement of the clients in the open community. Yet the rural community mental health social worker is ill prepared to address these issues, largely due to lack of training.

At the present time, few mental health professionals question the value of community-based treatment for those persons labeled mentally ill. Widespread controversy, however, surrounds how best to develop humane, effective, and economically feasible community-based treatment modalities. Whereas deinstitutionalization policy is based on the freedom of choice concept of treatment alternatives, the following characteristics of rural areas limit the extent to which this premise can be operationalized: the geographical vastness of rural areas, low population density, lack of such resources as adequate diagnostic, treatment, and referral centers, a paucity of residential placement alternatives and trained personnel, and rural residents' characteristic attitudes toward mental illness (Bachrach, 1977; Horejsi, 1977; Jeffrey and Reeve, 1978; Segal, 1973).

Deinstitutionalization involves a diminished focus on the mental hospital as the primary treatment locus. It entails instead an increased reliance on community-based facilities for treatment of the mentally ill, a return to the community of institutional residents who have been adequately prepared for this transition through socialization and vocational rehabilitation programs, establishment of a humane and appropriate residential environment, development of prevention programs for those individuals who are at risk of becoming institutionalized, and promotion of community acceptance of persons labeled mentally ill (Bachrach, 1977; Horejsi, 1977, Mittler, 1979). As this policy applies to social work practice, it dictates that the responsibilities of the mental health professional include such diverse activities as prevention, resocialization instruction, vocational rehabilitation, client advocacy, coordination of community services, public relations, consultation, and education—a task of overwhelming proportions at best, but especially in rural areas in which staff turnover and burn-out rates are disproportionately high. Additionally, some doubt exists as to whether or not schools of social work are adequately training their graduates to meet the demands of practice in these settings (Wodarski, Giordano and Bagarozzi, 1981).

A number of researchers feel that large-scale implementation of deinstitutionalization programs may have begun too soon. Political pressure to discharge vast numbers of patients into the community before an adequate system of community care could be developed and before results of pilot studies had been analyzed may have created program plans that have not been firmly based on empirical data (Mannino, Ott and Shore, 1977). The rush to deinstitutionalize these often weak and highly dependent individuals has frequently resulted in discharging them to environments even more impoverished and unstimulating than the hospital (Turner and Ten Hoor, 1978). Alone and unsupported, with atrophied coping skills and Social Security dollars in their pockets, former patients are frequently exploited by unscrupulous board and care home operators and urban criminal elements (Allen, 1976; Lamb, 1976; Mechanic, 1980; Silverstein, 1979). Fortunately, researchers, administrators, and clinicians have reacted to this sad state of affairs by endeavoring to assess the needs of this population and to develop community-based programs to meet those needs. The available literature, however, concerns primarily urban-based research and doubt exists as to whether or not many of these programs can be successfully replicated in rural communities. The following discussion examines the political, legal, and medical advances that have created the thrust toward community treatment. The current status of deinstitutionalization programs is discussed along with the issues that emerge when successful urban-based models are applied to rural settings. The implications of these findings as they pertain to social work training and practice complete the discussion.

HISTORY OF THE DEINSTITUTIONALIZATION MOVEMENT

A variety of social, legal, and medical advances have impelled the deinstitutionalization movement over the past 35 years. Although the community care concept has roots extending back to 13th century Flanders when the villagers of Geel housed mentally ill pilgrims who had travelled to the shrine of St. Dymphna, the modern trend toward deinstitutionalization probably began with the passage of the National Mental Health Act of 1947 that gave the federal government direct responsibility for assistance in research, training, and services in mental health (Huey, 1977; Kramer, 1977). Passage of this act stimulated a great deal of new clinical, field, applied, and administrative research and training of mental health personnel. As these new research findings were implemented in the field, the newly trained administrators and clinicians opened increasing numbers of outpatient clinics and inpatient units in general hospitals, assisting in the shifting of treatment locus from the state hospitals to the communities (Kramer, 1977).

The Mental Health Study Act, passed in 1955, established the Joint Commission on Mental Illness and Mental Health for purposes of evaluating and analyzing needs and resources of the mentally ill in order to make recommendations for a National Mental Health Program. The Commission's report led to President Kennedy's Message to Congress on Mental Illness and Mental Retardation in February, 1963. This message proposed a national program for mental health that called for the establishment of comprehensive community mental health centers, improved care in state mental hospitals, expanded research efforts, and increased support for training personnel for research and service. Passage of the Mental Retardation Facilities and Community Mental Health Center Construction Act in October 1963 further increased the range of treatment settings which shifted the emphasis from hospital to community treatment (Kramer, 1977). At this time, idealism was rampant and the deinstitutionalization machinery shifted into full gear (Mechanic, 1980).

Another significant variable giving impetus to deinstitutionalization was Medicare legislation granting disability payments under Social Security legislation to individuals who had been hospitalized in mental institutions. Passed in July, 1965, this legislation enabled former patients to pay for community treatment services and private residential facilities more easily (Blain, 1975).

In 1969, California passed the Lanterman-Petris-Short Act limiting involuntary commitment only to those individuals considered dangerous to themselves and others. Under this law, simply being psychotic and requiring treatment were no longer grounds for involuntary commitment. Passage of this legislation decreased by 99% the number of petitions for involuntary admission filed by the courts (Blain, 1975).

The Community Mental Health Centers Amendments of 1976 required state mental health authorities to develop and carry out plans to improve the quality of care in mental institutions, eliminate inappropriate placements in institutions, establish and enforce standards for operations of mental health programs and facilities, provide assistance in screening persons at risk of institutionalization, and provide after-care programs for ex-patients. Three of the seven essential new components added to the list of mandatory services had a direct bearing on services to long-term patients; assistance to courts and other public agencies in screening persons considered for referral to state mental health facilities, aftercare for those discharged from a mental health facility, and establishment of halfway houses for ex-patients (Lamb, 1976).

In 1977, President Carter established a Presidential Commission on Mental Health. The Commission's report argued for a greater investment in mental health services, as mental health currently received a disproportionately low percentage of all general health expenditures. The report also noted the need for more community-based services, as well as the need for those services to be more geographically, financially, and socially accessible and able to serve the needs of a variety of social and racial groups. The report also called for increased attention to chronic mental illness. This report, therefore, implied that further programs for the patient in rural areas needed to be developed (Mechanic, 1980).

The Commission's report led to the passage of the Mental Health Systems Act in 1980 which mandates an improved network of services for the chronic patient and promotion of preventive care. The bill also supports mental health advocacy services and seeks to eradicate the discriminatory practices of communities against deinstitutionalized patients (Mechanic, 1980).

Under the Reagan administration, mental health, along with most other social services, can be expected to take a back seat. Although it is uncertain at this time exactly how mental health will be affected, it seems doubtful that any new programs will be implemented unless such programs can be shown to be extremely cost effective and accountable, and to contain a strong evaluation component.

In addition to federal and state legislation, several important court cases have set precedents in such areas as the right of potential involuntary patients to procedural safeguards (*Lessard* vs *Schmidt*, 349 F. Supp. 1078, Ed. Wis., 1922); right to treatment (*Rouse* vs *Cameron*, 373 F. 2nd 451, D.C. Cir., 1966; *Wyatt* vs *Stickney*, 344 F. Supp. 373, M. D. Ala. 1972); the responsibility to use the least drastic form of care (*Lessard* vs *Schmidt*); the right of nondangerous individuals to freedom (*O'Conner* vs *Donaldson*, No. 74–8, 1975) and the right to treatment in the least restrictive alternative (*Dixon* vs *Weinberger*, 405 F. Supp. 974, D.C. 1975). These legal decisions have all had a significant impact on the de-institutionalization movement (Wodarski, 1980a).

The advent of the major tranquilizers in the 1950s provided yet another impetus for the change in locus of treatment. Psychotropic drugs provided both rapid stabilization of acute illness and symptom reduction in the chronic population allowing thousands of patients to be deinstitutionalized and preventing the institutionalization syndrome, which often accompanies long-term treatment, from occurring in many more. Chemotherapy continues to be a vitally important treatment modality in both hospital and community settings. After the first reports of therapeutic success with drugs, psychiatrists initially hoped that the chronic backward patient would become a phenomenon of the past. Unfortunately, the new tranquilizers were no panacea. Although the chronic schizophrenic's more pressing symptoms may be reduced or eliminated and social adjustment within the hospital improved, chemotherapy has not eliminated the necessity for hospitalization. Some patients fail to respond to psychotropic medication (Cochran, 1974). Freyhan and Merkel (1961) note that good clinical response to drug therapy does not guarantee a good clinical and social response once patients leave the hospital. These researchers found that mere symptom reduction does not ensure that a patient will recover motivation, ambition, and drive; nor that he or she will manifest an acceptable level of social skills. Furthermore, it was discovered that some patients can function adequately in their social and vocational roles even while manifesting a full-blown symptom constellation.

Discharge rates since the introduction of drug therapy are actually little different qualitatively from release rates achieved with such therapies as ECT and insulin. The available drugs are nonspecific in their actions in that they affect no known causal process (Klerman, 1961). The widespread use of the major tranquilizers has, however, made hospitalization periods briefer, if not less frequent. The effect has been that the public now perceives the hospital as a treatment center rather than a permanent home from which patients seldom, if ever, emerge (Klerman, 1961). Additionally, psychotropic medications can be prescribed and monitored on an outpatient basis. Administration of the older therapies usually required that the patient be hospitalized. Clearly, chemotherapy has been a major force in the gathering momentum of deinstitutionalization policy. Development of these "wonder drugs," combined with idealism in social policy and an increased emphasis on civil liberties, created a fertile soil in which deinstitutionalization has mushroomed. It was an idea whose moment had come, but time, experimentation, and personnel training were necessary before the goals implicit in the policy could be effectively realized.

A REVIEW OF PROBLEM AREAS IN DEINSTITUTIONALIZATION AND MAJOR SUCCESSFUL INTERVENTION STRATEGIES

As research practitioners have studied the special needs of the deinstitutionalized chronic patient, they have generally focused on identification of: 1) common characteristics of the chronic patients; 2) subgroups of chronic patients most likely to be rehospitalized; 3) problem areas in the patient's environment in which interventions are most likely to have a positive impact on community adjustment; and 4) types of interventions most likely to be successful.

The major characteristics common to chronic patients that have been identified are:

1. High vulnerability to stress   Even the minimal to moderate stress inherent in community life often causes relapse.
2. Lack of coping or everyday living skills   These individuals often depend heavily on their families, institutions, or aftercare programs for assistance in day-to-day living.

3. An inability to compete successfully in the job market This is largely due to lack of skills and work habits, poor interpersonal skills, and significant gaps in employment history.
4. Inability to establish and maintain close interpersonal relationships
5. Lack of either motivation or ability to seek help from or sustain rapport with mental health professionals
6. Tendency toward acting out agressive behaviors that interfere with their own well-being or that of others
7. Dependency needs that are exacerbated by fears of abandonment or engulfment, as well as an incapacity for autonomous functioning characterized by a need to seek external structure and control
8. Limited repertoire of problem solving techniques
9. Abnormal sensitivity to interpersonal relationships, physical environment, and cultural attitudes (Glasscote et al., 1971; Isenberg, Mahnke, and Shields, 1974; Lamb, 1976; Test and Stein, 1978; Turner and Ten Hoor, 1978)

Although most chronic mental patients share these characteristics, research practitioners began to notice that among the chronic population, certain subgroups manifest a higher rate of readmission to institutions. *Recidivism rates* were higher for schizophrenics than for nonschizophrenics, but it was found that schizophrenics who received aftercare services had a good chance of staying outside the hospital (Winston et al., 1977). Several studies have attempted to identify those patients most likely to be drop-outs of aftercare programs: males were more likely than females to discontinue aftercare services as were single rather than married individuals. Patients with less than a high school education were also considered to be at risk (Winston et al., 1977; Wooley and Kane, 1977). Researchers also discovered that the longer a patient can remain outside the hospital, the greater are his or her chances of making a successful long-term community adjustment. Return rates are believed to be highest during the first 3 months after discharge and the first month in the community was found to be particularly critical (Cunningham et al., 1969; Smith and Smith, 1979).

Numerous critics of institutional care have commented on the hospital's tendency to foster attitudes of dependency and passivity in patients which insidiously undermine their chances of making a successful adjustment to life in the community where autonomous and independent functioning is essential. During long years of hospital treatment, patients lose confidence in their ability to meet their own needs. Work and interpersonal skills atrophy and families emotionally divorce the patients; they truly become "dead to the world" (Boettcher and Schie, 1975; Denner, 1974; Lamb, 1976; Lipsitt, 1961; Test and Stein, 1978; Wright and Kogut, 1972). These criticisms not only had the effect of accelerating the deinstitutionalization movement, but also led to significant changes in hospital treatment programs, undermining the medical model concept that rehabilitation training should not be instituted until after symptomatology is eliminated (Fairweather et al., 1969). As researchers began to report on successful community-based treatment alternatives, the hospitals began to institute short-term, crisis theory oriented programs aimed at preventing the institutionalization syndrome (Huey, 1977; Test and Stein, 1978).

As the characteristics of the chronic, overly institutionalized mental patient were examined, it soon became evident that ex-patients required long-term, open-ended community training and support programs aimed at the major problem areas of socialization, establishment of supportive living programs, vocational rehabilitation, help for patients in becoming reintegrated into their families, and development of health maintenance and medication monitoring programs (Schinke, 1979; Schinke and Olson, in press; Test and Stein, 1978; Turner and Ten Hoor, 1978). Community-based intervention strategy development began to be perceived in terms of lessening the aggregate environmental demands placed on the client.

Socialization

A major advance to facilitate community maintenance, socialization training involves the acquisition or revival of skills in fundamentals of nutrition, meal planning and preparation, shopping, use of public transportation, money management and banking, leisure skills, essentials of grooming and personal hygiene, and knowledge of basic social amenities. It also focuses on the control or elimination of bizarre and/or aggressive verbal and motor behaviors and the development of interpersonal skills. Numerous researchers have suggested that socialization preparation is probably the single most important factor in maintenance of community placement (Anthony and Margules, 1974; Cochran, 1974; Lamb, 1976; Paul and Lentz, 1977). Because socialization is so essential, tremendous effort has been aimed at developing successful intervention strategies. A review of the literature suggests that in order to be successful, a socialization program should be community based, using non-mental health professionals whenever possible in order to provide a "normalizing" learning environment that facilitates generalization of skills. Also, it should be aimed at a specific socialization target, be long term rather than time limited, and should define specific treatment goals for each client (Lamb, 1976; Test and Stein, 1978; Turner and Ten Hoor, 1978; Wodarski, 1980b). Socialization programs differ in their approaches. The three most commonly employed models are the educational program, the social club, and the companionship program.

The Educational Model Lamb (1976) reported on the development of a Personal Growth Education course for ex-patients that was held as part of a local high school's adult education program. The course enabled patients not only to acquire socialization skills, but also to perceive themselves in a normal societal role (i.e., students in school). Gottesfeld (1976) mentions a successful skills educational program using volunteers and operating on a very limited budget ($150 a month in 1972) which trained ex-patients in self-care, current events, and use of public transportation. Furedy, Crowder, and Silvers (1977) devised a transitional socialization program in which patients and their families together formulated behavioral objectives and reviewed goal attainment at weekly group meetings. Patients and their families kept frequency counts between meetings in order to correctly assess the extent of behavioral change. Patients were taught daily living skills, money management, meal planning, use of city transportation, and recreational and social skills. The success of this program can be attributed largely to the use of behavior modification techniques and is consistent with a considerable body of literature suggesting that application of learning theory principles is the most successful, efficient, and cost-effective means of socialization skills training (Friesen, 1974; Furedy et al., 1977; Glasscote et al., 1971; Paul and Lentz, 1977).

Paul and Lentz (1977) conducted a highly ambitious and well designed study comparing milieu and social learning theory approaches. Two matched groups of severely debilitated chronic patients were housed in identical facilities and subjected to similar psychosocial rehabilitation programs. The social learning program maintained clear superiority over the milieu program with 90% of the social learning residents remaining continuously in the community after discharge at the time of the 1½ years followup, as opposed to 70% of the milieu group. However, only 50% of the hospital group with which both programs were compared maintained community placement. Moreover, cost effectiveness analysis found that the social learning program was the most effective and least expensive. Considered economically, during the project period it returned over three times the dollar savings of the hospital program and over 30% more dollar savings than the milieu program for the same dollars spent on treatment costs. Social learning therapy produced improvements across the board and clearly emerged as being the treatment of choice.

Results of the foregoing project demonstrated that how staff activity and attention are applied is much more important than how much occurs. In the area of adaptive behavior, both programs produced initial improvement in self-care, interpersonal, and communication skills. However, the communication of expectancies, group pressures, and practice in group problem solving and crises resolution in the milieu program led to no further improvement beyond activating the performance of dormant skills. In contrast, the social learning residents produced consistent, gradual increases in the acquisition of new skills. In the area of maladaptive behavior, social learning also emerged as more effective than milieu therapy for reduction or elimination of bizarre behavior. Such bizarre motor behaviors as rocking, repetitive movements, and blank staring were the most frequent observable class of "crazy" behavior. Social learning techniques for dealing with these problems primarily consisted of ignoring them and reinforcing incompatible adaptive behaviors. Bizarre dysfunctional cognitive behaviors (such as verbalized delusions and hallucinations, incoherent speech, and smiling without apparent stimulus) were reduced about equally in both milieu and social learning programs. These findings are in keeping with a considerable literature suggesting that cognitive functions, in general, tend to be more consistent within individuals, less variable across situations, and more modifiable through simple transmission of information (Paul and Lentz, 1977).

Social Clubs   Bell (1970), Lamb (1976), and Wechsler (1961) have commented on the rehabilitative effect of client participation in ex-patient social clubs. Besides providing social skills training, leisure time activity, and exposure to "normal" role models when community volunteers are used, these clubs also help clients to develop a support system, overcoming their very real feelings of isolation and alienation. Clubs can be led by members, professionals, or volunteers and may be highly goal oriented or strictly social. Belonging to a club may help the ex-patient cope with the sense of abandonment he or she may feel when no longer belonging to the hospital.

Companionship Programs   This model stresses the benefits of forming close one-to-one relationships between former patients and community members. Denner (1974) and Lamb (1976) comment on the positive modeling effects that occur when this model is implemented, but both researchers stress that the companions must encourage independence, utilize public transportation, and encourage the client to participate in the planning of the activities in order to help overcome apathy and dependence.

A variety of both formal and informal socialization programs can be extremely valuable in helping the long-term patient meet the normal demands of daily living. Formal programs with a learning theory approach can teach such basic living skills as the patient needs to provide confidence in one's ability to cope independently. Informal social clubs and companionship programs provide the opportunity to cement those skills and to practice the development of interpersonal relationships in a supportive, low-stress situation. Both kinds of experience are necessary to help the patient meet the inevitably stressful demands of normal life.

Supportive Living

Arrangement of adequate residential placements for ex-patients has been a major problem plaguing mental health professionals since the inception of the deinstitutionalization movement. Locating clean, comfortable, and affordable rooms for ex-patients is next to impossible in some communities. Many ex-patients are unable to live independently and need at least minimal supervision in order to remain in the community. Even when housing programs for these individuals are ongoing, numerous problems prevail. Many board and care homes are as effective in "institutionalizing" patients as are hospitals, due to lack of stimulation and rehabilitative treatment efforts. Buildings are often substandard, with numerous safety hazards existing, and clients are many times fed starchy, nutritionally unsound diets (Allen, 1976; Silverstein, 1979). "Mental health ghettos" evolve in the inner city due to local zoning ordinances, requirement for use permits, and other interpretations of various ordinances, all of which are designed to prevent the establishment of residential facilities in more attractive neighborhoods (Edelson, 1976).

In an effort to remedy this unfortunate situation, a variety of residential alternatives have been successfully developed, including cooperative apartments, group homes, family and foster care homes, foster care communities, halfway houses, and lodges (Earles, 1976; Fairweather et al., 1969; Goldmeir, 1975; Huey, 1977; Mannino et al., 1977). These programs differ extensively in the degree of supervision, size, and the extent to which the facility limits the number of choices the resident is free to make. Although space limits an extensive discussion of each of these residential models, comprehensive descriptions are available in the literature cited above. What this array of models does have in common is a commitment to stimulating, high-quality residential care.

Findings suggest that half-way houses are probably the best residential alternative, with one study reporting that 80% of half-way house residents make a successful community adjustment and that rehospitalization rates are lower for this population (Gottesfeld, 1976). Unfortunately, relatively few such facilities exist. These environments generally provide a rehabilitative, high-expectation milieu in contrast to the stultifying atmosphere common to most board and care facilities. Paul and Lentz (1977) note that patients often regress in functioning in the latter, with the highest regression rates being found in facilities that benefit financially for retaining ex-patients.

Although a wide variety of alternatives exist, the mental health practitioner encounters many difficulties in locating a placement. The worker must take a number of factors into consideration, such as the level at which the patient can function, the patient's treatment needs, and the patient's personality in relation to the personalities of the staff and other residents at a given facility. In addition, there is often a problem of timing. Perhaps no vacancy exists at the time it is needed, or perhaps the community does not offer the kind of residence the patient seems to require (Edelson, 1976). The size of the facility is another factor that should be taken into consideration. Cunningham et al. (1969), found that ex-patients placed in larger homes tend to remain in the community longer. Earles (1976) also found that schizophrenics were more comfortable in larger homes.

Interventions with Families

Although a substantial body of literature suggests that ex-patients should not be discharged to family members, such placements are often inevitable because of the lack of acceptable residential facilities. Byers, Cohen, and Harshbarger (1978) found that the best single predictor of recidivism was the person to whom the patient was discharged. Patients released to a spouse were the most likely to be readmitted and averaged the fewest number of days in the community between release and first readmission, whereas patients discharged to a sibling averaged the fewest number of days in the community during a 2-year period. Patients discharged to their children or a nonrelative comprised the most successful group. Leff (1976) noted that severely disturbed behavior among patients was reported for 30% of patients living with a spouse or parent and that these patients were readmitted at least once in the final 3 years of a 5-year follow-up. Nevertheless, as deinstitutionalization accelerates, and as alternative means supported through federal and state tax dollars diminish, more families will probably find themselves burdened with the responsibility of caring for their mentally disturbed relatives. Efforts should therefore be directed toward providing patients and their families with the services and support needed to make such placements as comfortable as possible for all concerned. Additionally, research indicates that a patient's relationship with the family can serve as an index of total social adaptability. A mature, cooperative attitude toward the family corresponds generally with successful social adaptation; whereas the patient who maintains a hostile or indifferent attitude toward his or her family usually exhibits poor social performance (Meszaros and Meszaros, 1961). Clearly, the complex emotional relationships existing in a family unit require special handling if a family placement is to be successful. Lamb (1976) indicates that the family members need contact with professionals who can understand their problems, answer their questions, and comprehend the stress involved in living with an ex-patient. In answer to this need, he recommends the use of diagnostic family interviews in day treatment programs. Such diagnostic interviews allow the staff to gain insight into the family's interactional patterns, which the patient may be unable to verbally describe. Family interview sessions should be ongoing if the patient and family are willing and if staff time allows.

Huey (1977) reports Aguilera's suggestion that family stresses arise, in part, because the family members eliminated the patient from their lives while he or she was in the hospital. The family must undergo a readjustment when the patient returns home. If the patient fails to adjust to the routine the family has established during his or her absence, the family may want the patient returned to the hospital. When a family wants a patient readmitted, the practitioner must learn to identify who is in crisis—the patient or the family. The family's attempt to have the patient readmitted may be a reaction to its own anxiety about the patient's possible disruptive behavior. When original symptom displays reappear, there is usually a correlation between change in the family's routine and the patient's resumption of abnormal behavior. The practitioner must determine what event precipitated the return to psychotic behavior and also whether or not the patient is taking prescribed medication.

Crisis resolution techniques include helping patients to understand the crisis and openly express their feelings, exploring coping techniques used in the past that can be used in the present, finding family members and friends in the environment who can support the patient, and planning with the patient ways to reduce the likelihood of future crises.

Lamb and Oliphant (1978) recount many of the stresses with which family members must cope when the patient lives at home. The schizophrenic's behavior is unpredictable, often socially embarrassing, and even violent at times. The patient's social withdrawal, inactivity, excessive sleeping, and lack of conversational skills provide little positive reinforcement for the family. In addition, the family experiences the stigma of having produced a schizophrenic. Many parents of schizophrenic children withdraw from their social contacts because of the guilt and stigma attached to their situation. The family also experiences trauma when confronted with the notion, prevalent in some psychiatric circles, that the entire family unit is sick and the patient simply happens to be the person labeled as ill.

These same authors report on the recent growth of family advocacy and mutual-support groups. Such groups help members feel less isolated. The group can share feelings, get each other through crises, work through guilt feelings, and learn to see themselves in a less self-condemnatory light. The groups also can provide for emotional catharsis. In addition, one study found that participation in groups facilitated individual casework. Family members felt less threatened by the exploration of sensitive material once they had aired their feelings in a group (Grinspoon, Courtney, and Bergan, 1961).

Group members can also share practical tips that make living with a schizophrenic easier. If professionals and the relatives can mutually agree on what a patient can achieve, and if the relatives can maintain emotional objectivity, they can apply pressure to counteract the patient's withdrawal. Patients must not be pushed to achieve beyond their capabilities, however, and they must be given the opportunity to exercise a good deal of control over their own behavior.

Relatives learn that it is often useless to contradict delusional ideas, but patients can be taught not to talk back to hallucinations in public. Relatives can also learn to expect a certain amount of withdrawal, which may be a necessary defense mechanism. Too much withdrawal, however, can lead to a form of institutionalism at home.

Family members are especially in need of support when the first psychotic break occurs. At that time, the family is particularly vulnerable and sensitive. They may feel guilty and wonder what they have done to "cause" such a thing to happen. Marital relationships also are strained during this time. Siblings of patients are often ignored or neglected while parental attention is focused on the "sick" member of the family. Practitioners should provide understanding and reassurance at this point. They should always explain to the relatives that schizophrenia is not merely the result of environment; heredity and biological factors are equally important (Lamb and Oliphant, 1978).

In certain cases, assertiveness training helps relatives set limits on the amount of crazy behavior with which they are willing to cope. It may also help them deal more effectively with the professionals they encounter (Lamb and Oliphant, 1978). As noted earlier, family members' cooperation and participation in formulating and monitoring behavioral objectives can be extremely significant in the success of socialization training.

Vocational Rehabilitation

Because an ability to compete successfully in the economic marketplace has long been an important criterion of success in American society, many researchers have directed efforts toward vocational training for ex-patients. An ability to successfully perform in the work world gives patients a sorely needed sense of mastery. Gottesfeld (1976) reports the Gibson et al. finding that when an experimental group of chronic patients were given work assignments commensurate with their skills and interests, the community re-entry rate was 37%, whereas only 18% of the control group were able to make a successful adjustment to the community.

Gottesfeld (1976) also describes a rehabilitation program in Virginia in which chronic patients in a state hospital received vocational training before entering a community residence and finding local employment. The majority of the group participants made a successful readjustment and very few group members were readmitted.

Kirk (1977) reports that the unemployed may constitute a special population at risk of readmission. Wooley and Kane (1977) note that patients with less than a high school education tend to evidence more recidivism and a higher rate of unemployment. Yet those patients who had been previously employed in professional and managerial positions may have an equally difficult time finding employment. Generally, those patients from semiskilled, labor, and agricultural fields have a higher probability of being rehired (Wooley and Kane, 1977).

Ex-patients often report that co-worker conflict, low pay, and lack of skills interfere with their ability to make a successful vocational adjustment (Peretti, 1974). Additionally, such patients have been found to hold unrealistic and grandiose expectations regarding their employment potential (Fairweather et al., 1969). Other major problem areas that have emerged include difficulties in interpersonal relations, phobic attitudes toward work in general, fear of failure, ineffective use of job interviews, projection of self-rejection to authority figures, oversensitivity to disappointment or inadequacy, inability to persevere toward task completion, and an inability to take orders (Greenblatt and Simon, 1959; Huey, 1977). Thus, social workers should be prepared to deal with these variables to ensure the success of community maintenance.

Despite the apparently acute need for vocational skills training, few opportunities for rehabilitation exist. Day treatment programs seldom maintain a sheltered workshop on the premises, and mental health centers and public vocational rehabilitation programs are often scarce (Gottesfeld, 1976). Such public agencies usually focus on the plight of the physically disabled and perceive the problems of the mentally disabled as belonging to the mental health system. In order to address these problems, numerous experimental programs have been developed. Researchers have generally found that in-house vocational rehabilitation programs should be designed to be as much like a genuine work environment as possible so that the patient can create an identity of themselves as a worker, rather than as a patient. Lamb (1976) found that behaviors varied considerably among patients in transition from day treatment to a sheltered workshop. Patients spent one-half day in each setting; because crazy behavior was not tolerated in the workshop, patients behaved like workers. In the morning, however, when patients attended the day center, they exhibited bizarre behavior never seen in the workshop. Apparently, the majority of patients can learn to behave like normal workers when it is required of them. Fairweather and his colleagues (1969) found that when patients were asked not to hallucinate on the job, they could comply, and began to hallucinate only when they were back in the truck on the way home after work. Thus, the supervisor's expectations have a substantial influence on the patients' work behavior.

Freisen (1974) argues that behavior modification techniques can be extremely useful in teaching work habits to patients. When patients are having a work problem, their behavior can be observed and the environment modified to remove those elements that encourage sick behavior. Token economies imitate the real world and help to accustom patients to working for secondary reinforcers. Tokens can be saved and spent as the patients wish, thus teaching them to postpone immediate gratification.

In addition to job and interpersonal skills, ex-patients also need to learn how to look for a job and how to behave on an interview. Furedy et al. (1977) included behavioral rehearsals to teach job-finding skills in their socialization program. Patients role-played job interviews and job-related social situations. Likewise, Anthony and Margules (1974) reported on a program designed to improve job seeking and interviewing. At the nine-week followup, 50% of the clients had been employed 30 days or more in contrast to 24% of the untrained group. Clearly, training in job seeking and interviewing imparts motivation and a sense of confidence to these chronic patients.

No discussion of innovations in vocational rehabilitation for the mentally ill would be complete without mentioning Fountain House in New York City. The center's transitional employment program, which has served as a model for vocational rehabilitation programs all over the country, places members on four- to six-month rotations in entry level positions in 54 New York City businesses. The key to this program is gradual transition from the residence to the employment context.

Medication Monitoring

Research literature suggests that drug therapy must remain a constant for many chronic patients if they are to survive in the community. Gross and Reeves (1961) note that the risk of relapse is considerably greater if medication is discontinued, at least during the first year after discharge. Kris (1961) states that certain patients may even require an increased dosage when they return to the community, due to the increased level of stress and excitement. Paul and Lentz (1977), on the other hand, feel that no changes in drug status should be made during the first few months after discharge, believing that such a change inhibits the transfer of behaviors learned in the treatment setting. At any rate, medication should be monitored carefully during the initial post-release period, particularly as certain patients—notably males and patients who are aggressive, paranoid, or hypomanic—resent taking medication and tend to discontinue doing so (Freyhan and Merkel, 1961).

A variety of experimental medication monitoring programs have enjoyed success. Gottesfeld (1976) reported that as many as 40% of patients may fail to report to office-centered therapy sessions, but that a goal-achievement-oriented home visit program for 20 after-care patients resulted in a recidivism rate of zero during the first 6 months. Staff members monitored drug ingestion during non-scheduled visits and dispensed rewards to those patients who continued medication. The investigators estimated that costs for the home visit group amounted to only about one-third the costs incurred by the control group who had a significant recidivism rate.

Isenberg et al. (1974) successfully implemented a weekly medication group for outpatients in a Massachusetts clinic. The authors noted that the patients' fears of being unable to regulate their dosages and of being dependent on the drugs lessened as they had the opportunity to discuss their feelings with others.

Test and Stein (1978), in discussing the importance of continued medication monitoring, note that certain studies suggest that medication is considerably more effective than psychotherapy in reducing recidivism. Indeed, insight-oriented psychotherapy may even hasten relapse in certain groups of patients (Lamb, 1976; Test and Stein, 1978).

By and large, the literature suggests that regular medication is almost essential for most chronic patients. Unfortunately, these patients typically lack the motivation necessary to continue self-medication or to maintain contact with after-care services. Thus, a requisite role for the rural community mental health social worker is to ensure that deinstitutionalized clients take their medication. Behavior modification programs, group meetings, and home-centered outreach programs may be essential—particularly for the high-risk groups mentioned earlier.

Despite its importance, drug therapy is no cure-all. Psychotropic drugs often create such side effects as extra-pyramidal symptoms and tardive dyskinesia, causing these patients to manifest such bizarre motoric behavior that normal community members may be shocked or repelled. Although these side effects can usually be counteracted by the administration of additional medication, it is nevertheless ironic that chemotherapy has created yet another barrier to community acceptance for the chronic patient.

EMERGING ISSUES IN RURAL DEINSTITUTIONALIZATION

Throughout history, artists and writers have romanticized country life as idyllic and carefree and, to some extent, these ingrained stereotypes of rural environments have stunted the development of research efforts aimed at meeting the special needs of rural mentally ill individuals. The back-to-nature ideology of the 60s and 70s further promoted the notion that pastoral life enhances rather than diminishes mental health. The evidence available now, however, suggests that rural communities tend to be characterized by higher than average rates of psychiatric disorder, particularly depression, and data from one study in Tennessee suggest that 12% of the rural population require psychiatric care (President's Task Force on Long-Term Care, 1978).

Rural individuals differ significantly from urbanites in their attitudes toward mental illness. They are more inclined to perceive the cause of mental illness as societal, citing such sources as the unsettled world situation, economic pressures and stresses within their county, and the failure of such traditional institutions as the church and family to provide necessary emotional support (Segal, 1978). Rural people frequently manifest a suspiciousness of outsiders and may be wary of mental health services, particularly when treatment demands that they disclose a substantial amount of personal information (Helton, 1977). This fear is not without realistic basis, as confidentiality is considerably more difficult to maintain in small communities (Horejsi, 1977).

Rural residents often have a fatalistic attitude toward life in general which is fostered by the fundamentalist religious beliefs common in these areas. They often have low expectations for even their "normal" family members and are unable to see the value of training and education for their mentally and/or emotionally disabled offspring (Helton, 1977; Horejsi, 1977). The President's Task Force on Long-Term Care (1978) notes that rural people have restricted opportunities to develop adequate coping mechanisms for facing stress and problem solving and have little faith that change is possible. Rural residents may, however, have higher tolerance for the idiosyncratic behavior of mentally ill persons. Segal (1973) mentions that rural patients were rated by their relatives as less helpless and more stable than were their urban counterparts. These same rural people were judged by their clinicians to be more adaptable, less impaired, and less perceptually disturbed than city patients in their manifestations of hostility and grandiosity. As a possible explanation, Segal (1978) suggests that the urban patient who is excited, hostile, and grandiose is more likely to land in a full-time hospital than is a rural patient who is manifesting the same symptoms. Urban patients exhibited more of the passive-type symptoms (helplessness, instability, and impairment) associated with the institutionalization syndrome and caused by longer and/or more frequent hospitalizations.

Rural patients are generally felt to be less of a source of distress to their families, despite the strong bonds of interdependency common to rural families (Helton, 1977; Segal, 1973). Meszaros and Meszaros (1961), however, feel that dependency problems are more severe among rural patients. They argue that geographic isolation and social isolation go hand in hand, causing the members of the family unit to be highly dependent upon the adjustment of each other, as interests and activities are often confined to the family itself. Therefore, family stresses and tensions are more apt to tip the emotional balance of rural patients.

A lack of adequate residential and treatment facilities further compounds the problems of chronically mentally ill individuals. Sparsely populated communities are frequently forced to place rural patients in urban after-care settings because of limited or nonexistent residential alternatives in their home communities. Unfortunately, these "transplants" experience heightened psychological and social problems in urban rehabilitation settings (Bachrach, 1977). Because the half-way house is a predominantly urban phenomenon, rural residents often must be discharged to their families which, as previously discussed, necessitates that clinicians be available for family counseling and crisis intervention. Yet this mode of intervention is rarely feasible due to geographic distance and transportation difficulties (Horejsi, 1977). Many impoverished rural residents do not own vehicles and although traveling teams of professionals are often used, travel time shrinks the federal budget dollars as the professional hours it buys are then proportionately diminished (Segal, 1973).

Staff attitudes also contribute to the problem of meeting rural clients' needs. Community mental health centers are often committed to primary prevention and treatment of life crises; treatment of the chronically mentally ill is frequently a low priority (Lamb and Edelson, 1976). The chronically mentally ill individual is not always a rewarding client, but practitioners' frustrations probably have more to do with a lack of appropriate clinical skills than with the client's degree of treatability. Behavior modification techniques have been demonstrated to be a successful treatment strategy with this population, yet most social workers have received their training in schools that stress a traditional psychoanalytically oriented treatment approach. Workers in community mental health centers understandably feel resentful and rejecting when called upon to provide services for vast numbers of chronic clients, as neither the workers nor their agencies have been adequately prepared to deal with this population (Feldman, 1978; Silverstein, 1979; Test and Stein, 1978). The demands of practice in rural areas are even more overwhelming. Breadth of duties and excessive travel causes staff burnout and high turnover. Yet rural communities can rarely afford or attract a wide variety of professionals with specialized skills. Practitioners may also suffer from loneliness and isolation, and lack of professional stimulation, supervision, and consultation (Horejsi, 1977).

IMPLICATIONS FOR PRACTICE AND TRAINING

If rural practice presents many problems for social workers, it also offers many challenges and potential rewards when practitioners have developed the necessary competencies.

1. One essential competency is the ability to train and supervise para-professionals and volunteers. Paraprofessional mental health workers currently, and will continue to, play an increasingly significant role in rural community mental health. Use of indigenous workers can be invaluable in remote areas in which recruitment of skilled professionals is difficult and funding for highly trained workers scarce (Horejsi, 1977). Paraprofessionals can be extremely valuable in outreach programs and can aid in early detection and intervention. Personnel who live among the people they treat and with the people who form a network of community caregivers can more easily keep a finger on the pulse of the community and support networks that are available (Dyck, 1974).

    Use of paraprofessionals has already become a trend in many urban day treatment centers; and preliminary findings have suggested that they may actually have fresher, more optimistic attitudes toward chronic patients' potential than do professional staff members (Gottesfeld, 1976; Wright and Kogut, 1972). Obviously, graduate level social workers will be needed to provide consultation, education, and supervision in order to ensure that these workers have the adequate skills and training to carry out these tasks.

2. The ability to coordinate and mobilize existing community resources is an essential competency rural social workers must develop. Numerous authors have noted that one major problem in effective implementation of de-institutionalization exists because no one agency at any level of government has been clearly charged with responsibility for comprehensive assessments of mental health services, for appropriate community support activities, such as planning and implementing a system to assure needs are met, and for monitoring the quality of both institutional and community programs. Consequently, many of the people most seriously in need of service "fall through the cracks" (Gottesfeld, 1976; Horejsi, 1977; Smith and Smith, 1979; Turner and Ten Hoor, 1978). Social work practitioners must use their relationship skills to cultivate bonds not only with existing public agencies, but with such leaders of the indigenous helping network as physicians, teachers, ministers, volunteer groups, and service clubs (Horejsi, 1977). Service clubs are often the prime movers in rural American communities. Although they may lack professional knowledge and sophistication in the mental health field, community leaders and influential people capable of motivating community support are often members of such organizations and can be extremely helpful if the social worker can learn to break down the needed tasks into components that the members can handle (Horejsi, 1977). Community leaders can also help the worker gain knowledge of local folklore which may have a bearing on the community's acceptance of essential programs (Horejsi, 1977).

A few of the contributions volunteer, church, and service organizations can provide include transportation for clients, respite care in their homes, fund raising activities, and local business contacts for work that clients can complete in sheltered vocational rehabilitation settings. The social worker who is skilled in community organization, public relations, and community education techniques can capitalize on the rural community's characteristic slant toward helping the person rather than curing the illness (Segal, 1973).

The social worker in rural community mental health must also strive to overcome interagency conflict and bias. Comprehensive mental health care can be developed by drawing on local resources. Johnson and Nelson (1972) report on a program in Iowa comprised of the psychiatric unit of a general hospital, a locally supported mental health center, a private group practice, and a half-way house for alcoholics. Long-term care and partial hospitalization services are provided by a nearby county home with a separate psychiatric unit. This coordinated system has resulted in a continuing drop in the area's admissions to the state hospital and substantial financial savings for the counties involved. This program model can be applied to many rural areas. The elements on which to build a high quality comprehensive program are available if imagination and foresight are utilized.

3. As previously noted, the available literature resoundingly supports the use of behavior modification techniques in socialization training, vocational rehabilitation, family interventions, and medication monitoring (Friesen, 1974; Furedy, et al., 1977; Glasscote et al., 1971; Paul and Lentz, 1977). Social workers dealing with the chronic population have a responsibility to provide their clients with the most effective treatment strategies available; and behavior modification has been shown to be not only the treatment of choice, but also the most cost-effective, a major consideration in rural areas in which travel expenses rapidly gobble up federal budget allotments (Paul and Lentz, 1977).

SUMMARY

Social, legal, and medical advances since World War II have caused the deinstitutionalization movement to snowball; and mental health professionals may now be wondering whether or not they have created a monster. There are no simple techniques for dealing with the chronic population. Indeed, the term *chronicity* implies that the programs serving this population must be long-term and open-ended (Turner and Ten Hoor, 1978). The numbers of chronic clients, in both rural and urban areas, are expected to increase while available federal monies decrease (Silverstein, 1979). This chapter has attempted to cite successful programs and techniques and to discuss the issues and implications for practice as they apply to the rural chronic population. The emerging profile of the successful rural-based implementer of deinstitutionalization strategy suggests that he or she: is familiar with the characteristics of the rural chronic population; is skilled in learning theory-based intervention strategies and applies them to the five major problem areas of socialization, supportive living, family intervention, vocational rehabilitation, and medication monitoring; effectively trains and supervises paraprofessional workers; and skillfully utilizes existing helping networks and coordinates community services.

Schools of social work have a responsibility to the chronic population to train their graduates to meet the challenges of implementation of deinstitutionalization strategies in rural areas. Practitioners must be equipped to assess the variety of factors that influence the return of clients to their original communities, and once returned, what maintenance factors operate to enable them to carry out this critical aspect of community mental health practice. Specific emphasis should be on delineating the use of natural and community support networks to provide essential mental health services to high risk, underserved populations such as the aged, minorities, and and high-risk children and adolescents in rural areas.

The focus of a comprehensive deinstitutionalization program in a rural area is provision of services through a balanced service system. Through this focus, practitioners assess how clients can benefit from a system that emphasizes continuity of care, remedial education, community alternatives when possible, coordination of services, acquisition of social skills necessary for community reintegration and maintenance, and use of specific criteria for community placement decisions, such as the client's ability to attend to personal needs, demonstrated or expressed willingness to share in housekeeping and maintenance tasks, if employable—a plan for employment, plans for involvement in constructive daytime activity in the community, and reasonable responsibility about medication. As an essential aspect of the rural mental health training project described in this text, students are taught treatment technologies that help clients acquire requisite social skills. Students also learn how to manipulate environmental resources necessary for their clients to function in a complex society.

In the rural mental health training project, emphasis has been on the development of materials to enable community mental health trainees to utilize efficacious and cost effective assessment procedures to isolate physical, psychological, and social factors leading to successful placements. The following are emphasized: 1) assessment of individual attributes, such as dependence, social skills, and economic resources, and community attributes, such as homogeneity of population, social cohesion, and employment possibilities; 2) evaluation of the individual's intimate environment, for example, family and primary groups that often play a part in the genesis and maintenance of problematic behaviors, and the assessment of whether or not such groups will help to support and maintain functional and more desirable behavior changes once they have been instituted; 3) preparation of the community in terms of enlistment of social networks such as family, peers, ministers, and public employees to provide necessary support; 4) preparation of the individual in terms of emphasizing appropriate social behaviors that will be rewarded and will facilitate integration into the social structure of the community; 5) educating the individual about support services available and whom to contact, and gradually introducing the individual to the new living context and to appropriate available support systems, that is, significant others, family members, friends, church members, and so forth; 6) maintaining placement, that is, monitoring placement and making necessary alterations to facilitate successful placement through the use of relevant diagnostic aids, for example, determining whether the individuals are maintaining themselves physically and socially in terms of going to work or receiving appropriate medical care and experiencing frequent social interactions to prevent social isolation, depression, and so forth (Brook, 1976; Fields, 1975; Keskiner, 1977; Lamb, 1976; Levine and Kozloff, 1978; Miller, 1977; Morrissey, 1965; Segal, 1973; Swann, 1973; Wood, 1976).

REFERENCES

Allen, P. 1976. A bill of rights for citizens using outpatient mental health services. In H. R. Lamb (ed.), Community Survival for Long-term Patients, pp. 147–170. Jossey-Bass, San Francisco.

Anthony, W. A., and Margules, A. 1974. Toward improving the efficiency of psychiatric rehabilitation: A skills training approach. Rehabil. Psychother. 21:104–105.

Bachrach, L. L. 1977. Deinstitutionalization of mental health services in rural areas. Hosp. Community Psych. 28:669–672.

Bell, A. Z. 1970. Social clubs help prevent readmission. Hosp. Community Psych. 21:161–162.

Blain, D. 1975. Twenty-five years of hospital and community psychiatry. Hosp. Community Psych. 26:605–609.

Boettcher, R. C., and Schie, R. V. 1975. Milieu therapy with chronic mental patients. Soc. Work, 20:130–134.

Brook, B. 1976. Community families: An alternative to psychiatric hospital intensive care. Hosp. Community Psych. 27:195–197.

Byers, E. S., Cohen, S., and Harshbarger, D. D. 1978. Impact of aftercare services on recidivism of mental hospital patients. Community Ment. Health J. 14:26–34.

Cochran, B. 1974. Where is my home? The closing of state mental hospitals. Hosp. Community Psych. 25:393–401.

Cunningham, M. K., Batwinik, W., Dolson, J., and Weickert, A. A. 1969. Community placement of released mental patients: A five-year study. Soc. Work 14:54–61.

Denner, B. 1974. Returning madness to an accepting community. Community Ment. Health J. 10:163–172.

Dyck, G. 1974. The effect of a community mental health center upon state hospitalization. Am. J. Psych. 131:433–436.

Earles, T. 1976. Building a state-wide supportive living program. Paper presented at the 25th Institute on Hospital and Community Psychiatry of the American Psychological Association, September, Atlanta, Ga.

Edelson, M. B. 1976. Alternative living arrangements. In H. R. Lamb (ed.), Community Survival for Long-Term Patients. Jossey-Bass, San Francisco.

Fairweather, G., Sanders, D., Maynard, H., Cresler, D. L., and Bleck, D. S. 1969. Community Life for the Mentally Ill: An Alternative to Institutional Care. Aldine Publishing Co., Chicago.

Feldman, S. 1978. Promises, promises or community mental health services and training: Ships that pass in the night. Community Ment. Health J. 14:83–91.

Fields, S. 1975. Breaking through the boarding house blues. Innovation Summer:2–10.

Freisen, D. D. 1974. The use of behavior modification techniques with the mentally ill. In R. E. Hardy and J. G. Cull (eds.), Modification of Behavior of the Mentally Ill: Rehabilitation Approaches, pp. 15–35. Charles C.Thomas Publishers, Springfield, Ill.

Freyhan, F. A., and Merkel, J. 1961. Clinical and social aspects of compensatory drug treatment. In M. Greenblatt, D. Levinson and G. Klerman (eds.), Mental Patients in Transition: Steps in Hospital-Community Rehabilitation. Charles C. Thomas Publishers, Springfield, Ill.

Furedy, R., Crowder, M., and Silvers, F. 1977. Transitional care: A new approach to aftercare. Hosp. Community Psych. 28:118–122.

Glasscote, R. M., Cumming, E., Rutman, I. D., Sussex, J. N., and Glassman, S. M. 1971. Rehabilitating the Mentally Ill in the Community: A Study of Psychosocial Rehabilitation Centers. Publication of the Joint Information Service of the American Psychiatric Association and the National Association for Mental Health, Washington, D.C.

Goldmeir, J. 1975. New Directions in Aftercare: Cooperative Apartment Living. A report for the Mental Health Study Center, National Institute of Mental Health, Adelphi, Md., Professional Services Contract No. 158536.

Gottesfeld, H. 1976. Alternatives to psychiatric hospitalization: A review of the literature, 1972–1975. Community Ment. Health Rev. 1:4–10.

Greenblatt, M., and Simon, B. 1959. Rehabilitation of the Mentally Ill: Social and Economic Aspects. Publication No. 58 of the American Association for the Advancement of Science. Washington, D.C.

Grinspoon, L., Courtney, P. H., and Bergan, H. M. 1961. The usefulness of structural parent's group in rehabilitation. In M. Greenblatt, D. Levinson and G. Klerman (eds.), Mental Patients in Transition: Steps in Hospital-Community Rehabilitation, pp. 229–260. Charles C Thomas Publishers, Springfield, Ill.

Gross, M., and Reeves, W. P. 1961. Relapses after withdrawal of atractic drugs: An interim report. In M. Greenblatt, D. Levinson and G. Klerman (eds.), Mental Patients in Transition: Steps in Hospital-Community Rehabilitation, pp. 313–326. Charles C Thomas Publishers, Springfield, Ill.

Helton, S. 1977. Deinstitutionalization in a rural community. In R. K. Green and S. A. Webster (eds.), Social Work in Rural Areas: Preparation and Practice. pp. 298–302. University of Tennessee School of Social Work, Knoxville.

Horejsi, C. R. 1977. Rural community-based services for persons who are mentally retarded. In R. K. Green and S. A. Webster (eds.), Social Work in Rural Areas: Preparation and Practice, pp. 368–379. University of Tennessee School of Social Work, Knoxville.

Huey, K. 1977, The chronic psychiatric patient in the community: Highlights from a conference in Boston, Hosp. Community Psych. 28:283–290.

Isenberg, P. L., Mahnke, M. W., and Shields, W. E. 1974. Medication groups for continuing care. Hosp. Community Psych. 25:517–519.

Jeffrey, M. J., and Reeve, R. E. 1978. Community mental health services in rural areas: Some practical issues. Community Ment. Health J. 14:54–62.

Johnson, D. L., and Nelson, H. L. 1972. Providing comprehensive mental health services with local resources. Hosp. Community Psych. 23:279–281.

Keskiner, A. 1977. Determinants of placement outcomes in the foster community project. Dis. Nerv. Syst. 38:439–443.

Kirk, S. A. 1977. Who gets aftercare? A study of patients discharged from state hospitals in Kentucky. Hosp. Community Psych. 28:109–113.

Klerman, G. R. 1961. Historical baselines for the evaluation of maintenance drug therapy of discharged psychiatric patients. In M. Greenblatt, D. Levinson and G. Klerman (eds.), Mental Patients in Transition: Steps in Hospital-Community Rehabilitation, pp. 34–45. Charles C Thomas Publishers, Springfield, Ill.

Kramer, M. 1977. Psychiatric Services and the Changing Institution Scene, 1950–1985. NIMH, BHEW Publication No. (ADM) 77–433, Superintendent of Documents, U.S. Government Printing Office, Washington, D.C.

Kris, E. B. 1961. Prevention of rehospitalization through release control in a day hospital. In M. Greenblatt, D. Levinson and G. Klerman (eds.), Mental Patients in Transition: Steps in Hospital-Community Rehabilitation, pp. 155–162. Charles C Thomas Publishers, Springfield, Ill.

Lamb, H. R. 1976 Community Survival for Long-Term Patients. Jossey-Bass, San Francisco.

Lamb, H. R., and Edelson, M. B. 1976. The carrot and the stick: Inducing local programs to serve long-term patients. Community Ment. Health J. 12:137–144.

Lamb, H. R., and Oliphant, E. 1978. Schizophrenia through the eyes of families. Hosp. Community Psych. 29:803–806.

Leff, J. P. 1976. Schizophrenia and sensitivity to the family environment. Schiz. Bull. 2:566–574.

Levine, S., and Kozloff, M. A. 1978. The sick role: Assessment and overview. In R. H. Turner, J. Coleman and R. C. Fox (eds.), Annual Review of Sociology. Annual Reviews, Inc., Palo Alto, Calif.

Lipsitt, D. R. 1961. Institutional dependency: A rehabilitation problem. In M. Greenblatt, D. Levinson and G. Klerman (eds.), Mental Patients in Transition: Steps in Hospital-Community Rehabilitation, pp. 34–45. Charles C Thomas Publishers, Springfield, Ill.

Mannino, F. V., Ott, S., and Shore, M. P. 1977. Community residential facilities for former mental patients: An annotated bibliography. Psychosoc. Rehabil. J. 1:1-43.

Mechanic, D. 1980. Mental Health and Social Policy. Prentice-Hall, Englewood Cliffs, N.J.

Meszaros, A. F., and Meszaros, E. S. 1961. Integration of the discharged schizophrenic patient within the family. In M. Greenblatt, D. Levinson and G. Klerman (eds.), Mental Patients in Transition: Steps in Hospital-Community Rehabilitation, pp. ·218–229. Charles C Thomas Publishers, Springfield, Ill.

Miller, M. 1977. A program for adult foster care. Soc. Work 22:275–279.

Mittler, P. (ed.) 1979. Proceedings of the 5th Congress of the International Association for the Scientific Study of Mental Deficiency: Frontiers of Knowledge in Mental Retardation Vol. 1. University Park Press, Baltimore.

Morrissey, J. 1965. Family care for the mentally ill: A neglected therapeutic resource. Soc. Serv. Rev. 39:63–71.

Paul, G. L., and Lentz, R. J. 1977. Psychosocial Treatment of Chronic Mental Patients. Harvard University Press, Cambridge, Mass.

Peretti, P. O. 1974. Precipitating factors of readmission of psychiatric patients. Community Ment. Health J. 10:89–92.

President's Commission on Mental Health. 1978. Vol. 2 and 4—Task Panel Reports, February.

President's Task Force on Long-Term Care. 1978. Government Printing Office, Washington, D.C.

Schinke, S. P. 1979. Staff training in group homes: A family approach. In L. Hamerlynck (ed.), Behavioral Systems for the Developmentally Disabled: II. Brunner/Mazel, Inc., New York.

Schinke, S. P., and Olson, D. G. Home remediation of subacute sclerosing panencephalitis. Educ. Treat. Child. In press.

Segal, J. 1973. The Mental Health of Rural America: The Rural Programs of the National Institute of Mental Health. DHEW Publication No. (HSM) 73-9035. Washington, D.C.

Segal, S. 1978. The Mentally Ill in Community Based Sheltered Care: Study of Community Care and Social Integration. Wiley-Interscience, New York.

Silverstein, M. 1979. Deinstitutionalization and the chronic mental patient. In A. J. Katz (eds.), Community Mental Health: Issues for Social Work Practice and Education, pp. 92–101. Council on Social Work Education, New York.

Smith, C. J. and Smith, C. A. 1979. Evaluating outcome measures for deinstitutionalization programs. Soc. Work Res. Abstr. 15:23–30.

Swann, R. 1973. A survey of a boarding-home program for former mental patients. Hosp. Community Psych. 24:485–486.

Test, M. A., and Stein, L. I. 1978. Community treatment of the chronic patient: A research overview. Schizophr. Bull. 4:350–363.

Turner, J. C., and Ten Hoor, W. J. 1978. The NIMH Community Support Program: Pilot approach to a needed social reform. Schizophr. Bull. 4:319–348.

Wechsler, H. 1961. The ex-patient club: A general survey and case study. In M. Greenblatt, D. Levinson, and G. Klerman (eds.), Mental Patients in Transition: Steps in Hospital-Community Rehabilitation, pp. 104–113. Charles C Thomas Publishers, Springfield, Ill.

Winston, A., Pardes, H., Papernik, D. S., and Braslin, L. 1977. Aftercare of psychiatric patients and its relation to rehospitalization. Hosp. Community Psych. 28:118–121.

Wodarski, J. S. 1980a. Legal requisites for social work practice. Clin. Soc. Work J. 8:90–98.

Wodarski, J. S. 1980b. Procedures for the maintenance and generalization of achieved behavioral change. J. Sociol. Soc. Welfare, 7:298–311.

Wodarski, J. S., Giordano, J., and Bagarozzi, D. 1981. Training for competent community mental health practice: Implications for rural social work. Paper presented at the Annual Meeting of the Council on Social Work Education. March, Louisville, Kent.

Wood, P. 1976. A program to train operators of board-and-care homes in behavioral management. Hosp. Community Psych. 27:767–770.

Wooley, R. R., and Kane, R. L. 1977. Community aftercare of patients discharged from Utah State Hospital: A follow-up study. Hosp. Community Psych. 28:114–118.

Wright, A. L., and Kogut, R. S. 1972. A resocialization program for the treatment of chronic hospitalized schizophrenic patients. Dis. Nerv. Sys. 33:614–616.

This chapter was written with the assistance of Ms. Vicki Young, M.S.W., and Jeff Giordano, Assistant Professor of Social Work.

Chapter 4

Implementation
of Change Strategy

How, Where, By Whom, Why,
How Long, and On What Level?

SERVICE DELIVERY MODELS

In recent years there have been numerous radically different models proposed and attempted for the delivery of mental health services in rural areas. Each has been an honest attempt to meet the unique demands and needs of the populations in these underserved areas. The overwhelming need has, in many instances, forced many professionals to attempt to be everything to everyone. The demands of this type of generalist practice, coupled with the demand for services with limited funding and staffing, leaves little time, money, and staff for research in rural mental health service delivery and practice (Clayton, 1977). Most service delivery models have evolved from an individual or group attempt to find a better way to deliver services, at times in an almost trial-by-fire atmosphere. Thus, there exist wide variations in delivery models found in rural areas with little regard for the differences within the individual rural areas. There is little question of the difference between the wide open spaces of the western states and the rural areas of the Appalachian Mountains region, and between the wilderness of Alaska and the poor, rural areas of the Southeastern states. It should suffice to say that these differences also play a major role in explaining the wide variation in models.

It may prove helpful at this point to elucidate a definition of the term *model*. As described by Mahoney and Hodges (1969), the term model is not a fixed or rigid concept but indicates a pervasive theme with the possibility of a multiplicity of variations on any one theme. To these authors, model indicates a general sense of direction or leaning. For the purposes of this chapter, this definition is most appropriate and useful.

In reviewing the literature available on the subject of rural service delivery models, there seems to be a continuum of models developed, more or less, from three central themes. It is these three pervasive themes, the traditional or medical model, the consultation or indirect service model, and the combination or public health model, that are discussed in terms of their relevancy for rural areas with certain characteristics.

The Traditional or Medical Model

The traditional direct service model is the oldest and most extensively used of the three general models, its major emphasis stemming from the pervasiveness of the traditional medical model of mental disease and treatment (Wodarski and Bagarozzi, 1979). This medical model still provides the general frame of reference for many of the programs for training mental health professionals. Hollingsworth and Hendrix (1977), in a study of a number of rural mental health centers in a four-state area, found that individual psychotherapy was the primary treatment method of choice in most centers. This office-centered, private practice model is simply one variation of the traditional or medical model.

The traditional model associates mental health centers with general hospitals and with traditional staff including nurses and psychiatrists (Daniels, 1967). Certain rural programs are built around the state hospital with the staff of the hospital following the patients into the community for the provision of aftercare services (Huessy, 1972a). Huessy (1972b) indicates that a major obstacle to the development of rural mental health programming is the tendency for state administrative staff to try to duplicate in rural areas the same kinds of services and facilities as exist in urban areas. This approach does not allow for the geographic and cultural differences between the two areas to be taken into account in planning services.

Ramage (1971) provides a fairly representative view of a rural community mental health program organized from a traditional model. He states:

> The center should have at its base of operations, facilities for brief inpatient care, outpatient care, aftercare, and day care of patients. However, heavy emphasis should be placed on decentralizing services into the outlying counties, communities, and neighborhoods and on tailoring the program of services to meet the needs of the people in the communities in which they are located. This decentralization should be viewed as an extension of the center. There should be a direct telephone line from all outreach facilities to the center with consultation and service facilities immediately available at the center. The mental health center itself, in effect, should be the neighborhood or regional outreach clinic.

This description embraces a seeming preoccupation with facilities as opposed to programs and services. This facility orientation is most prevalent in the traditional model, and of much less importance in the consultation or combination models.

An example of the facility orientation was reported by Kiesler (1969) in his discussion of program development in Minnesota following the State Enabling Act for Mental Health Programs. Most implementation efforts in the state had immedi- ately become facility oriented. They focused on a mental health center as a psychiatric service facility staffed by professionals employing direct diagnostic and treatment methods to solve mental health problems in the community.

A similar type of facility orientation is found in a discussion of the proposal for the Saskatchewan Plan in Canada (Rands, 1960). The proposal called for dividing the province into regions with populations of about 75,000 and building in each region a small mental hospital to provide all the psychiatric services for the region. The hospitals were to be comprised of treatment cottages housing 30 patients each. The general intent of the plan was to provide geographically local accessibility to mental health services. Both the facility orientation and the identification with the hospital and the medical model are consistent with the traditional model of service delivery. Also consistent with this model is the Swift Current Health Region's use of a full-time clinic in the major city of the region and monthly part-time clinics in three other locations (Rands, 1960).

Another example comes from Wisconsin (Erickson and Macht, 1970), a state which utilizes a county mental hospital system that is composed of 36 small mental hospitals instead of five or six large ones. In this system, outpatient care is provided primarily by medical facilities with a medical model orientation. The general hospitals also participate in the system by providing inpatient psychiatric units which, in effect, provide the services on an even more local basis.

Variations on the general theme of the traditional model can be found in most areas of the country. In Wyoming, for example, Tranel (1970) reports the efforts of a small group of people in one area initiating a part-time, two-night-a-week, outpatient clinic using donated space in the local general hospital. In Massachusetts (Sills, 1975), it was proposed to turn the state mental hospital in one area over to the community programs for the purpose of integrating the systems. Unfortunately, due in part to disagreements over staff and resource allocations, the attempt was unsuccessful and the traditional relationship and programs were reinstituted.

An interesting variation discussed by Tranel (1970) outlines the placement of Wyoming mental health professionals singly in outlying areas to provide direct services and the referral of patients to the base center for inpatient care when necessary. In addition, a psychologist and a psychiatrist travel to the various sites on regular tours to provide both direct services to patients and consultation to the outstationed professionals. This type of model is intended to allow for unique program differences to develop within different communities and areas.

In brief, the traditional direct service model is characterized by a facility orientation, often directly connected to the state hospital system, and utilizing the medical model as a general orientation for the delivery of services. Individual psychotherapy or counseling is the standard treatment mode with the majority of treatment provided directly by trained, professional mental health personnel. Administration for these programs will often fall to physicians or psychiatrists, which ultimately perpetuates the medical model theme. The professionals are perceived as the experts on mental illness and the population is remanded to their care for the mental health needs of the community. This model is not especially adaptable or effective for those rural areas in which a paucity of mental health professionals is the rule, in which there are no centers of population, and travel to satellite clinics is extensive. In response to this ineffectiveness for some rural areas, other practitioners attempted to establish an indirect service model. This model has been identified as the consultation or indirect service model.

The Consultation or Indirect Service Model

One of the major forces in the development of the consultation model of service delivery for mental health in rural areas has been the large catchment area size and the relatively small professional staff allocations to these same areas. In certain areas, the consultation model was instituted following unsuccessful attempts to establish a more traditional direct service model (Halpern and Love, 1971). It is possible to get an idea of what is involved in a consultation model from the general comments of authors using this model to deliver mental health services in rural areas.

Tranel (1970), in reviewing the delivery of services to small rural communities, believes that particular attention should be given to the indirect service model because the full range of direct services by professional mental health personnel will probably not be available to these areas in the foreseeable future and even if it were available the communities are not prepared to use the services. Eisdorfer, Altrocchi, and Young (1968) indicate that, given a paucity of mental health professionals in a given community, the best way to initiate a mental health program is through consultation with people in the community who are already responsible for handling mental health problems as an integral part of their routine professional functioning. They indicate the strong point of this approach is that it allows for a maximum amount of flexibility for the program in meeting the needs of the community. Moreover, supportive of this approach, Edgerton and Bentz (1969) and Edgerton, Bentz, and Hollister (1970) state that means must be found to utilize the manpower from all human service programs that exist in rural areas, as scarce as they are in comparison with their urban and better financed counterparts.

A more extensive discussion of the consultation model is provided by Daniels (1967). He states that the goal of this model is to develop, mobilize, and seek cooperation among existing community resources and structures. The consultant provides indirect mental health services to the people where they live and work by utilizing available resources and structures rather than creating a whole new state-wide direct mental health services structure. He views the mental health worker's role as providing primarily consultation, education, data collection and subsequent analysis and interpretation, and community organization. Daniels outlines the advantages of the indirect service model as opposed to the traditional direct service model. These advantages are:

1. Existing resources and structures are utilized and coordinated.
2. Services are provided where people are in the communities.
3. The approach deals with both visible and concealed mental disorders.

4. Uneconomical parallel mental health structures are not created.
5. Because it is differently staffed, it is more mobile and flexible.
6. Such indirect services truly facilitate preventive psychiatry.
7. There is increased community participation and enthusiasm with this approach.
8. Novel programming is facilitated through the heterogeneous and broad-based participation.
9. There is a greater possibility for research.

Further insight into the actual mechanics of the consultation model may be gained from the presentation of a program as it was developed.

Libo and Griffith (1966) describe a program plan as it was outlined for rural New Mexico when it was decided to utilize a consultation approach and to develop local resources. It was decided that the most feasible approach was to place qualified and experienced professionals in various locations from which they could serve as extended territory leaders in community development and as consultants in mental health. The state division of mental health placed one mental health professional in each outlying district of the state and gave the practitioner the responsibility for developing an indigenous program tailored to local needs, customs, and resources. According to Libo and Griffith, the individual professionals were to provide four services:

1. Consultation to health, welfare, education, recreation, correction, rehabilitation, religious, industrial, and other agencies and individuals on the mental health aspects of their programs and the mental health needs of those they served
2. Guidance to community agencies and organizations in planning and establishing mental health services
3. Dissemination of information concerning available mental health facilities, practitioners, and reference materials
4. Conducting education, orientation, and training programs in mental health for professionals and lay groups.

It is important to note that, according to this model, the consultant provides no direct services to clients.

There are potential drawbacks or hazards to the model, not the least of which is the effect of community expectations (Tranel, 1970). In many cases, public expectations are that a mental health treatment program will provide the same services as the state hospital, only closer to home. It is this community assumption that all things will be the same except for travel time and distance that has the potential for creating massive resistance to any effort to establish a consultant approach in certain areas. Tied in with this notion, Wedel (1969) reports that frequently unsophisticated caretakers, in their anxiety, wish more immediate answers to problems rather than a more lengthy path of inservice training and self-discovery. Consultation that heavily emphasizes recognition of the unsophisticated consultee's feelings will be met with resistance if the consultee expects practical help. Timing also becomes a critical factor in the success or demise of a consultant-type program. Attempts to place premature demands on a community without sufficient cultivation of the population and existing programs and personnel will prove disastrous for a consultant and his or her program.

Eisdorfer et al. (1968), although supportive of the consultation indirect service model, note that in selected instances, direct clinical services may be very valuable to the community and to the development of consultation programs. Mental health consultants must not only be expert clinicians, but must be willing to use their clinical skills directly when appropriate. It is this type of thinking that has led other practitioners to develop a model that combines aspects of both the traditional direct service model and the consultation indirect service model. This combination model is mainly referred to as the public health model.

The Combination or Public Health Model

Some practitioners were not comfortable with either the traditional direct service model or the consultation indirect service model but could appreciate the merits of each. The general focus of these practitioners is to evaluate the needs of an area, decide on the task at hand, and then do whatever is necessary to address the task. This idea is implicit in the notion that the mental health professionals are not the guardians of mental health, but should be regarded as agents of the community, among others, in developing and conserving its human resources and in restoring to more effective functioning people whose performance has been impaired (Smith and Hobbs, 1966).

It has been previously established that rural areas are substantially different from urban areas, and it naturally follows that practice tasks in these areas should also be different. These different needs, resources, and tasks call for specialized intervention tactics tailored to these particular aspects of rural life. An example of this was expressed by Tranel (1970) in his discussion of a different view of direct services. It is his belief that direct services must provide sufficient attention to environmental manipulation and perhaps less attention to problems of inter-personal interactions in rural areas because rural individuals expect concrete services. Although somewhat foreign to many practitioners, this approach may well increase the effectiveness of a given program for a given area. To further illustrate this point, Gurian (1971) remarks that rural community mental health even leads psychiatrists away from the traditional medical model.

Jones, Robin, and Wagenfield (1974), in a study involving 20 mental health centers, found a general movement away from the strict traditional model to more of a public health model that includes modifying the environment to enhance mental health along with the direct services. In looking at the centers with regard to their outreach proclivity, or the amount of time and energy they were willing to invest in other than direct services, these investigators found that rural centers are twice as motivated in this area as their urban counterparts.

This combination, or public health model as it is sometimes called, often incorporates the notion of an interdisciplinary team with members who have quite diverse backgrounds working toward the common goal of community mental health. Members are recognized for their specific expertise, whether they are physicians, psychologists, nurses, social workers, home-health aides, teachers, housewives, senior citizens, or concerned citizens willing to volunteer, and each of their skills is utilized in a holistic approach to treatment. In various areas, the public health model is facilitated by the placement of mental health services within the local health department. Thompson and Bell (1969) explore one such program in which the county board of supervisors came to acknowledge the importance of the health department in the provision of mental health services by placing its new mental health program in the same department, making the public health director also the director of mental health services. For this particular program in this rural area, 85% of the program time was allocated to direct outpatient treatment and only 15% to consultation, information, and educational services.

Thompson and Bell (1969) also report on a center in Grand Rapids, Michigan, that used a radically different combination model for service delivery. This center provided 85% of their service in the form of consultation as virtually the entire service to a sparsely populated area with only 15% of patients referred actually being admitted to direct service and being seen at the center. The remainder were managed entirely by the referring professionals with the supportive consultation of the staff of the center. These two radically different programs exemplify the flexibility inherent in the public health model. Through utilization of aspects of both direct and indirect services, effectiveness of service can be enhanced while avoiding many of the criticisms of the two other models.

Some of the key issues involved in the development of a public health model program were experienced by Kiesler (1969) in a rural tri-county area in Minnesota. They were originally faced with community expectations for a traditional mental health center and worked to shift the focus to a public health model orientation. The professional staff attempted to allocate a major portion of their time to consulting with existing mental health service providers in the community in addition to providing traditional clinical services. They found that they had to deal with the reluctance on the part of the natural service providers to keep their cases once the professionals were introduced into the community. Their preference was to unload their cases on the professionals for treatment, potentially jeopardizing the consultative alternative approach and inundating the professionals with clients. Without the persistance of the professionals, the community expectations would have been realized and a traditional mental health center would have been established for this area.

In summary, for the purposes of this review, three main themes have been presented. The reader should bear in mind the somewhat arbitrary and artificial distinction designed for the theoretical perspective it affords. In reality, programs and models fall on a continuum and are, therefore, rarely if ever found in a pure form. The objective of this discussion is to provide tools for examining the general orientation of a given program in a particular rural area.

TREATMENT SETTING

Structural barriers to effective intervention are created when a client who exhibits a problematic behavior in one social context, such as school, is provided behavioral change strategies in another social context, such as a child guidance clinic, family service agency, or community mental health center (Kazdin, 1975, 1977; Stokes and Baer, 1977; Wodarski, 1975, 1980). Data indicate that, if possible, therapeutic intervention should be provided in the same setting in which problematic behaviors occur. If therapeutic change strategies are implemented in other contexts the probabilities are reduced that learned behaviors can be sufficiently generalized and maintained.

In light of the previous discussion, there is little doubt that the general model of a program will affect the type of setting that will be used for the delivery of services. Along with this, the available resources, community needs, and community expectations also play a major role in the determination of setting. These issues, among others, will be elaborated later in this chapter. Initially, there is a need to address issues such as the definition of setting, why social workers should be concerned with the issue of settings, and what are the current types of settings found in rural community mental health.

It is much too simplistic to define setting as simply "where services are provided." Although setting does involve the location of the service in the community, it also includes the type of service to be provided, the physical facility, staffing issues, the population to be served, and the image within the community. The range of issues involved in setting is exemplified in a discussion of the notion of deinstitutionalization by Bachrach (1977). Deinstitutionalization involves the transferring of the responsibility for patients away from the traditional large state hospital and concurrently establishing localized, community-based mental health services and programs. Bachrach states that there are three basic assumptions in the deinstitutionalization model. The first is that community-based care is preferable to institutionalized care for most, if not all mental patients. The second is that the community is both able and willing to assume responsibility and leadership in the care of the mentally ill. And the third of these assumptions is that the functions of the mental hospital can be assumed successfully by community-based facilities.

There is no doubt that the deinstitutionalization model was designed primarily with the urban centers in mind. They have available a range of treatment alternatives and settings that do not exist in rural areas. Rural areas often have only one center and sometimes only one staff member or service provider. As a result, rural patients are often placed in urban facilities simply because the facilities and programs do not exist in their home communities. Deinstitutionalization utilizes programs such as inpatient programs, rehabilitation services, outreach services, transitional services, outpatient services, halfway houses, emergency services, residential programs, and myriad other programs and services in an effective total program package. It is totally unrealistic to expect rural areas to have the financial or manpower resources to develop a program of this nature, let alone the population size or density to justify the existence of such an intricate program design.

While acknowledging the importance of considerations in the determination of setting for rural community mental health services and programs, the reader may ask of what concern this is to social workers. Research suggests that social workers, in light of the impetus toward the community mental health philosophy, will become increasingly involved in more community organization and planning roles, such as consultants, coordinators, political advisors, and adult educators, along with the traditional direct treatment role of practitioners (Berg, Cohen, and Reid, 1978). No longer is the social worker's role limited to the front-line, direct service tasks and viewed as synonymous with the do-gooder public welfare worker image of the past. Social workers are branching out into all areas of community service with increased responsibility for program development and management. It is becoming more and more common to find social workers as executive directors of community agencies and programs. As an example of this, in the community mental health center network in Ohio, social workers represent the single most prevalent professional group among the executive directors of the more than 80 programs in existence.

To expand on a point mentioned earlier, setting is not synonymous with facility. Smith and Hobbs (1966) state that facilities should be planned to fit a program and not vice versa. New physical facilities will necessarily be required, but the mistake of constructing large, congregate institutions should not be repeated. Small units of diverse design reflecting specific functions and located near users and near other services are indicated, and often can be constructed at a lesser cost than a centralized unit linked to a hospital. Each community should work out the pattern of services and related facilities that reflects its own cultural styles, problems, resources, and solutions. The facility will play a greater or lesser role in the determination of setting depending on the model of the program but should not be the primary factor in the determination of setting if the program is to be most effective. The only time it should be of major import is when it directly affects the accessibility of the service to the clients (e.g., planning a program for nonambulatory clients on the fourth floor of a building without an elevator).

In rural areas there does exist an advantage with regard to ease in facility procurement as compared to urban areas. According to Huessy (1972a), the availabilty of fairly cheap real estate will help in the development of facilities in rural areas, especially for halfway houses and boarding homes. Many rundown properties offer the opportunity to start services with a minumum of capital investment. This advantage should help negate the need for program planners to become facility-oriented and should allow services to take precedence in determining program setting for rural areas.

Before elaborating the actual considerations in determination of setting for rural mental health service delivery, it should prove beneficial to discuss present settings, why they are used, and their benefits and drawbacks. In looking at examples of settings, it will become apparent that types of settings are closely tied into a specific model and may not be especially adaptable to other models. It is suggested that the reader keep the models in mind while examining these settings, as they affect the development and programming of the settings.

Traveling Clinics

Traveling clinics were one of the earliest types of noninstitutional settings to be used for delivery of community mental health services to rural areas. The general notion is for a team of professionals to travel to outlying areas on a periodic basis to provide both direct and indirect services to clients and communities (Hopple and Huessy, 1954; Huessy, 1972a, b). The traveling team, many times comprised of state hospital staff, provides on a one-day-a-week to one-day-every-two-months basis diagnosis and treatment to clients, consultation and education to various agencies' staffs, and organizational development of its own resources and services to the community. One notable problem with this approach is that there can be a total lack of continuity (Huessy, 1972b). Community follow-up of clinic recommendations may be haphazard and patients in acute need often have to wait too long to receive the services of the professionals.

One way of dealing with this problem is to establish a cooperative relationship between an agency in the community and the mental health clinic base. This association with an existing agency in the area provides a place for patients to turn for help until the team travels back to the community (Hopple and Huessy, 1954; Huessy, 1972a). Huessy (1972a, b) describes a better alternative, the establishment of at least a small part-time clinic (satellite) which would have at least one local staff member or, better yet, one full-time local staff member. He posits that a linkage would result in much higher levels of relevant service being delivered to the community.

Numerous variations of the traveling clinic setting or theme have been described in the literature. For example, in Alaska, the two-way radio is used between a paraprofessional in the community and a professional consultant at the mental health clinic base (Huessy, 1972a). This is used in conjunction with a professional who periodically visits the outlying areas by plane. Another variation of the traveling clinic approach is to provide day care or day treatment services as addressed by Shires (1977). She introduces the idea of a traveling day hospital, analogous to the mobile library which brings a sample of the amenities of the city library to small communities at limited times. With this approach, a van transports a clinical team from the psychiatric hospital and then from one small town to the next, using suitable locations in each community to provide the essential partial hospitalization services.

Inpatient Service Settings

This requirement of the Comprehensive Community Mental Health Centers Act is more easily met by rural providers than that of partial hospitalization. Inpatient services are usually provided in one of four settings. The first and easiest setting, in terms of facility availability for communities, is the use of the state hospital for provision of the service. A consideration in the feasibility of this approach involves the accessibility of the state hospital to the consumers of the service area. This aspect has been discussed previously with regard to utilization of the state hospital relative to distance between the facility and potential consumers.

A second type of setting is the development and use of smaller regional psychiatric facilities that may or may not be linked directly to the state hospital. This approach relieves the rural area of the total financial burden of this costly service. This participatory plan often serves several counties or catchment areas and each subunit contributes to the operating cost of the facility based on a rate of utilization. Unfortunately, with this type of approach, the communities or catchment areas exert very little control over the facility, much like their relationship with the state hospital, even though the facility is often considerably closer than the state hospital.

A third type of inpatient service setting is dependent on the availablity of a medical facility or general hospital in the community. If a hospital is present, an agreement may be possible whereby the hospital will provide inpatient beds for little or no financial consideration if the mental health center is willing to either wholly or cooperatively staff the unit. This can be an especially attractive alternative if both the hospital and the mental health center are funded by the county commissioners or supervisors in the catchment area. Cost efficiency is almost always desirable and, in this case, can contribute to effective, locality-oriented, and -controlled inpatient service delivery.

The last and potentially most expensive setting for inpatient services in rural areas is for the mental health center to establish its own independent inpatient unit or facility. The sparse population combined with limited funding and staff may prove prohibitive for implementation of this type of alternative. It would be difficult for most rural areas to justify, considering the type of facility that would be necessary combined with 24-hour staffing of the type required for the provision of adequate inpatient care.

Huessy (1972a) raises an important concern regarding the whole issue of inpatient services on a local level. He believes that the establishment of local inpatient services should be scrutinized closely as it may serve to increase hospitalizations out of convenience rather than out of necessity. It may discourage the mental health staff from trying to resolve crises in the community because the inpatient alternative exists and would definitely have to be viewed as a disservice to both the clients and the community.

Outpatient Service Settings

Outpatient services are often considered to be the very foundation on which community mental health programs were originally established. These services are delivered in a wide variety of fashions—ranging from the 50-minute hour of the private practice type model to the monthly medication checks and periodic case management contacts of the public health model. As has been noted earlier, the consultation model provides no direct services to consumers, but the consultees of the mental health professional would utilize a mode within the above-mentioned range. It is comparatively easy to identify the range of service delivery methods, whereas providing an all-inclusive description of the various possible settings within which the service may be delivered is next to impossible.

One of the most outstanding virtues of outpatient services is the ease with which they can be provided in almost any setting. There are almost no restrictions or prohibitions regarding the environment or setting, except for those imposed by each practitioner and his or her personal preferences. The setting may be a formal office in a mental health center, in the client's home, in a school, in a traveling automobile, on a street corner, in the middle of a corn field, or almost any other imaginable setting. Outpatient services could even be provided in the stadium stands during a major league baseball game, although this setting would probably be less desirable than other possibilities.

This brings up the issue of the desirable qualities of an outpatient service setting, wherever it may be in the community. Ideally, the setting would be such that the client feels safe and secure from immediate harm. When this is the case, the client will be less concerned with the surroundings and more able to concentrate on those issues for which he or she is seeking services. For example, a client who is fearful of riding in automobiles may be so distracted by traveling to a counseling session that he or she is unable to discuss or concentrate on the presenting problem. The client's inability to discuss the presenting problem in this situation may be viewed by the professional as resistance to treatment on the part of the client with resulting frustration for both and little progress in treatment until the traveling fear is brought out and dealt with.

A second desirable quality involves the notion of a distraction-free environment. One example of an environment infested with distraction is the previously mentioned stadium during a baseball game. Another, more subtle, distracting environment may be found fairly often when visiting clients in their own homes. A radio, television, or the presence of children may seriously affect the client's ability to concentrate on the treatment issues and problems. One more issue involved in home visits to clients is the presence of other family members and friends. The client may feel extremely uncomfortable or even refuse to discuss some problems or issues in the presence of others, especially if those persons are involved in or contributing to the problems or issues. In a setting other than the client's home, the issue of other persons in close proximity, either friends or strangers, may still prove to detract from the openness and ability to concentrate on the part of the client.

Although most of this review has centered around the setting issue for outpatient services from the client's position, the therapist, counselor, or case manager likewise has certain obligations to consider in regard to setting. It is his or her responsibility to recognize and eliminate the environmental distractions whenever possible to ensure the most effective treatment possible under the conditions (Wodarski, 1981; see also chapter three). Even more important, it is imperative that the clinician choose a setting that will ensure maintenance of the client's integrity and confidentiality in an ethical and professional manner.

Partial Hospitalization Settings

Partial hospitalization, by design, is a type of alternative to inpatient care or can be a type of linking or transitional service between the hospital and the community. The intent of the service is to provide a more sheltered environment for clients without having to use an inpatient facility or setting. As has been previously discussed, these services are directed toward those clients needing more support and supervision than is available in outpatient care, but, at the same time, not appropriate for or in need of the restrictive environment of inpatient care. There are two basic types of partial hospitalization programs, residential and nonresidential.

The nonresidential programs are, in many ways, an extended form of outpatient care or services. These programs often involve 5-day-a-week contact with clients for 2 to 8 hours per day. The clients take part in individual and/or group counseling, activities, arts, crafts, resocialization training, education, social skills development, or any combination of these depending on the needs of the clients and the design of the program. In many agencies, the program is operated as part of their aftercare program and is housed in a basement, large room, or building proximate to the center. The general intent of the programs is to increase the social functioning of the clients in a structured environment while maintaining them in the community. Client distance from the center and transportation difficulties are prohibitive factors to the wide-spread utilization of these programs in many rural areas.

Residential programs, on the other hand, are being increasingly utilized in rural areas as a means of providing partial hospitalization services. These programs are client live-in arrangements and include settings such as boarding homes, nursing homes, family care residential facilities, intentional families, halfway houses, lodges, and group homes or hostels (Fikany, 1975). A comprehensive discussion of these settings and their use is provided by Estelle Fikany (1975) of the Fort Logan Mental Health Center in Denver, Colorado. She describes boarding homes as privately owned homes that offer specific daily living services including bed and board for a fixed sum. The setting allows for considerable independence on the part of the client often accommodating nonpsychiatric individuals. A client in this type of setting will usually be receiving supportive outpatient services from the center and will be employed in many cases.

Nursing homes are described as usually corporate-owned, profit-making medical facilities that may provide care to psychiatric patients with physical illnesses or infirmities. Unfortunately, in many areas, geriatric psychiatric patients with a chronic mental condition are dumped into nursing homes for want of alternative suitable settings in the community. Although they are frequently used in this way as residential care settings, the nursing homes are primarily designed to provide either skilled or intermediate nursing care for patients with physical rather than mental problems, thus they are not prepared to handle the needs of clients with psychiatric problems.

The family care homes are private homes licensed as residential facilities that are supervised by center staff but are operated by individuals or families in residence. As opposed to boarding homes, these homes are more communally or family-oriented settings with increased support and supervision of both activity and medication due to the residents' impaired capacity for self-care. In many cases, clients are concurrently involved in day care activities, either in the home or at the mental health center. The key features of family care homes are structure, supervision, and support in a family-type protective living environment.

According to Fikany, the intentional family consists of two or more clients living together in an apartment or house, sharing the financial expenses of rent, utilities, and food, which in turn allows them to have more monies available for clothing, entertainment, and transportation. The apartment or house is selected and maintained by the clients with a minimum of support and supervision from the center staff. Roommates are selected based on individual preferences attempting to complement the strengths of the individuals while minimizing the total effect of each individual's weaknesses. This setting helps maintain individual independence while encouraging a healthy interdependence between the roommates.

The halfway house is a short-term residential facility, a transitional facility for clients awaiting placement in another program or setting, for clients recently discharged from psychiatric hospitals, or for clients in need of a supportive environment before becoming financially independent. A trained staff member is on duty at all times and will supervise medications for those clients incapable of self-administration. The halfway house is also used for clients in crisis but is inappropriate for inpatient services. This facility is, in many ways, a type of observation and referral setting for clients in transition.

The lodge is described as a cooperative living-working group setting designed for clients needing psychiatric and vocational treatment. Through the use of sheltered workshop activities, the clients learn work skills and habits in a structured and supervised setting. The group is responsible for decision-making and self-governance within the structure of the setting, one which has many of the features of the boarding home-type setting. The group home or hostel setting is similar to the lodge but does not have the cooperative work and vocational opportunities of the lodge. The group homes and hostels have a resident supervisor but the clients are self-care and desire a group living situation while they pursue employment and life activities.

Emergency Service Settings

Emergency care or services are usually provided through one or a combination of the previously mentioned settings. Analogously referred to as crisis intervention, the extent of emergency services is dependent upon the availability of the other service settings and is geared to the specific needs of the area. For example, emergency services may be limited to center staff taking turns on-call through the use of an after-hours telephone system or an automatic switching device in the center's telephone system for an area with little demand for crisis intervention services. With this type of service system, the staff member on call would either have to handle the emergency over the phone, make a home visit in an attempt to resolve the crisis, or arrange for inpatient or other supportive services unless this can be postponed until the next working day when an in-house appointment can be arranged.

In certain areas, the general or psychiatric hospital may handle the emergency care for the area either with or without center staff involvement in the service delivery. For those centers which operate a halfway house or their own inpatient facility, the delivery of emergency services is usually funneled through these programs. Regardless of the relative simplicity or sophistication of the setting, the intent is the same, to provide immediate crisis intervention to clients and families in an attempt to minimize the crisis or conflict in the early stages of development. As has been discussed earlier, the traveling clinics afford the least opportunity for effective crisis intervention unless they are cooperatively involved with an existing agency in the community.

Consultation and Education Service Settings

In light of the examples contained in the discussions of the consultation and public health models of service delivery, there is little need to describe the consultation and education services in detail here. The setting for these services could loosely be described as anywhere anyone is interested and willing to listen. More practically, however, this translates into settings such as schools, civic clubs and organizations, churches, social service and other agencies, fraternal organizations, and myriad other organizations and locations. Consultation can be a one-on-one encounter or a group activity, depending on needs, resources, and program design. The intent is to provide useful information and techniques to non-mental health professionals who are coming in contact with persons with psychiatric and emotional problems in the course of their daily activities.

Education also can be an individual or group activity and should be an ongoing process for all mental health programs. Media campaigns utilizing radio, television, or newspapers have proven to be effective educational tools with which to reach large portions of the population for educational purposes. Centers also frequently utilize films, slide presentations, and printed materials and brochures in their educational program efforts. Many states, counties, and cities also have mental health days, weeks, or months designed to promote awareness of and education about mental health issues and services. It is not uncommon to find a mental health fair held during these designated periods to provide a setting for the distribution of this information.

The opportunities are numerous for inventiveness and experimentation in these areas. It has not been very many years since mental health was an unspoken subject and is just now coming "out of the closet" and into the everyday lives of the citizens of the communities, both rural and urban. This relatively recent development hopefully will bring out the creativity and initiative of the mental health professionals and others interested in mental health for the development of new and better ways to educate the general population and thus destroy the damaging myths of mental illness through the presentation of facts. Such approaches are particularly relevant for rural areas due to the lack of information constituents have about mental distress.

Nonessential Service Settings

As has been reviewed, the nonessential but desirable services under the Community Mental Health Centers Act of 1963 include diagnostic services, rehabilitative services, precare, aftercare, training, research, and evaluation. These ancillary services are usually provided in one of the above mentioned settings and it will be left to the practitioner to individually explore the variety of implementation methods available.

The review has centered on the various settings typically used in the delivery of mental health services. It is important to appreciate the variety of possibilities available and their role in the considerations for the determination of setting for programs in rural community mental health. For the purpose of providing a different perspective on setting, it might prove helpful to examine a service system and the variety of settings used for the delivery of mental health services in one rural area.

A Rural Service System

Williams (1975) describes a rural mental health service system designed to serve a large area in southeastern Utah. This system utilizes two central offices, nine satellite clinics, a psychiatric wing for inpatient services in one community, and a general hospital in another. There is heavy reliance on extensive outreach activities, in-service training, school programs, alliances with other agencies, and the use of two-way radio communication while covering the territory in four-wheel-drive vehicles. Emergency care is provided by the main center, as is partial hospitalization services on a 5-day-a-week basis. Additionally, inpatient care has been contracted for with various hospitals that provide two or more beds each on a per-use basis for psychiatric inpatient treatment to complement the existing inpatient services.

Williams discusses specific variations in programming and setting that are a direct result of the needs and attitudes of the populations in the different areas they serve. For example, traditionally, an outreach worker was a practitioner that the client went to in a rural area. Now the outreach worker goes out to the clients, in many instances involving hours of driving by the staff members. In one particular situation involving the attitudes and norms of one group, the center staff felt it imperative to provide services compatible with the Navajo Indians' desire to work out their problems among themselves. In order to help facilitate this desire, the staff members and outreach workers traveled to the locations and provided a variation of outpatient group treatment that Williams identifies as "camp therapy."

Another significant variation of setting and programming was established to meet the unique needs of the Chicano population in a manner that was consistent with their attitudes and values. The Chicanos had been hesitant about going to a mental health center for treatment, especially when they perceived the center as being located in an area dominated by another ethnic group. To increase service accessibility, the center staff provided services through the development and use of a "Chicano cottage," an old house supplied by the county commissioners specifically for this purpose, that was located in an area with a high concentration of Chicanos.

As is demonstrated by this service system example, there are many factors to be considered in the determination of treatment setting for delivery of rural mental health services which will ensure the appropriate utilization rate. These considerations are the next area for discussion.

CONSIDERATIONS IN THE DETERMINATION OF SETTING

Numerous considerations in the determination of setting for rural community mental health programs should have become apparent throughout this discourse. In the discussion of differences between urban and rural areas, many considerations were alluded to without the in-depth attention that will be provided here. The sections on models and types of setting likewise dealt peripherally with these considerations. This section serves to organize and present the major and relatively universal considerations in the determination of setting.

Considering the differences between various rural areas, it would be impossible to develop a comprehensive listing of considerations that would be both precise and, at the same time, universal. To approach the issues involved in the determination of setting, major areas of concentration and the various concerns in each of these areas will be reviewed. The foremost goal is best described by Daniels (1967) as determining the specific characteristics and needs of a given area and developing programs that are consistent with these.

Location of the Facility

The first consideration regarding location is geographic accessibility. Lee, Gianturco, and Eisdorfer (1974) note that geographic considerations often present substantial obstacles to rural clients and this, in turn, negatively affects utilization of the services. Several authors have addressed issues of geographic barriers such as the issue of the highway system and its effect on service delivery (Gurevitz and Heath, 1969; Klein, 1965). The main arteries, connecting roads, and interconnecting highway system should be examined to ensure that the facility is reasonably accessible from all directions. For example, if a center were located in a settlement next to a river and had responsibility for serving the populations on both sides of the river, there would hopefully be a bridge directly linking the settlements on the two sides of the river. Requiring the residents from across the river to drive long distances to cross the river in order to receive services would be demonstrative of poor planning and would severely limit the accessibility of services. Similar types of issues also arise where hills, mountains, and coastal ridges are present (Gurevitz and Heath, 1969).

Another basic requisite involves the establishment of the central base for public mental health services (Gurevitz and Heath, 1969). There is often a temptation to establish the base facility in either the county seat or the largest population center in the area. This may not lend itself to accessibility for the total service area, especially when the county seat or largest population center is located in one corner of the service area. Tranel (1970) states that consideration must be given to the ways population settlements are dispersed in the area. Gurevitz and Heath (1969) add that a determination must be made as to whether or not the location will support a mental health facility. Their points are well taken but must be tempered with an acknowledgment of the implications of physical and top-ographical characteristics of the area and the prompt availability of and easy access to services for the entire service area (Gurevitz and Heath, 1969; Klein, 1965; Lee et al., 1974).

In an area in which this dilemma between centers of relatively dense population and area-wide accessibility exists, a solution may be found in the development of satellite or neighborhood clinics. This type of approach provides for more visibility as well as geographic relevance (Lee et al., 1974). With the availability of the variety of service settings that have been discussed previously, the needs of different areas can be accommodated with relative ease given a flexible and innovative program with responsive leadership.

Isolation and transportation difficulties are another significant issue associated with accessibility (Bachrach, 1977; Halpern and Love, 1971). With large service areas and sparse populations, special attention must be given to programs and locations designed to impact on the isolation issue. This isolation is partly due to distances between the population centers as well as between neighbors in many outlying areas. Another confounding factor is the lack of dependable personal transportation available to clients in many cases and, as a rule, a total absence of public transportaion (Gurevitz and Heath, 1969). One method of dealing with this issue is to utilize outreach activities and home visits as major components of the service program for the center. A different method is for the center to obtain a van or bus for the purpose of bringing clients to the center for treatment appointments and other activities on a regular basis.

Eisdorfer et al. (1968) suggest that in a new program in an area in which people are not oriented toward mental health problems it is better for the mental health professional to travel to the area than to have the clients travel a long distance to take advantage of the services. As has been discussed earlier, Tranel

(1970) adds that the distance people must travel to obtain services is a significant factor in their usage. Travel distances of 40 to 60 miles seems to be the practical limit for clients in rural areas. Again, a number of variations in setting design can be utilized to keep travel distances for clients within reasonable limits while increasing client utilization of the services.

A significant issue in many areas is the need for separation of mental health services from those of public aid or welfare (Buxton, 1973). Often there is a stigma attached to welfare agencies that would negatively affect client utilization of mental health services located in the same building. By reason of proximity, the center's services may be viewed by the general populace as only for welfare clients or may give rise to any number of other derogatory connotations. Although this type of program cohabitation may appear fiscally sound and attractive, the cost with regard to accessibility and public response may far outweigh any possible administrative or fiscal gains.

Finally, the issue of location may not be totally left to the discretion of the program planner or administrator. For example, as Clayton (1977) points out, in certain areas local politicians may threaten to cut off financial support to the program if a facility is not located within their specific jurisdiction. This, along with other types of community pressure, can play a significant role in determining the location of the center in any given area.

The Target Population

Due to the nature and characteristics of rural areas, the delivery of services to people where they live must obviously be programmed differently (Tranel, 1970). There must be the development of a service pattern that takes into account the sparsely populated areas and the increasing shortages of specialized personnel available to rural areas (Gurevitz and Heath, 1969). Given these prefatory disadvantages, the program planner is not at liberty to expend great amounts of time, energy, and resources in the determination of the most effective pattern of service delivery through repeated experimentation. The target population must be quickly but accurately identified and a program of services designed to readily engage and serve that population with as little delay as possible.

There are many issues involved in the determination of target population, including the establishment of smaller, locality-oriented service districts within the total service area that are reflective of that smaller district's population and needs. For example, Libo and Griffith (1966) found major contrasts between the districts in one area with regard to cultural, economic, and geographic factors. They also found that this entailed substantial differences in the distances the practitioners would have to travel to serve their territories. The need to be specifically concerned with the identification of the target population is also addressed by Ramage (1971). He states that certain ethnic groups in many rural areas have greatly influenced the customs, mores, and values as well as the political, professional, social, and cultural aspects of life, emphasizing even further the necessity of implementing a new and different approach to delivery of mental health services to these areas. An understanding of the contributions to a given area or influence of ethnic and other significant groups is extremely important as a consideration in determining the target population and is much more of a critical factor in rural areas than it would be in a more densely and diversely populated urban area.

The previously reviewed issue of locations may also inadvertently affect the center's ability to engage and serve the target population even after the target population has been identified. For example, if a region is not assessed carefully, only those clients who can travel easily may be served and the service will fail to reach the lower socioeconomic segments that live farther away from the center (Huessy, 1972a). Several authors (Gurevitz and Heath, 1969; Halpern and Love, 1971; Klein, 1965) have also indicated concerns regarding how any given location will affect the type of clientele that will utilize the services. One of these concerns is the problem of becoming overinvolved or overidentified with one subgroup of the population. The location of the service or facility will ultimately be interpreted in one place or another by the existing perspective and attitudes of the various subgroups with minority groups consistently identifying the facility with the existing power structure in the community.

For these reasons, among others, there is a critical need to carefully assess the area for the determination of target populations and the location of services and facilities aimed at these specific populations. Mistakes at this point could readily prove fatal to the program's effectiveness in a given area. It seems almost impossible to avoid negative attention or feedback from some of the subgroups in the area, but there are ways to minimize the negative identifications on the part of these subgroups. As was discussed earlier in the section on settings, Williams (1975) pointed out various ways one center modified its service delivery patterns for the purpose of engaging the subgroups found in their service area.

Still another possible resource for the minimization of the negativeness is inherent in the overall interactional pattern that exists in most rural areas. Tranel (1970) posits that the mental health professional should recognize that each community develops its own particular method of handling persons who demonstrate undesirable kinds of behavior. An awareness of this and a willingness to work within this framework, combined with the highly personalized quality to the pattern of care delivery systems found in most rural areas, will provide more of an opportunity to engage potentially resistant subpopulations. This one-on-one type of contact may well be the key to success in these situations when combined with positive "advertising" by way of the community grapevine.

BY WHOM SHOULD CHANGE BE DELIVERED?

We have little evidence to suggest what personal characteristics of social workers involved in rural community mental health facilitate the delivery of services to clients. Based on the accumulated literature one could pose general hypotheses, for example, workers should be reinforcing individuals with whom clients can identify; they should possess empathy, unconditional positive regard, interpersonal warmth, and verbal congruence; they should be able to use appropriate vernacular and dress, and know cultural customs of the area; and they should exhibit confidence, credibility, acceptance, trust, verbal ability, and physical attractiveness (Carkhuff, 1969, 1971; Carkhuff and Berenson, 1967; Corrigan et al., 1980; Fischer, 1975; Keefe, 1975; Mutschler and Rosen, 1977; Suinn, 1974; Truax and Carkhuff, 1967; Vitalo, 1975; Wells and Miller, 1973; Wodarski, 1981). Likewise, Rosenthal (1966), Rosenthal and Rosnow (1969), and Goldstein (1980) have suggested that the worker's expectation of positive change in clients is also necessary. Additional research suggests that a behavioral change agent should have considerable verbal ability, should be motivated to help others change, should possess a wide variety of social skills, and should have adequate social adjustment (Berkowitz and Graziano, 1972; Gruver, 1971). Thus, development of such skills will enable practitioners to better serve clients. It is evident that rural practitioners must be accepted as members of the community and its power structure. To facilitate acceptance, the worker must not remain aloof, but rather be personable and involved in community activities.

If the community mental health worker chooses to employ a child's parents, teachers, peers, or others as change agents they must realize that they will have to assess at the very least how motivated these individuals are to help alleviate the dysfunctional behavior and how consistently they will apply change techniques, what means are available to monitor the implementation of treatment to ensure that it is appropriately applied, and if the chosen change agent possesses characteristics such as similar social attributes, similar sex, and so forth that could facilitate the client's identification with him or her (Bandura, 1969, 1977; Tharp and Wetzel, 1969; Wodarski, 1981). It is important that the practitioner possess the ability to relate not only to individuals, but also to families, community groups, and to key figures in the community's power structure. Therefore, a social worker must be trained to use a variety of treatment modalities and in various nontraditional settings. Such a worker would be prepared to function in a variety of contexts, would be willing to work at times other than the traditional agency time frame of 8 to 5, and so forth.

In order to deal with the question of who should be the change agent in the rural setting, let us again briefly review the attributes of rural America. The Bureau of Census defines rural America as farm and nonfarm population who reside in the country or in communities of less than 2500. Voting patterns show that rural areas prefer traditionally established patterns and conservative values. There appears to be more resistance to change (Weber, 1976). Rural areas show a preference for minimal governmental involvement, local control, a sense of independence and self-reliance, and privacy. Importance is placed on the family, institutions like school and church, and local organizations which usually provide the locus of community activity (Weber, 1976).

In light of this picture of rural America, who should be the change agent in rural mental health? There has been no clear delineation made through research of what chacteristics are necessary for those who are involved as change agents. If we accept the qualities mentioned earlier, empathy, unconditional positive regard, interpersonal warmth, verbal congruence, confidence, acceptance, trust, verbal ability, a variety of essential communication skills, and physical attractiveness, as being important for the change agent to possess, then who is best suited for that work? We know the change agent should become part of the community, should know how the power structure functions and be functionally integrated into the community and that the client's identification can be facilitated by the proper choice of change agent.

Psychotherapists in the past have been trained primarily as physicians, psychologists, and social workers and not just as change agents. Each of the graduate disciplines has its own distinctive content, training goals, settings and values. Aspects of training appropriate for rural areas constitute a relatively small part of the training to which these master's and doctoral level people are exposed (Garfield, 1977).

In 1960 a significant pilot study was initiated in the Adult Psychiatry Branch of the National Institute of Mental Health to explore one means of alleviating the shortage of trained workers in the mental health field. The major objective of the study was to assess whether nontrained individuals could be trained in a short period of time to reduce the shortage of change agents and to curtail the cost of the provision of basic services. The persons chosen to be trained in this project were eight women in their 40s who formerly had been in the home caring for their families. The training of these women was oriented toward exposing them to a variety of theories and practices with the intention of helping them find their own style of therapy, making use of their own personalities and skills. With this focus on intensive training in psychotherapy, the project hypothesized that in a relatively short time the trainees would be qualified to work with clients in therapy (Rioch et al., 1963).

The outcomes of this training effort were positive. Blind raters who knew nothing of the project gave the group an average rating for therapeutic skills. Moreover, ratings from instructors and supervisors in placement confirmed these data. No trainee was rated below satisfactory, with the average rating being good. In looking at the change in the patients they served, none changed for the worst. Sixty-one percent showed change from slight to marked (Rioch et al., 1963).

The Susanville experiment is another of the classic studies in the training of lay mental health workers. Susanville is a town of 8,000 located in northern California. It had no mental health facilities, and was professionally isolated. Attempts had been made to hire consultants to come into the area, but in 1969 a plan of community self-help was devised. Adult lay members and high school students were trained to work with families selected for having problem children in schools or for being under stress. The trainees were chosen for their listening skills, for not being opinionated, and for being empathetic. The training, which consisted of 70 hours of role play and supervised practicum work, lasted 7 weeks. The trainees then worked with problem families using a communication model. This pilot project was of a short, 7-week duration, but in interviews with the client families and with the lay counselors, there was reported success. Eleven of the 15 adult trainees expressed an active interest in continuing working with families and consulting with each other and the occasional professional consultant. Of the seven high school trainees, five were planning to continue seeing students under the direction of their high school counselors (Beier, Robinson, and Micheletti, 1971).

In a similar study conducted by Carkhuff and Truax in 1965, results suggest that in a relatively short training period of 100 hours "both graduate students and lay hospital personnel can be brought to function at levels of therapy nearly commensurate with those of experienced therapists" (Carkhuff and Truax, 1965).

In a critical review of 34 studies, ranging from single case studies to reports on large-scale, multi-family training programs, Berkowitz and Graziano (1972) looked at the use of parents as behavior therapists for their own children in the home. This approach is an attempt to overcome major limitations of traditional child psychotherapy as viewed by behavior therapists, that is, therapy has to occur in an office, only by a professional, and for a long period of time. Because traditional therapy generally occurs 1 hour a week in a setting far removed from the child's natural environment, the therapist may never directly observe parent-child interaction or the behavior that brings the child to the clinician's office in the first place. In their conclusions, the authors state,

> In light of the available evidence, there is little doubt that behavioral techniques can be effectively applied to children's problem behaviors through the training of their parents. The direct and practical coping with the everyday realities of the disorganized family's situation may be an important therapeutic need currently not met by most child therapists. This entire development provides a new framework for clinical intervention, which, in addition to therapeutic value, has important implications for future use in a systematic and prevention-oriented model of mental health intervention (Berkowitz and Graziano, 1972, p. 64).

A corresponding study conducted in two Iowa rural communities where nonprofessionals were trained as lay counselors indicates that lay persons with a good grasp of social relationships can be trained to serve effectively as counselors. Extensive professional training is not required to deal with many emotionally disturbed children and adults or even with chronic mental patients (Kelley et al., 1977).

The article that presents the greatest question on professional training as a means of preparing clinicians for work with clients is one by Fischer (1975) who reviewed the training of MSW-level graduate students. A randomly selected experimental group was given special training in empathy, warmth, and genuineness. The ratings done by the practicum instructor showed a negative relationship between the independently rated level of empathy and academic grades. The higher the level of student's empathy, the lower his academic grades tended to be!

Data on warmth and genuineness followed the same pattern. It may be a myth that years of intellecutal, cognitively-oriented educational programs provide proper preparation for being a successful change agent. Fischer stated it as follows:

> This is not to say that intellectual activities are not important ingredients in professional training. But a large segment of the criteria for selection of students for professional programs, the training of students, and the evaluation of their competence are geared toward qualities that may be, at best, only weakly related, and at worst, antithetical to the qualities of effective helpers (Fischer, 1975, p. 122).

Vitalo (1975) argues for finding people to match functions. In looking for effective change agents with clients, he indicates that traditional credentials including degrees or diplomas have no established validity. These advanced degrees have no demonstrated value as indicators of capability. The only meaningful criteria for the assignment of responsibilities within the mental health service delivery system is what a person can deliver.

The research cited above indicates that the bestowing of an academic degree does not prepare one with the skills necessary for work as a change agent in mental health. It follows that the same would hold true for the rural area. In following Vitalo's suggestion of finding people to match functions, let us look at the skills that a worker must possess to function effectively in the rural setting.

SKILLS NEEDED FOR RURAL MENTAL HEALTH WORK

A change agent within the rural mental health setting may be described as the proverbial jack-of-all-trades. Unlike the urban counterpart, who sees people on a regular basis in a comfortable office, the rural worker may spend a good deal of work time away from the office interviewing a potentially suicidal person at the jail, visiting a home-bound elderly client who needs a medication evaluation, or making contact with a worker at the welfare services concerning a shared client. Typically, the rural worker may be in one part of his or her catchment area one day of the week and in another part the next.

In an area in which there are few social services available for clients, there is a demand for rural workers to be capable of autonomous work. The rural worker must be a self-starter because he or she is less likely to receive supervision or team backup that can be experienced in an urban setting. Workers must be able to develop their own personal guidelines and an adherence to them (Ginsberg, 1969).

An additional way the rural change agent must be self-motivated is in terms of professional growth and stimulation. The worker does not have access to the professional contacts and stimulation that occur naturally during coffee breaks in large organizations. It is up to individual workers to expand their contacts and skills through attending workshops and reading the current literature (Ginsberg, 1969).

The rural worker must know how to create and use social services that are not, in the traditional sense, viewed as social services. The local sheriff may be the county's answer to Travelers' Aid by housing transients in jail overnight. The worker must know how to identify a structure of services that is hidden. It is the role of the rural worker to assess the strengths of the structure and to assist it in improving, rather than viewing it as nonprofessional and something to disregard (Ginsberg, 1969).

In the rural setting it is important for the worker to be able to establish trust. Personal trust supercedes issues of competence, and an individual can function as a useful worker only if he or she is deemed trustworthy. It may be of more benefit to have coffee with the director of the welfare system locally or to exchange fish stories during this trust-building time than to introduce imaginative programs (Jeffrey and Reeve, 1978). This time spent may be more cost-effective than first meets the eye because the rural art of doing business is person-to-person.

The rural practitioner must have the capacity for quickly building relationships with all types of people in all types of roles. Although rural workers may have the opportunity to develop long-term relationships with certain clients, a number of their contacts will be irregular, due to the wide areas served by rural agencies. It is important that the practitioner be able to make the occasional contact count. The worker must be able to work with the client in such a way that the service continues under the auspices of existing organizations that fill the roles of social agencies (Ginsberg, 1969).

An important requisite to survival in the setting is to set goals in accord with the needs of the client group the worker serves. Rural workers face their share of unmotivated clients with multiple needs that are exacerbated by the scarcity of services. If the worker sees the goal as "personality reorganization" for these clients, he or she will rapidly become discouraged with lack of success. The rural worker may need to frame success for a client in small increments such as helping a female client see that being beaten by a husband is not a normal part of everyone's life, and supporting her appropriate anger. This step alone may not improve her situation but may be the first in her discovery of alternatives to her situation and her own strengths in pursuing such alternatives (Jeffrey and Reeve, 1978).

Kiesler (1969) and Tranel (1970) state that to work effectively in the rural setting rural workers must identify themselves with the area by becoming residents. According to Kiesler (1969, p. 119):

> Not only our personal attributes but also our interests, our life styles, our drinking habits, our marriages, our children, our religious practices, our politics, and our positions on various issues of current concern had to be cataloged before we could become personally predictable enough to be trusted with more than technical professional questions. Only when professionals have lived in rural areas long enough to emerge as citizens with as much personal stake in the future of the community as anyone else can their community begin to make full use of their capabilities . . .

The rural worker confronts the accompanying element of this high visibility mentioned above. The practitioner must be able to deal with the loss of personal privacy and be able to exercise control over social contacts (Riggs and Kugel,

1976). This leads to role-juggling. When an acquaintance of the mental health worker visits, it may not be clear as to whether he or she comes as client, friend, or member of a committee on which both of them serve. During a single encounter, the worker may have to adapt to all three situations. This requires a good sense of timing (Bachrach, 1977).

The rural worker must be able to assess the norms of the rural community so as to avoid violating those norms and offending people, particularly those in the power structure. Anonymity is almost impossible in the rural area, and separation of one's private self from one's work is nearly as impossible. Overt violation of local norms can lead to painful confrontations. There is nowhere to hide for the rural worker in violation (Ginsberg, 1969).

In 1974, Gertz, Meider, and Pluckhan conducted a survey of 215 rural community mental health centers across the United States. Part of the survey had to do with the qualities and skills needed by rural workers. From the 92 responses the skills were categorized as academic preparation, personal qualities, general abilities, and those requirements unique to the rural setting.

In terms of academic preparation, the disciplines of training mentioned were the usual ones of psychology, social work, and psychiatry, with the addition of anthropology. Specific skills mentioned were in the areas of individual, group, and family counseling. Knowledge of community resources was considered beneficial.

The three most often mentioned personal qualities were good communication skills, the ability to function autonomously, and the ability to make and maintain good interpersonal relationships. Another significant ability noted was that of tolerating isolation while still remaining visible to the community.

General abilities listed were those skills in teaching, consultation, public relations, management, and problem-solving. Assessment skills in recognizing the social network of the area, social planning skills, and those having to do with community organization were also mentioned.

In looking at the uniqueness of the rural setting and preparation for it, the questionnaire's respondents noted that a knowledge of rural politics and power structures and the ability to develop informal patterns of communication with leaders in the community was necessary for effective functioning of the staff. Recognizing informal pressure groups that exert control in the area is more important. Other requisite skills listed that have special importance for the rural worker are "familiarity and empathy with the particular cultures, socioeconomic levels, values and mores of rural residents" (Gertz et al., 1975, p. 817). Additional staff attributes noted were acceptance of the conservative rural ethic and a grasp of the demographic characteristics of the area.

Accumulated research indicates that the rural change agent is not formed through academic degree-bestowing programs. The agent is someone with basic skills in working with clients in a helping fashion and basic skills that enable him or her to assess and work with the local power structure, communicate effectively in a rural culture, and to work autonomously, often in an innovative fashion. The literature also indicates that the way to gain acceptance for mental programs within the rural setting is through an informal network of getting things done. This speaks highly for training local lay people to work as rural mental health agents. Research indicates that they certainly could provide basic competent therapeutic services as rural mental health agents. Moreover, they would bring the advantage of already understanding the culture, accepting the norms, knowing the power structure of the area, and having knowledge that should facilitate the isolation of the best change agents. Likewise, they could bring to the program the element of personal trust in the known rather than expertise imposed from the outside. One possible problem in hiring the local person is the reluctance of people in the community to seeking help from one already known to them for years. Confidentiality fears may be higher. It is posited that for rural areas bachelor's-level practitioners provide direct services and master's-level practitioners provide specialized micro and macro interventions and that lay community members can be trained to provide basic services. Thus, the functions of a change agent are conceptualized on a continuum from basic to intermediate to advanced skills.

RATIONALE FOR SERVICE PROVIDED

The rationale for offering a program should be based primarily on empirical grounds. Research indicates that rural individuals want concrete and time-limited service; thus, the task-centered model for individuals and groups is the method of choice. In urban areas many programs are already established. In rural areas in which services are sometimes nonexistent the practitioner has greater responsibility for program development. The decision-making process should reflect that the community mental health workers have considered what type of agency should house the service, that they have made an assessment of the organizational characteristics of the treatment context, and that the interests of the agency personnel have been considered in planning the service. Practitioners are made aware that a number of additional questions should also be posited to ensure the provision of relevant services. How can the program be implemented with minimal disruption? What new communication structures must be added? What types of measurements can be used in evaluating the service? What accountability mechanisms must be set up? And what procedures can be utilized for monitoring execution of the program (Feldman and Wodarski, 1974, 1976; Wodarski and Feldman, 1974)? These may be particularly difficult for the rural worker because they may be operating out of several different geographic contexts.

DURATION

Few empirical guidelines exist regarding how long a service should be provided; that is, when client behavior has improved sufficiently, in terms of quality and quantity, to indicate that services are no longer necessary. Such criteria should be established before the service is to be provided and these should indicate how the program will be evaluated. The criteria should enable workers to determine whether or not a service is meeting the needs of the client. Moreover, they should help reveal the particular factors involved in deciding whether a service should be terminated. The more complete the criteria, the less this process will be based on subjective factors. In answering such questions, practitioners realize that theory, intervention, and evaluation are all part of one total interventive process in community mental health. For rural practice a short term model of intervention seems appropriate because clients want to deal with concrete items that are relevant to their current functioning.

LARGER UNITS FOR SOCIAL CHANGE

Even broadly defined social policy decisions can directly affect the behaviors that will be exhibited by clients. For example, certain economic policy decisions (e.g., those pertinent to teenage employment, rural area development, and other social phenomena) have a determinate effect on behaviors that clients will exhibit in the future. Likewise, a decision to adopt a full employment policy would ensure that each child is provided with adequate housing, education, justice, mental health and social services, and so forth.

If, following a community analysis, a worker decides that a client is exhibiting appropriate behaviors for his or her social context and determines that a treatment organization or institution is not providing adequate support for appropriate behaviors, or that it is punishing appropriate behavior, the community mental health worker must then decide to engage in organizational or institutional change. This may involve changing a social policy or current bureaucratic means of dealing with people, or employing other strategies. In order to alter an organization the worker will have to study its components and assess whether or not he or she has the power to change these structures in order that the client can be helped. Practitioners see that, whereas in social work practice the primary focus has been on changing the individual, future conceptualizations should provide various means of delineating how human behavior can be changed by interventions on multilevels. The obvious question that will confront community mental health social workers is how to coordinate these multilevel interventions.

Interventions at the macro-level are increasingly more critical because follow-up data collected 5 years later on antisocial children who participated in a year-long behavior modification program, which produced extremely impressive behavioral changes in the children, indicate that virtually none of the positive changes were maintained (McCombs et al., 1977, 1978). Possibly, maintenance could be improved when change is also directed at macro-levels which would provide the necessary support for changed behaviors. However, macro-level intervention for rural practice may be resisted unless the power structure supports it. Moreover, specific criteria as to when this avenue and others are to be used by the change agent are yet to be developed.

SUMMARY

This conceptual focus which emphasizes specificity of the training decisions for *Implementation of Change Strategy: How, Where, By Whom, Why, How Long, and On What Level* will help practitioners to make service specific diagnoses. It will also help define the boundaries of service, not only between social workers in community mental health, psychologists, and psychiatrists, but also among BSW-, MSSW- and DSW-trained practitioners. Specification and clarification of competencies in community mental health for BSW- and MSSW-trained practitioners should clarify how services should be structured. Such innovation and streamlining of services will increase the mental health resources through better utilization of personnel with little additional cost.

What knowledge should be conveyed at the BSW as opposed to the MSSW level in rural community mental health must be isolated. Data from the rural community mental health project indicate the probable outcome will be the training of MSSW personnel as supervisors of BSW workers who will be those primarily involved in direct services to deinstitutionalized individuals. MSSW practitioners will possess advanced treatment skills and macro-level skills of needs assessment, planning, administration, and management. DSWs must be trained in research and evaluation. This requires a thorough knowledge of research design and evaluation that includes a working knowledge of statistics in order to provide empirical support to the programs designed for clients. Additionally, research indicates lay individuals can be trained to provide basic services. Such a balanced service system provides essential reintegration and maintenance services, thus reducing costs and increasing human life years.

REFERENCES

Bachrach, L. L. 1977. Deinstitutionalization of mental health services in rural areas. Hosp. Commun. Psych. 28:669–672.

Bandura, A. 1969. Principles of Behavior Modification. Holt, Rinehart and Winston, New York.

Bandura, A. 1977. Social Learning Theory. Prentice Hall, New Jersey.

Beier, E. G., Robinson, P., and Micheletti, G. 1971. Susanville: A community helps itself in mobilization of community resources for self-help in mental health. J. Consult. Clin. Psychol. 36:142–150.

Berg, L. K., Cohen, S. Z., and Reid, W. J. 1978. Knowledge for social work roles in community mental health: Findings of empirical research. J. Educ. Soc. Work 14:16–23.

Berkowitz, B. P., and Graziano, A. N. 1972. Training parents as behavior therapists: A review. Behav. Res. Ther. 10:297–317.

Buxton, E. B. 1973. Delivering social services in rural area. Pub. Welfare 31:15–20.

Carkhuff, R. R. 1969. Helping and Human Relations. Holt, Rinehart and Winston, New York.

Carkhuff, R. R. 1971. Training as a preferred mode of treatment. J. Counsel. Psychol. 18:123–131.

Carkhuff, R. R., and Berenson, B. G. 1967. Beyond Counseling and Therapy. Holt, Rinehart and Winston, New York.

Carkhuff, R. R., and Truax, C. B. 1965. Training in counseling and psychotherapy: An evaluation of an integrated didactic and experiential approach. J. Consult. Clin. Psychol. 29:333–336.

Clayton, T. 1977. Issues in the delivery of rural mental health services. Hosp. Community Psych. 28:673–676.

Corrigan, J. O., Dell, D. M., Lewis, K. N., and Schmidt, L. E. 1980. Counseling as a social influence process: A review. J. Counsel. Psychol. 27:395–441.

Daniels, D. N. 1967. The community mental health center in the rural area: Is the present model appropriate? Am. J. Psych. 124 (Suppl.): 32–37.

Edgerton, J. W., and Bentz, W. K. 1969. Attitudes and opinions of rural people about mental illness and program services. Am. J. Public Health 59:470–477.

Edgerton, J. W., Bentz, W. K., and Hollister, W. G. 1970. Demographic factors and responses to stress among rural people. Am. J. Public Health 60:1065–1071.

Eisdorfer, C., Altrocchi, J., and Young, R. F. 1968. Principles of community mental health in a rural setting: The Halifax County program. Community Ment. Health J. 4:211–220.

Erickson, G. D., and Macht, A. J. 1970. Providing local services for rural counties. Hosp. Community Psych. 21:128–129.

Feldman, R. A., and Wodarski, J. S. 1974. Bureaucratic constraints and methodological adaptations in community-based research. Am. J. Community Psychol. 2:211–224.

Feldman, R. A., and Wodarski, J. S. 1976. Inter-agency referrals and the establishment of community-based treatment programs. Am. J. Psychol. 4:269–274.

Fikany, E. 1975. Philosophy for Community Placement (Fort Logan Mental Health Center, Denver, Colorado). Paper presented at the Ohio Department of Mental Health and Mental Retardation Continuing Education Program—Alternatives to Institutionalization, May, Dayton.

Fischer, J. 1975. Training for effective therapeutic practice. Psychother. Res. Pract. 12:118–123.

Garfield, S. L. 1977. Research on the training of professional psychotherapists. In A. S. Gurman and A. M. Razin (eds.), Effective Psychotherapy: A Handbook of Research. Pergamon Press, New York.

Gertz, B., Meider, J., and Pluckhan, M. L. 1975. A survey of rural community mental health needs and resources. Hosp. Community Psych. 26:816–819.

Ginsberg, L. H. 1969. Education for social work in rural settings. Soc. Work Educ. Rep. Sept:28–32, 60–61.

Goldstein, A. P. 1980. Relationship enhancement methods. In F. H. Kanfer and A. P. Goldstein (eds.), Helping People Change. Pergamon Press, New York.

Gruver, G. G. 1971. College students as therapeutic agents. Psychol. Bull. 76:111–127.

Gurevitz, H., and Heath, D. 1969. Programming in a new region. In H. R. Lamb, D. Heath, and J. F. Downing (eds.), Handbook of Community Mental Practice. Jossey-Bass, Inc., San Francisco.

Gurian, H. 1971. A decade in rural psychiatry. Hosp. Community Psych. 22:56–58.

Halpern, H., and Love, R. W. 1971. Initiation community consultation in rural areas. Hosp. Community Psych. Sept:274–277.

Hollingsworth, R., and Hendrix, M. 1977. Community mental health in rural settings. Prof. Psychol. 8:232–238.

Hopple, L. M., and Huessy, H. R. 1954. Traveling community mental health clinics: Their extratherapeutic aspects and functions. Ment. Hyg. 38:49–59.

Huessy, H. R. 1972a. Rural models. In H. H. Barten, and L. Bellak (eds.), Progress in Community Mental Health, Vol. 2. Grune & Stratton, Inc., New York.

Huessy, H. R. 1972b. Tactics and targets in the rural setting. In S. E. Golann and C. Eisdorfer (eds.), Handbook of Community Mental Health. Appleton-Century-Crofts, New York.

Jeffrey, M. J., and Reeve, R. E. 1978. Community mental health services in rural areas: Some practical issues. Community Ment. Health J. 14:54–62.

Jones, J. D., Robin, S. S., and Wagenfield, M. O. 1974. Rural mental health centers—Are they different? Int. J. Ment. Health 3:77–92.

Kazdin, A. E. 1975. Behavior Modification in Applied Settings. Dorsey, Homewood, Ill.

Kazdin, A. E. 1977. The Token Economy. Plenum Press, New York.

Keefe, T. 1975. Empathy and social work education: A study. J. Educ. Soc. Work 11:69–75

Kelley, V. R., Kelley, P. L., Gauron, E. F., and Rawlings, E. I. 1977. Training helpers in rural mental health delivery. Soc. Work 22:229–232.

Kiesler, F. 1969. More than psychiatry: A rural program. In M. F. Shore and F. V. Mannino (eds.), Mental Health and the Community: Problems, Programs, and Strategies. Behavioral Publications, New York.

Klein, D. C. 1965. The community and mental health: An attempt at a conceptual framework. Community Ment. Health J. 1:301–308.

Lee, S. H., Gianturco., D. T., and Eisdorfer, C. 1974. Community mental health accessibility: A survey of the rural poor. Arch. Gen. Psych. 31:335–339.

Libo, L. M., and Griffith, C. R. 1966. Developing mental health programs in areas lacking professional facilities: The community consultant approach in New Mexico. Community Ment. Health J. 2:163–169.

McCombs, D., Filipczak, J., Friedman, R. M., and Wodarski, J. S. 1978. Long-term follow-up of behavior modification with high risk adolescents. Crim. Just. Behav. 5:21–34.

McCombs, D. Filipczak, J., Rusilko, S., Koustenis, G., and Wodarski, J. S. 1977. Follow-up on behavioral development with disruptive juveniles in public schools. Paper presented at the 11th Annual Meeting, Association for the Advancement of Behavior Therapy, December, Atlanta, Ga.

Mahoney, S. C., and Hodges, A. 1969. Community mental health centers in rural areas: Variations on a theme. Ment. Hyg. 53:484–487.

Mutschler, E., and Rosen, A. 1977. Influence of content relevant and irrelevant client verbalizations on interview effect. J. Soc. Serv. Res. 1:51–61.

Ramage, J. W. 1971. A basic philosophy in developing a rural mental health program. Public Welfare Fall:475–477.

Rands, S. 1960. Community psychiatric services in a rural area. Canad. J. Publ. Health 51:404–410.

Riggs, R. T., and Kugel, L. F. 1976. Transition from urban to rural mental health practice. Soc. Casework 57:562–567.

Rioch, M. J., Elkes, C., Flint, A. A., Usdansky, B. S. Newman, R. G., and Silber, E. 1963. National Institute of Mental Health pilot study in training mental health counselors. Am. J. Orthopsych. 33:678–689.

Rosenthal, R. 1966. Experimenter Effects in Behavioral Research. Appleton-Century-Crofts, New York.

Rosenthal, R., and Rosnow, R. L. (eds.) 1969. Artifact in Behavioral Research. Academic Press, New York.

Shires, J. 1977. A traveling day hospital. Soc. Work Today 8:16–18.

Sills, M. 1975. The transfer of state hospital resources to community programs. Hosp. Community Psych. 26:577–581.

Smith, M. B., and Hobbs, N. 1966. The community and the community mental health center. Am. Psychol. 21:499–509.

Stokes, T. F., and Baer, D. M. 1977. An implicit technology of generalization. J. Appl. Behav. Anal. 12:349–367.

Suinn, R. M. 1974. Traits for selection of paraprofessionals for behavior-modification consultation training. Community Ment. Health J. 10:441–449.

Tharp, R. G., and Wetzel, R. J. 1969. Behavior Modification in the Natural Environment. Academic Press, New York.

Thompson, C. P., and Bell, N. W. 1969. Evaluation of a rural community mental health program. Arch. Gen. Psych. 20:448–456.

Tranel, N. 1970. Rural program development. In H. Grunebaum (ed.), The Practice of Community Mental Health. Little, Brown & Company, Boston.

Truax, C. B., and Carkhuff, R. R. 1967. Toward Effective Counseling and Psychotherapy: Training and Practice. Aldine, Chicago.

Vitalo, R. L. 1975. Guidelines in the functioning of a helping service. Community Ment. Health J. 11:170–178.

Weber, G. K. 1976. Preparing social workers for practice in rural social systems. J. Educ. Soc. Work 12:108–115.

Wedel, H. L. 1969. Characteristics of community mental health center operations in small communities. Comm. Ment. Health J. 5:437–444.

Wells, R. A., and Miller, D. 1973. Developing relationship skills in social work students. Soc. Work Educ. Rep. 21:60–73.

Williams, M. M. 1975. A rural mental health delivery system. Hosp. Commun. Psych. 26:671–674.

Wodarski, J. S. 1975. Requisites for the establishment, implementation, and evaluation of social work treatment programs for anti-social children. Paper presented at the Annual Program Meeting of the Society for the Study of Social Problems, August, San Francisco.

Wodarski, J. S. 1980. Procedures for the maintenance and generalization of achieved behavioral change. J. Sociol. Soc. Welfare 7:298–311.

Wodarski, J. S. 1981. Role of Research in Clinical Practice. University Park Press, Baltimore.

Wodarski, J. S., and Bagarozzi, D. A. 1979. A review of the empirical status of traditional modes of interpersonal helping: Implications for social work practice. Clin. Soc. Work J. 7:231–255.

Wodarski, J. S., and Feldman, R. 1974. Practical aspects of field research. Clin. Soc. Work J. 2:182–193.

Chapter 5

Prevention

An Idea for Which the Time Has Come

One major implication of the community mental health approach to intervention is the effect it has upon the traditional role of the social worker and to the time when intervention should be undertaken. The community mental health approach stresses the teaching components of the intervention process to obtain the goals of the preventive approach. Emphasis is on helping clients learn how to exert control over their own behaviors and the environments in which they live. Community mental health clinicians do not take a passive role in the interventive process. They use their professional knowledge, expertise, and understanding of human behavior theory and personality development in their dealings with clients. They are capable of applying a wide variety of interventive techniques derived from behavioral science to produce desirable changes in community structures. Because the training of social workers equips them to evaluate scientifically any treatment procedure that they have instituted, there exists the capability for continual evaluation of the treatment process. In keeping with their active role, mental health clinicians focus attention upon prevention as a major treatment consideration. They share their knowledge of principles and techniques of human behavior with their clients. They may offer their expertise to prospective parents in the area of child rearing practices and management techniques drawn from behavioral science theory, or they may offer their services to individuals involved in intimate interpersonal relationships who require guidance in the areas of problem-solving, conflict management, or improvement of communication skills. For educators and individuals who work with groups of children or institutionalized adults, social workers can help implement programs for increasing group and individual performance and social participation as well as offer concrete guidelines for management of problematic behaviors. In this new approach the social worker's role is one of prevention rather than remediation.

In rural areas the preventive approach has been limited. This chapter elucidates possibilities and practicalities of preventive endeavors in the rural community.

PREVENTION DEFINED

Whereas a major preoccupation of mental health programs across the country appears to be crisis intervention and direct therapy, a more serious approach to reducing recurring problems, and to detecting signs of future problems, is coming into focus. These programs, aimed at prevention, may be the key to mental health in the 1980s. As there is a gradual shift away from the band-aid, after the fact, approach to mental health, programs designed to prevent more serious consequences of present and/or future mental health problems, or to prevent the recurrence of mental distress, are beginning to emerge in rural, as well as in urban areas.

Prevention is defined as the act of discouraging a problematic behavior or illness before it actually happens, or before it becomes a problem. The term *prevention* will subsequently be used to indicate the prevention of mental problems. A working definition of mental problems should set standards against which preventive activities can be judged. This definition must particularly pertain to rural communities. Mental problems in rural areas may differ in each particular area, and are quite likely to differ from mental problems in urban areas. Let us start with a general definition of mental health, as well as of mental problems.

Gerald Caplan (1974) describes mental health as a dynamic process rather than a stable, individual quality. To determine an individual's state of mental health, one must make a judgement of the individual's internal stability and equilibrium. Mental problems, therefore, may be noticeable fluctuations in the mental health process (Caplan, 1974). But how, exactly, might one judge internal stability or mental health? What specific criteria does one use? Is there a specific list that composes the qualities of a healthy mind? Generally, behaviors are a key to an individual's state of health. Mental problems, therefore, can be detected through undesirable or ineffective behaviors. These behaviors result when a person either cannot cope with life's problems or attempts to cope, but obtains undesirable results (D'Zurilla and Goldfried, 1971). Undesirable behaviors are usually unpredictable (Whittman, 1977). Caplan elaborates that the prime difference between healthy and sick is predictability and variability of adaptive behaviors in healthy individuals. Problem behaviors are indications of rigid and restrictive quality and an inability to deal appropriately with developmental tasks (Caplan, 1961). Thus, problem behaviors tend to vary and to be unpredictable, but by whose standards? This is an especially important point in rural areas. Behaviors that would elsewhere be considered bizarre and destructive may be a natural occurrence in rural areas. Therefore, an agency must establish its standards for measuring mental dysfunction in specific types and degrees for a particular area (Caplan, 1974).

Several factors may influence, or bring on, maladaptive behaviors. These factors can include economic distress, racism, and unemployment, all characteristic of rural areas (Whittman, 1977). These factors should be taken into account and dealt with as part of the problem gestalt.

APPROACHES TO PREVENTION

Preventive programs should focus on reducing the number of individuals who will need services in the future if no ameliorating activities occur. These preventive programs should reduce the number of mental problems (as measured by behaviors) within the community, reduce the number of recurring mental problems in an area, and prevent individuals with mild mental problems from deteriorating (Gottesfield, 1972). The ultimate goal of preventive programs should be to eliminate or alleviate the known causes of mental problems, such as poverty, incest, and unemployment in rural areas (Caplan, 1974). Moreover, preventive mental health programs must teach alternate ways of dealing with environmental conditions (alternatives to undesirable behaviors). For example, programs could focus on the development of social skills, or on acquisition of cognitive and emotional skills for reducing stress in one's own life (Rae-Grant, Gladwin, and Bower, 1966). Essentially, preventive mental health programs must achieve two objectives. Each program must develop knowledge of factors that predispose the individual to mental distress and it must organize the community system to use this specific knowledge in its programs aimed toward altering such factors. Prevention of mental distress encompasses, therefore, a massive array of programs, services, and information.

There are, of course, several types of preventive approaches that indicate the use of different types of treatment. Prevention of mental disorders can be classified into three basic types. *Primary prevention* is a focus on reducing altogether the number of individuals with mental problems in a community. *Secondary prevention* keeps present mental problems from becoming worse, or shortens their duration. *Tertiary prevention* refers to the process of helping people who have had emotional problems, but who are currently adequately functioning (Caplan, 1974).

Extensive research has been conducted to discover the actual components of life crises in an effort to understand and modify factors that contribute to mental health or mental illness (Caplan, 1974). These components, which may be considered in reference to preventive programs, can be classified into three categories: physical, psychosocial, or sociocultural. Deficits in any one of these three areas may reduce the natural human coping patterns, thereby reducing the ability to deal successfully with life span developmental tasks, and leading ultimately to mental illness. What is encompassed in the three categories of needs? Physical needs seem fairly self-explanatory. Human beings need adequate food, water, sleep, shelter, and sensory stimulation. Reduction in any of these needs for a prolonged period of time can lead to the individual exhibiting undesirable behavior. Psychosocial needs include the need for affection, emotional and intellectual development, and positive identity formation. Processes such as severe illness, divorce, or the death of a family member can certainly affect the mental health of an individual. Finally, sociocultural needs are initiated by the community's social structure. These requisites include an adequate educational, economic, and social system. Again, deficiencies in these systems can affect the person's mental functioning (Gottesfield, 1972). These factors or needs influence all three types of prevention techniques and the indicated methods of treatment.

Primary prevention deals with universal patterns influencing people's lives. Primary prevention is concerned with methods of reducing the overall incidence of mental illness. Two specific foci of primary prevention include teaching individuals to cope with stress and reducing stress in the actual environment (Gottesfield, 1972). A good example of primary prevention of physical need deficits could be testing newborns for PKU to prevent mental retardation and providing parents nutrition education. Primary prevention of psychosocial need deficits could focus on teaching mothering skills to pregnant women. A last example links primary prevention with sociocultural needs, as in an educational system. Counseling provided to college freshmen may prevent occurrences of mental illness during crisis periods.

Secondary prevention takes on a different approach to the problems of mental illness. Secondary prevention is aimed at early detection of existing mental problems. Such a focus necessitates the organization of a helping system for select candidates within the community (Caplan, 1974). Medication prescriptions for clients known to be mentally distressed is an example of secondary prevention from a physical perspective. Crisis intervention centers, home visits, and family counseling are examples of psychosocial secondary preventive measures. Secondary sociocultural prevention is present in school systems in the form of psychological testing and counseling services, and in mental health centers in the form of educational classes or groups.

Tertiary prevention deals with individuals who have had previous mental problems. The goal is to maintain the individual in the community and to prevent problems from recurring. Community organization and planning is essential for tertiary prevention programs (Gottesfield, 1972). The effort here is to reduce the recidivism rate of individuals who have been hospitalized. Tertiary prevention programs try to ensure that those who have recovered will be aided, not hampered, by the community to which they return (Caplan, 1961). Continued medication and referrals for additional services are examples of physical tertiary prevention services. After-care counseling, follow-ups, and day treatment programs are all types of psychosocial tertiary prevention. Finally, educational programs, legislative bills, and workshops aimed at changing society's view of mental illness are programs contained in tertiary sociocultural models.

CRISIS PERIODS

All three types of prevention recognize the importance of crisis periods during a human lifetime. A short-term crisis can be described as a short period of time during which an individual is at risk in terms of psychological or emotional imbalance due to the adaptive stress (Caplan, 1974). Deaths, divorces, and financial or natural disasters are all high-risk situations during which individuals may lose their coping capacities. A primary prevention program would focus on studying the components of crisis and later using those factors in preventive programs. A secondary prevention program would strive for early identification and detection of the crisis situation to prevent recurrences or full-blown difficulties (Rae-Grant et al., 1966). A program based on the tertiary model would focus on former patient referrals and out-patient crisis centers as methods of intervention.

Crisis periods are of vital importance, especially in rural areas, because they may represent a turning point in the health of an individual. Crisis periods may be an excellent point of entry for the rural community mental health social worker. Studies have shown that individuals are more likely to be influenced by help while they are in a crisis situation (Caplan, 1974). The first step is to make sure that help is available during a crisis period. This point is especially critical in rural areas in which there are often substantial distances to travel, lack of professionals, and long waiting lists for services (Gottesfield, 1972). The next step is to make sure that the assistance given is quality counseling. Individuals are substantially confused during crises. They may work out their own methods of dealing with crisis, which can include postponing the solution, developing maladaptive behaviors for coping, or developing psychological symptoms as a result of a crisis situation (Gottesfield, 1972). Any such coping method—either adaptive or maladaptive—developed by the family or the individual tends to become a part of the natural coping process and will be used in dealing with problems in the future. Thus, it is important to develop appropriate coping methods and problem solving skills for dealing with stressful situations during the time in which the person is in crisis (Gottesfield, 1972).

In summary, there are three different types of prevention, each calling for slightly different methods of intervention. There are a number of situations that necessitate preventative programs, and numerous suggestions for these programs. Essential to all preventative work is the concept of crisis. Crises should be prevented, if at all possible, through appropriate use of coping skills and early intervention. Such crises must be attended to as early as possible for preventive programs to be successful.

PREVENTION IN RURAL AREAS

Of major interest here are preventive mental health programs in relation to the rural community. There are several community aspects unique to rural mental health. These aspects include reputation and location of the mental health center, community view of mental health in general, procedures and language used in the center, and fees charged for services.

Center Reputation

Perhaps the most important contribution to the success of rural mental health prevention programs is the reputation that the center establishes within the community. This point relates directly to the characteristics of the client population. Individuals in rural areas are not openly receptive to counseling treatment methods, and much less receptive to prevention programs. Being concrete thinkers, "sick" to a rural resident almost always means physically sick. Mental health has not yet received the attention, the publicity, or the educational focus in rural areas that it has in more densely populated regions. Country folks often have little or no use for "mental services." Often rural folks are resistant to receiving treatment, or to visiting a mental health center. They can be very skeptical of outside professionals—outside, meaning not from within the community.

Extensive public relations work *must* be done before any rural program is initiated and must continue while the program is in operation. Rural individuals place faith in proven products. In essence, the mental health center will have to prove itself, at first by showing results and advertising services and programs, especially preventive programs, because they tend to be rather vague. Programs should be thoroughly outlined to the target groups within the community.

Church groups, women's service organizations, and men's service or fraternal associations are potential gold mines to help initiate community public relations. One advantage to being in a rural community is that the smaller the population, the less anonymity, and the greater the likelihood that community support will be very strong once it develops. An additional advantage is in having local community members on the staff. Local staff or members of the boards of directors constitute resources that cannot be underestimated. Local staff members are not only likely to increase clientele referrals, but will also serve as valuable public relations agents. One of the first steps is to practice increased public relations in a straight-forward fashion, with as many familiar faces as possible. Such individuals should be used to gain support for prototypes of preventive approaches such as those found in courses on parental effectiveness, sex education, vocational and marital enrichment, interpersonal skills training, and so forth.

Location and Physical Characteristics of the Center

The physical location of the mental health center is vital to the success of preventive programming. First of all, a community mental health program must be in the community. A program in a city or elsewhere outside the community in all probability will not reach the target groups. People must be able to get to the center to benefit from its programs. The rural center must be accessible in all types of weather. Rural roads are not likely to be safe in snow storms or floods. A house on top of a hill may have sparse clientele in the winter months. Transportation in general may present problems. Bus systems are generally very limited or non-existent in rural areas. Office hours must be adjusted to fit client schedules. No matter how beneficial a program may be, it cannot be of much use if people cannot get to the facility or do not know about it.

The more homey the building, the better, for the clients will feel more at ease. Rural individuals are not likely to flock to huge, impersonal cement-block buildings. Likewise, the physical surroundings of the mental health center should reflect the local color of the clientele.

Finally, there must be a widespread, instant referral base for rural prevention programs. Such referral systems are virtually nonexistent in many rural areas, but are vital to reach populations. Interagency alignments are essential to facilitate the development of such referral networks.

Client-Worker Relationships

Characteristics of the rural client are sharply different from those of the typical urban client. Many of these rural folks may have low levels of education, but it is very important that they be treated with respect and dignity, mixed with appropriate warmth and friendliness. Perhaps the single most important factor is language. In many instances it is quite likely that there will be an imbalance between the educational levels of the staff and of the clientele. The professionals must talk in terms that the client can understand. Clients must be able to understand professionals to have trust in them, to build a relationship with them and to benefit from treatment. In addition, the types of treatment and procedures used by the center should be geared to the client population. Obviously, an alcoholic with a 4th-grade education is not going to get into intensive psychotherapy. The key here is to balance the treatment with the client and with the social assessment.

Aims of Preventive Programs

Rural mental health programs must be *success oriented*. Rural individuals must be highly motivated to participate in preventive programs. They must be able to see what direct impact the program can or will have on their lives. The goals must be acceptable, attainable, realistic, and often concrete for clients to be truly motivated to participate. This is especially true of prevention programs, because their goals are generally vague and long term. Goals should be broken into simple, attainable steps, in which success is a fairly guaranteed entity.

For example, the preventive approach to medicine offers exciting possibilities for community mental health workers. Prevention of coronary heart disease is illustrated by efforts to identify high risk individuals and apply health care programs designed to decrease weight and increase exercise, stop smoking, reduce serum cholesterol, and teach effective management of stress (Meyer and Henderson, 1974).

Program Cost

The last factor to be mentioned with specific reference to rural programs is the cost. Although there are numerous exceptions, the typical rural client coming into a public mental health facility does not have the money needed for hours of therapy or for group training sessions. Many of these clients are farmers, small businessmen, retired people, or common laborers. Sliding fee scales are almost essential to any mental health service, but particularly in rural areas, and especially for prevention programs. Prevention takes longer than, for example, crisis intervention, which runs up a larger bill. Thus, even if the rural community supports the program, has access to it, and understands the techniques involved, if they cannot afford the services the services are almost useless.

SPECIFIC PREVENTIVE ACTIVITIES

Many types of preventive activities can be undertaken in rural areas. For example, in planning programs for adolescents the following topics would be relevant:

1. Nutrition education
2. Social skills training
3. Adequate health care: smoking, sexuality, consumption of alcohol
4. Job securement and maintenance
5. Resolving parental conflict
6. Problem solving techniques.

Programs are available to facilitate implementation of all the above. For excellent reviews see Gilchrist, 1981; Schinke and Blythe, in press; Schinke, Blythe, and Gilchrist, 1981; Schinke, Gilchrist, and Blythe, 1980; and Wodarski et al., 1980.

In a more specific example, adolescents identified as high risk in terms of coping with the daily problems of living could be taught a problem solving approach based on the work of D'Zurilla and Goldfried (1971), Goldfried and Goldfried (1975), Schinke (in press), and Spivack and Shure (1974). The general components emphasized are:

1. How to generate information
2. How to generate possible solutions
3. How to evaluate possible courses of action
4. Ability to choose and implement strategies through the following procedures:
   a) General introduction to how the provision of certain consequences and stimuli can control problem-solving behavior
   b) Isolation and definition of a behavior to be changed
   c) Use of stimulus control techniques to influence rates of problem solving behavior
   d) Use of appropriate consequences to either increase or decrease a behavior
5. Verification of the outcome of the chosen course of action.

Adolescents having difficulty in securing employment and social interaction could benefit from the two programs outlined below.

Vocational Enrichment Program   The vocational program is based on the work of Azrin (1978), Azrin, Flores, and Kaplan (1975), and Jones and Azrin (1973). The general components emphasized are:

1. Group discussions involving strong motivation for vocational enrichment. These discussions involve mutual assistance among job seekers, development

of a supportive buddy system, family support, sharing of job leads, and widening the variety of positions considered.

2. Employment securing aids, such as searching want ads, role playing interview situations, instructions in telephoning for appointments, procedures for motivating the job seeker, developing appropriate conversational competencies, ability to emphasize strong personal attributes in terms of dress and grooming, and securing transportation for job interviews.

The Social Enrichment Program   This program is based on the work of Lange and Jakubowski (1976) and involves interpersonal skills training and development of assertive behavior for appropriate situations. Specific elements that are emphasized include:

1. How to introduce oneself
2. How to initiate conversations and continue them
3. Giving and receiving compliments
4. Enhancing appearance
5. Making and refusing requests
6. Spontaneous expression of feelings
7. Appropriate use of nonverbal distance, body language, face, hand and foot movement, and smiling.

Let us now narrow the focus of this chapter to a more specific area of preventive services that are desperately needed in rural areas. A narrower focus should provide a more accurate picture of what can realistically be accomplished in the field of prevention. The problem to be focused on in the remainder of this chapter is child abuse and its prevention through specific techniques. Accumulated literature indicates this is one of the major social problems in rural America.

PREVENTIVE APPROACH TO THE PROBLEM OF CHILD ABUSE

Some background information on the subject of child abuse will be helpful in interpreting the preventive aspects pertinent to the discussion. Child abuse has been termed *the battered child syndrome*. It can be defined as an instance in which a child has suffered serious physical punishment that may show up as broken bones, swelling, bruises, or unusual cuts. This physical assault on the child is inflicted by the parents or by parent-figures (Paulson and Blake, 1969). These assaults need not be frequent to be termed child abuse; they can entail situational abuse by the parents when the family is under great stress (Roth, 1975). A psychosocial environment that does not facilitate the development of competencies in terms of self image, ability to interact with others, academic skills, and others that relate to the completion of life span developmental tasks can be considered emotional abuse (Wodarski, 1981).

The first case of child abuse was reported in 1874. At that time there were no organizations or legal means to protect children from their families. Neighbors of the abused child appealed to The Society for the Prevention of Cruelty to Animals to provide protection for this young victim. Shortly afterward, in 1875, the Society for the Protection of Children was established (Paulson and Blake, 1969). Since that time, statistics have been computed as to the number and frequency of incidences, actions have been taken against known child abusers, and a substantial number of studies have been completed researching the causes of child abuse. Very little has been done, however, in the area of actually preventing child abuse.

It is evident that child abuse is a serious national problem. The number of cases reported to protective agencies in the year 1974 alone ranged between 50,000 and 60,000. An estimated additional 2 million cases of child abuse go unreported each year. Moreover, it is estimated that 50% of all children's visits to the emergency room are due to some form of physical abuse (Wonklestein, 1976). In one small county of rural Georgia, 88 cases of suspected child abuse have been reported over a 5-month period.

Who are these abused children? Most abused children are very young, frequently less than 1 year old (Spinetta and Rigler, 1972). Younger children with greater attention needs and less mobility constitute the greatest percentage of abused children (Young, 1966). Thus, abuse occurs when the children are at greatest risk (Wodarski, 1981).

Numerous factors can be mentioned as possible causes of child abuse. An attribute in the child, such as a physical or psychological abnormality, may elicit abusive behavior from the parents (Belsky, 1970). Sociological factors that may influence child abuse include disorganization of the family, urbanization, rapid social change, lack of employment possibilities, and new technology, all of which put wear and tear on the family system. In many cases there is an increasing demand for success and achievement, although not all people are ready to meet these demands. Isolation of families in rural areas seems to be a social factor contributing to child abuse. Also, a lack of an extended family or community interaction appears in case after case of child abuse (Garbarino, 1977). This is especially noticeable in rural areas (Bybee, 1979). Socioeconomic stress is also a predominating factor (Garbarino, 1977). A final contributing factor to child abuse is the parent's history. Most abusing parents have been abused themselves (Spinetta and Rigler, 1972). Abusive parents often view their children as reminders of their own unhappy past (Galston, 1975). Abusive parents frequently treat their children as if they were older than they are, and expect far too much from them. They typically expect these children to provide the love and security they missed as children themselves (Spinetta and Rigler, 1972). In addition, the typical abusive parent feels unprepared and uncomfortable in dealing with the parental role (Schrier, 1979). Not only do abusive parents feel that they have missed out on having loving parents themselves, but they have no suitable role models once they become parents. The combination is deadly, literally.

Recent research shows that abusive parents' feelings seem to stem back to just after the birth of the child, or, in certain cases, before the birth. One study found that abusive mothers were afraid of hurting their children while they were pregnant, usually during the fourth to seventh months of pregnancy (Wonklestein,

1976). Other studies have shown that pregnancy was a problem for abusive mothers. Many had trouble "making peace" with their own bodies, during and after pregnancy (Galston, 1975). Recent studies have successfully predicted the potential for child abuse from the time of birth of the child victim. Interviews and observations in the delivery room provided information that assigned mothers to levels of "risk of abuse" according to the birth weight of the children. There was a positive correlation of high-risk mothers and abusive acts on low birthweight children (Gray et al., 1979). Thus, preventive activities are shifting toward newborn babies and their parents, and especially to young parents (Elmer, 1979).

Prevention of Abuse

The critical question remains, can child abuse be prevented? If so, how? Recognizing the underlying causes of child abuse helps focus on the types of prevention programs. One point that becomes disturbingly clear is that most of the programs aimed at preventing child abuse fall far short of their goal.

How can a program prevent child abuse? What can be done to or with child abusers? Should expectant couples be required to sign a contract promising never to abuse their children? Should mothers-in-law be required to live within the house as monitors? Should all those who have abused their children, or who act like they are going to, be sterilized? A comprehensive approach to the problem may provide the best means of altering the incidence of abuse.

To substantially reduce the incidence of child abuse in rural areas will require massive community changes. Attitudes toward children and child development must change. Ideally, corporal punishment in the home should be stopped and family planning should be accepted (Resnick and Sweet, 1979). There must be an increase in educational programs to members of the community who may come in contact with evidence of child abuse (Bybee, 1979) and in community support and protection for the children in that particular community area (Light, 1973). In addition, parents and prospective parents should be educated about stages of child development, that is, what to expect of and how to deal with children at various stages (Light, 1973). Thus, prevention of child abuse must be a comprehensive effort . . . one supported by mass media, the community, the professional world and the legislators. The focus of prevention must be aimed directly at parents of future parents, first, because they are the abusers, and because they have almost total control over their children's lives for the first 6 years. Here is where prevention must begin (O'dell, 1974).

There are several methods of treating abusive parents and abused children. Treatment often focuses on providing counseling for either party or both. It can also include removing the child from the home, or drawing up behavioral contracts for reducing parent's abusive behavior. Treatment is not equal to prevention, however, and subsequently the focus must shift.

The first step in prevention is to identify high-risk populations or families. This can be done by hospital staff, church officials, school faculties, mental health staff, and by practitioners within the Department of Family and Children Services

(Resnick and Sweet, 1979). Additionally, potential abusers can be identified through the Child Abuse Registry (Gray et al., 1979). Ideally, a prevention program could be initiated as early as high school. Educational classes and programs on child rearing, child management, and child development could be initiated in high schools across the country as a prerequisite to graduation. Providing the opportunity for teenagers to spend time volunteering in day care centers, securing direct interactional experience with children, is another approach (Light, 1973). More realistically, a prevention program must rely on other agencies and institutions for referrals of potential child abusers. This is a limited beginning, but it is a beginning nonetheless. The next step is to provide services for the potential child abuser. The type of services preferred and the type to be presented in this chapter are classes on child management training, and/or behavioral techniques. Reasons for this particular approach with reference to rural areas are provided later in this chapter.

Emphasis on Child Management Training and Behavioral Techniques in the Prevention of Child Abuse

There have been numerous studies linking behavior management techniques to treatment and prevention of child abuse. Identification of specific, observable problem behaviors is essential, as well as identification of specific coping skills for parents (Belsky, 1970). Parents can learn what to expect in terms of behaviors from children at different stages of life. They learn to consistently reward children for good behaviors, and to use stimulus control to alter children's misbehaviors (Mastria, Mastria, and Hawkins, 1979; Polkov and Peabody, 1975; Resnick and Sweet, 1979; Tracy and Clark, 1974; Wodarski and Bagarozzi, 1979). Contingency contracting, discrimination training, and assertiveness training are all parts of such a preventive approach. Time-out procedures frequently are used (Polkov and Peabody, 1975). Keeping charts of observable behaviors has been determined to be quite a successful practice in preventing misbehaviors by parents and children (Tracy and Clark, 1974). Modeling of appropriate behaviors by an instructor in class is important to demonstrate acceptable role models (Belsky, 1970). Behaviors are broken into small, achievable steps. Videotaped sessions of interactions between parent and child have been used successfully in prevention programs (Mastria et al., 1979). Classes emphasizing reinforcement of anger control have also been used in conjunction with preventing child abuse (Resnick and Sweet, 1979). Such classes have focused on role playing, listening skills, and even homework assignments for parents (Rinn and Markle, 1977). Special attention has been focused toward improving the consistency of parenting skills, as that factor seems to be linked to child abuse (Resnick and Sweet, 1979). Paul S. Graubard in his book, *Positive Parenthood*, emphasizes the importance of parents' recognizing and reinforcing their children's strengths more than their drawbacks or weaknesses (Graubard, 1977). In fact, a special training procedure has been developed by Dr. Thomas Gordon (1970) of behavior management techniques for parents. In his book, *Parent Effectiveness Training*, Dr. Gordon outlines a specific course (usually eight weekly sessions, each 3 hours long) for target parents. The course covers parent-child communication, guidelines for listening skills, and a no-lose method for solving conflicts (Gordon, 1970). The behavior management approach may be appealing and successful because it focuses on what to teach and tells one how (Graubard, 1977).

What are some of the advantages to behavioral approaches, in general, and specifically, in reference to rural areas? Gelfand and Hartman (1968) state that there are several advantages to behavioral management classes. These include: that the practices are empirically based; the number of individuals dealt with at one time is large; the training period is relatively short-term in nature; the training requires a small professional staff; the training is not based on a sickness model; and lastly, a large percentage of childhood problems can be broken into specific behaviors suitable for change by this training (O'dell, 1974).

Why should such training be appropriate for rural areas? There are numerous reasons. Perhaps the most important concerns the language used. Behavior management can be presented in easily understandable, frequently observable terms. Clients of average intelligence and below average education can understand the basic concepts. Rural people need terms and procedures that they can easily grasp, that they can relate to, and that are relevant to their everyday lives. They do not need to be bothered with fancy therapy techniques. Likewise, a majority of people receiving public mental health services could not understand the fancy terminology used in psychotherapy or Gestalt therapy.

Next, the classes break problems and behaviors into small, observable, countable steps. In other words, easy success for parent and child is the key feature of this program. This increases participation and motivation as well as understanding. The programs are relatively short in duration and can serve several families at once, which reduces the cost and increases the served population. Moreover, the classes can be held at night for working parents. Parents can share feelings, interact with and observe role models of other parents, and are likely to benefit from the support derived from being in a group. A skilled leader of such classes does not have to be highly trained or highly paid. He or she can be someone from the community, and a successful parent as well. No special equipment is needed to teach these skills. Finally, and of utmost importance, such a program provides a positive approach. It involves no burden of guilt for parents. In fact, classes are very beneficial to all parents because no "sick" label is attached to participants. This encourages participation, dedication, and communication about such a program in a positive, proud way. Behavior management represents the new look of child abuse prevention in rural areas. An example of a program used in rural areas is presented in this chapter.

SUMMARY

A major challenge to the community mental health approach is the question of the timing of intervention. The community mental health approach places great emphasis on the teaching components of the interventive process with social workers attempting to help clients learn how to exert control over their own behaviors and the environments in which they live. This becomes difficult when rural individuals possess a characteristic fatalistic perspective (Ginsberg, 1971). On the other hand, however, they possess a trait considered to be a general prerequisite for the use of preventive approaches; that is, assumption of responsibility for one's life.

The community mental health approach to social work practice offers much promise for the social work profession. It provides a view of the person that is optimistic. Social workers realize that community health is mass-oriented rather than individual-oriented, and it seeks to build health from the start rather than to repair (Chu, 1974; Kelley, Snowden, and Munoz, 1977; Whittman, 1977). In recognition of the critical role of prevention in improving the mental health of all citizens, it has been suggested that a special staff be set up in each mental health center just for prevention programs (Rae-Grant et al., 1966). Such a set-up would be costly, but the impact in the long run would be substantial.

REFERENCES

Azrin, N. H. 1978. A learning approach to job finding. Paper presented at Association for Advancement of Behavior Therapy, November, Chicago.

Azrin, N. H., Flores, T., and Kaplan, S. J. 1975. Job-finding club: A group-assisted program for obtaining employment. Behav. Res. Ther. 13:17–27.

Belsky, J. 1970. A theoretical analysis of child abuse remediation strategy. J. Clin. Child Psychol. 7:117–120.

Bybee, R. 1979. Violence toward youth: A new perspective. J. Sociol. Issues 35:1–14.

Caplan, G. 1961. Prevention of Mental Disorders in Children. Basic Books, New York.

Caplan, G. 1974. Support Systems in Community Mental Health: Lectures on Concept Development. pp. 111–215. Behavioral Publications, New York.

Chu, F. D. 1974. The Madness Establishment. Grossman, New York.

Collins, J. D. 1971. The effects of the conjugal relationship modification method on marital communication and adjustment. Unpublished doctoral dissertation: The Pennsylvania State University.

DeRisi, W., and Butz, G. 1975. Writing Behavioral Contracts. Research Press, Champaign, Ill.

D'Zurilla, T., and Goldfried, M. 1971. Problem solving and behavior modification. J. Abnorm. Psychol. 78:106–126.

Elmer, E. 1979. Child abuse and family stress. J. Sociol. Issues 35:60–71.

Galston, R. 1975. Preventing the abuse of little children. Am. J. Orthopsych. 3:372–381.

Garbarino, J. 1977. The price of privacy in the social dynamics of child abuse. Child Wel. 56:565–567.

Gelfand, D. M., and Hartman, D. P. 1968. Behavior therapy with children: A review and evaluation of research methodology. Psychol. Bull. 69:204–215.

Gilchrist, L. D. 1981. Social competence in adolescence. In S. P. Schinke (ed.), Behavioral Methods in Social Welfare. pp. 61–80. Aldine Publishing Company, New York.

Ginsberg, L. H. 1971. Rural social work. Encycl. Soc. Work, 2:1138–1144.

Goldfried, M., and Goldfried, A. 1975. Cognitive change methods. In F. Kanfer and A. Goldstein (eds.), Helping People Change. Pegram Press, Inc., New York.

Gordon, T. 1970. Parent Effectiveness Training. Plume, New York.

Gottesfield, J. 1972. The Critical Issues of Community Mental Health. pp. 123–137. Behavorial Publications, New York.

Graubard, P. 1977. Positive Parenthood. Bobbs-Merrill, New York.

Gray, J., Cutler, C., Dean, J., and Kempe, H. 1979. Predicting and preventing child abuse and neglect. J. Sociol. Issues 35:127–139.

Jones, R. J., and Azrin, N. H. 1973. An experimental application of a social reinforcement approach to the problem of job finding. J. Appl. Behav. Anal. 6:345–353.

Kelley, J. G., Snowden, L. R., and Munoz, R. F. 1977. Social and community intervention. In M. R. Rosenzweig and L. W. Porter (eds.), Annual Review of Psychology, Annual Review, Inc., Palo Alto, Calif.

Lange, A. J., and Jakubowski, P. 1976. Responsible Assertive Behavior. Research. Press, Champaign, Ill.

Light, R. 1973. Abused and neglected children in America: A study of alternate policies. Harv. Educ. Rev. 43:556–596.

Mastria, E. O., Mastria, M., and Hawkins, J. 1979. Treatment of child abuse by behavioral intervention: A case report. Child Welf. 58:253–263.

Meyer, A. J., and Henderson, J. B. 1974. Multiple risk factors: Reduction in the prevention of cardiovascular diseases. Prevent. Med. 3:225–236.

O'dell, S. 1974. Training parents in behavior modification: A review. Psychol. Bull. 81:416–433.

Paulson, M. J., and Blake, P. 1969. The physically abused child. Child Welf. 48:86–95.

Polkov, R. L., and Peabody, D. 1975. Behavioral treatment for child abusers. Int. J. Offend. Ther. Compar. Criminol. 19:100–102.

Rae-Grant, Q. A. F., Gladwin, T., and Bower, E. M. 1966. Mental health social competence, and the war on poverty. Am. J. Orthopsych. 36:652–664.

Resnick, P., and Sweet, J. J. 1979. The maltreatment of children: A review of theories and research. J. Sociol. Issues 35:40–59.

Rinn, R., and Markle, A. 1977. Parent effectiveness training: A review. Behav. Rep. 41:95–109.

Roth, F. 1975. A practice regimen for diagnosis and treatment of child abuse. Child Welf. 54:268–273.

Schinke, S. P. Social competency training for disturbed preadolescents. J. Soc. Serv. Res. In press.

Schinke, S. P., and Blythe, B. J. Cognitive-behavioral prevention of childrens' smoking. Child Behav. Ther. In press.

Schinke, S. P., Gilchrist, L. D., and Blythe, B. J. 1980. Role of communication in the prevention of teenage pregnancy. Health Soc. Work, 5:54–59.

Schinke, S. P., Blythe, B. J., and Gilchrist, L. D. 1981. Cognitive-behavioral prevention of adolescent pregnancy. J. Counsel. Psychol. 28:451–454.

Schrier, C. J. 1979. Child abuse: An illness or a crime? Child Welf. 58:237–240.

Spinetta, J., and Rigler, D. 1972. The child abusing parent. Psychol. Bull. 77:296–304.

Spivack, G., and Shure, M. B. 1974. Social Adjustment of Young Children. Jossey-Bass, San Francisco.

Tracy, J., and Clark, E. 1974. Treatment for child abusers. Soc. Work 19:338–342.

Whittman, M. 1977. Application of knowledge about the prevention in social work education and practice. Soc. Work Health Care 3:37–47.

Wodarski, J. S. 1980. Procedures for the maintenance and generalization of achieved behavioral change. J. Sociol Soc. Welf 7:298–311.

Wodarski, J. S. 1981. Treatment of parents who abuse their children: A literature review and implications for professionals. Child Abuse Negl. 5:351–360.

Wodarski, J. S., and Bagarozzi, D. 1979. Behavioral Social Work. Human Sciences Press, New York.

Wodarski, L. A., Adelson, C. L., Tidball, M. T., and Wodarski, J. S. 1980. Teaching nutrition by teams-games-tournaments. J. Nutr. Educ. 12:61–65.

Wonklestein, A. 1976. Evolution of a program for the management of child abusers. Soc. Casework 57:309–310.

Young, L. 1966. An interim report on an experimental program for protective services. Child Welfare 45:373–381.

EDUCATING POTENTIAL CHILD ABUSERS IN RURAL AREAS: A CURRICULUM FOR SOCIAL WORKERS

The object of this curriculum is to train rural mental health workers to teach high-risk parents behavior management techniques as a means of preventing child abuse. These techniques can be used on parent as well as on child behaviors.

Referrals

The main thrust of any preventive program must be identification of the target group. The first area in which the trainer of the group, the rural social worker, must attain competency, therefore, is in discovering suspected child abusers in the community.

The worker must be aware of indicators of incidences of abuse and must continually monitor such indicators. Competency in detecting child abuse can be tested through a quiz of the checklist of indicators and of practical application of those indicators. In other words, does the trainer know what to look for, what to overlook, or what to report regarding child abuse? Adequate knowledge of these indicators on a written quiz may be one test of competency, but the test must go further than to just measure the worker's knowledge. The trainer will not ensure an effective program if he or she does not use the principles in practice settings. Competency, especially in this area, is hard to judge. A decrease in the number of recurring child abuse cases and of recurring abuse reports in the community can be used to measure success or failure of the trainer's ability to detect child abuse.

Weighing heavily on the successful prevention of child abuse are community referrals. Competency in establishing adequate referral systems can be judged by the following:

Does the trainer have community contacts

within the court system?
within the educational system?
with the Public Health Department?
with the Department of Family and Children Services?
with other local Mental Health Centers?
with hospitals in the area?
with Family Planning Clinics?
with local doctors?
with local Drug and Alcohol programs?
with Day Care Centers in the area?

If the answer to any of these questions is no, then the trainer must establish such contacts. It becomes evident then that a considerable amount of groundwork must be done before the implementation of any training.

Content Knowledge

Subsequent instructions apply directly to services or training rendered by the community mental health social worker. These instructions are similar to those outlined by Gordon (1970) in his book, *Parent Effectiveness Training*. Certain of the steps have been simplified and broken down to increase understanding on the part of the rural clientele. In addition, a great deal of information has been gathered from Graubard's (1977) book, *Positive Parenthood*.

The techniques in which a participant must possess competency include the following: reinforcement, punishment, time-out, stimulus control techniques, listening skills, and application of all of these. First, parents must understand the meaning of *reinforcement*, what constitutes postive reinforcement, how to use it, when to use it, and how to get results. The importance of consistency must be stressed in reference to reinforcement. Methods to test for competency in this area include written or verbal quizzes, class exercises, class examples, role model examples, and the use of videotapes. The ability of the individual to understand and apply these principles in the classroom will be judged by the instructor. Emphasis will be placed on mastery of the skills, instead of passing or failing. To be judged competent, the participant must: 1) make 70% or above on all of the quizzes; 2) demonstrate mastery of the positive reinforcement techniques in four or more class examples; 3) participate in two or more class exercises; 4) attend class regularly; and 5) make a videotape with the child and the trainer-observer in the room, using behavior modification techniques. Four to six sessions should be spent concentrating on reinforcement techniques, because they are critical to any intervention program. In the seventh session, the concept of shaping should be introduced to the class, explained, and demonstrated. Testing for competency with regard to shaping can be accomplished through role plays with other class members, role plays with children, written and verbal quizzes, and class exercises. Competency can be judged in a manner similar to that explained above.

The technique of *punishment* is likewise very important to behavior modification. After the concept of reinforcement has been mastered by all, punishment techniques should be introduced. Parents must be able to sense when and when not to use punishment. They should understand the dynamics of punishment, as well as be able to differentiate various kinds of punishment for different situations. Competency can be judged through written/verbal quizzes, group exercises, lists of behaviors that call for the use of punishment, and charts kept on how often punishment is used at home (See Tables 1 and 2). Again, competency will be judged by the trainer according to these criteria: attendance at sessions, 70% or better scores on quizzes, lists of behaviors turned in to the counselor, participation in group discussion, and exercises.

Time-out procedures constitute an important aspect of successful behavior modification. Parents must understand the concept of time out and when to apply it. Competency can be judged through: 1) quizzes, 70% or higher; 2) group discussions in which each member presents a problem for which time out would be the appropriate intervention; 3) making a list of acceptable instances to use time out; and 4) making a complete list of resources that the parents can use for time out activity. *Stimulus control techniques* for altering behavior can be reviewed in Chapter 4 of Wodarski and Bagarozzi's (1979) text entitled *Behavioral Social Work.*

The last step in instruction and clinical application centers on *listening skills.* The majority of clients need to learn to listen to their children. They must practice listening to each other before they can listen to their children. The parents participate in group presentations on listening, in two-person exercises on listening skills, and in group listening exercises. Competency in this area can be judged by: 1) attendance at meetings; 2) successful two-person exercises; 3) participation in at least two group listening exercises; and 4) through an interview with the trainer.

Clients must master these techniques before attempting to change their children's behaviors. In addition, clients may know the principles like the back of their hands, but they will not be able to use them if they are not practiced at home. Practice is vital to the success of the program, and it must be tested and thoroughly monitored.

Implementing the Program

The first step is to be able to correctly define a problem. The client must be able to recognize a problem, and then to break it down into observable, measurable behaviors. The problems to be worked on must be real to each family and specific to each family's needs. Competency for defining problems is measured by: 1) input into the group discussions about problem behaviors; 2) oral presentation and analysis of a problem; 3) compiled lists of age-specific problems that are common to one or more families; and 4) oral or written quizzes. The client must describe at least one problem to the trainer, pass the quizzes (70% or better), participate in group discussions of problem behaviors, and present one problem behavior to the group. Competency will be judged by the trainer, and in group situations, by the group members.

The next step is in who owns up to the problem. Parents must be able to recognize and separate their problems from their children's. Competency in this area will be judged on the basis of group participation, role plays, and a quiz (written or oral) and will be determined by the trainer or, when appropriate, by the group.

A final, and most important step, is the implementation of principles in the home. All of what the parents have learned must be implemented and practiced at home for any success to occur. Competency will be judged by several methods. Each client must describe a real problem behavior at home, define it, own up to it, break it down, decide what to do about it, and then follow through with the implementation. Problems will be presented to the group and trainer for feedback. Behavioral contracts will be drawn up. Charts on children's behaviors will be maintained. Where possible, videotapes of parents interacting with their children should be made. Children will come to class at a designated meeting so parents can practice programs within sight of the group and the trainer. Finally, the trainer will make home visits to each of the houses to observe the parents in action to provide the requisite feedback necessary to correctly implement the techniques.

Competency in this most vital area will be judged by the instructor and the group and will include the following: 1) The client must describe at least one problem to the class, define it and present a treatment plan. 2) Behavior contracts will be written and signed by parent and child (if the child is over 7); progress or changes will be brought up before the trainer and the group. 3) Behavior charts marking increases or decreases in behaviors and the type of intervention must be presented and approved by the group and trainer. 4) One videotape (to be reviewed by the trainer) of a successful intervention between the parent and the child will be presented to the trainer. 5) Children must attend three classes; parents will be observed by the trainer while interacting with the children. 6) There must be at least three successful home visits. Success is defined as observing at least one appropriate interaction and implementation of one or more behavior modification techniques. Also, target behaviors are altered as a result of the intervention.

OUTLINE OF EACH PROGRAM SESSION

Presession I

The success of the program is often judged through home visits. One visit should take place before the training begins, if possible, to provide baseline data. The trainer then has an idea of the baseline activity of the trainees, as well as the existing parental structures and discipline procedures. These visits are strongly urged, but not totally necessary.

Session I

The first session must be an informal, information sharing, trust-building session. Many of the clients may have been forced, or strongly encouraged, to participate in the group. In any event, almost everyone will be feeling anxious, perhaps threatened, reluctant, and/or angry that they have to be there. The trainer must not rush into the training. There must be genuine effort and participation from the parents for this program to work. Therefore, it is extremely necessary for the trainees to feel at ease and accepted. The trainer should spend some time at the beginning of the session just chatting with the group, perhaps providing coffee and/or iced tea and baked goods to stimulate interaction. The following should be included in the first session:

1. Praise or thanks for coming to the first meeting
2. Introduction of the trainer in a personal, straightforward manner

3. Introduction of parents and encouragement of interaction between them in loosely structured, nonthreatening ways
4. A successful or positive experience for each couple during the first night is very important—whether the parents are voluntary or involuntary clients
5. Discussion of children with regard to problems, appropriate behaviors at developmental stages, past histories, and so on
6. Late in the meeting—a basic outline of the course, with reference to the clients as students or trainees
7. Talk about any transportation problems, the need for any changes in times or dates of meetings, problems with childcare during meetings (the worker can facilitate a joint sitter for the families or a childcare service)
8. Discussion of fees, with an explanation of the sliding fee scale, including its purpose as well as problems associated with it
9. A phone number for emergencies with encouragement to use it
10. If rewards are to be given to parents, the reward system can be determined by finding out what will be appreciated or appropriate for each client (examples are course credit, money, prizes at the end, or a certificate).

Most important, the trainer must become established as a friend to participants. Open the lines of communication. Make sure they leave feeling good about themselves, the trainer, and the program.

A test to judge competency in this area includes a checklist. Did the trainer follow all of these suggestions? The trainer may be rated by an observer to determine competency. Also, the trainer could be rated by the group. Also, role taken at the second session could indicate how successful the instructor was in the first meeting.

Session II

In the second session the trainer needs to begin introducing basic behavior modification principles. The key word here is simplicity. The principles must be broken down into very small, simplistic terms. The steps should be broken into easily attainable goals and presented in plain, simple language.

The first principle to be introduced is reinforcement. This is a vital part of the behavior modification system, and it must be understood thoroughly for any success to be realized in the training. The trainees must understand what reinforcement is, how it works, and when and how to use it. The trainer should gather clients around a table and talk facing all of them in a casual manner. The trainees should be able to face each other and feel comfortable talking to each other. The trainees should be provided with paper and pencils. A blackboard is helpful, also. The instructor should explain reinforcement verbally to the group, using the blackboard for diagrams and examples.

The following is an example of a lesson plan for use by the trainer. First, ask the trainees what they think reinforcement is. Get everyone to answer or provide input into the discussion. Then elucidate: reinforcement increases behavior. It makes behavior happen more often. The technical definition states that reinforcement is an event that happens just after a behavior occurs that increases the chances of that behavior happening again. Stress that the key point is reinforcement makes behavior more likely to happen. If the reinforcement does not increase the behavior, then you are not really reinforcing anything. Now, stress that reinforcement can be many things. It can be candy, food, attention, money, a kind word, praise, and so on. Ask the group for examples of what would be reinforcing to them. What would make them exhibit a behavior more often? Write the examples on the board. Talk about them. Talk about the behaviors that will increase as a result of such reinforcement. Then give these examples, or some similar to these.

1. If Betty gets a piece of candy for completing her homework after supper, she is being reinforced for doing her homework. The candy is the reinforcement. The behavior being increased is completing homework. Draw this diagram:

    Betty..sitting quietly..finishes homework .... candy
        (behavior)   (reinforcement)

    Discuss the diagram and the situation.

2. If Bobby makes his bed each morning, he gets to play softball with his father from 5 to 6 each evening. The reinforcement is playing ball with Dad. The behavior that is increasing is the bed-making. Draw this diagram:

    Bobby makes his bed .... an hour of baseball with Dad
        (behavior)   (reinforcement)

    Discuss it.

3. If Mom gives Billy a big hug and kiss each day that he comes home from school clean, Billy is being reinforced for coming home clean. The hug and kiss are the reinforcment. The behavior being increased is coming home clean. Draw this diagram:

    Billy comes home clean .... hug and kiss from Mom
        (behavior)   (reinforcement)

    Discuss it.

Then have each person identify one behavior to be changed and a reinforcement to be used to change it. Go around the room and get individuals to describe the situation they would like to change, and how. You draw the diagrams, or let them draw one for their situation. Discuss each example in terms of the behavior diagram and the reinforcement.

Close the session with a review of the meaning of reinforcement. Set the meeting time for the next session. Get feedback from the group on how they felt about this session. Were you too fast? Too slow? Make it personal.

Session III

Assemble the group around a table with pencils and paper. Spend adequate time talking about major problems or upsets that have occurred in the past week. Then review the last session. What is reinforcement? Ask for answers from the group. Retrace briefly what happened from the last session. Then draw this diagram on the blackboard:

Suzy completes one household chore (dishes)..............30 minutes of TV time

Ask what Suzy is being reinforced for doing. Make sure that if a participant does not understand, you go over the example, pointing out both the behavior and the reinforcement. Then ask for a problem behavior from the group and diagram it. Ask for examples of reinforcement and when to give the reinforcement. Discuss this.

Break into teams of two people. Give each team a problem behavior to be worked out in written or in oral form. Reconvene the group and ask each team to discuss their problem, behavior, and reinforcement.

There are a few important points to be made here by the instructor. First, for reinforcement to be effective, it must be positive. The child or parent must view the reinforcement as something good, an item to work for. For example: giving Johnny spinach as a reinforcement for doing his homework when he does not like it, is not likely to increase his homework behavior. Also, different behaviors may require different sizes or values of reinforcement. For example, one cannot offer a piece of candy as a reward for good grades for an entire school term. The reward must fit the behavior or task. Next, and most important, the reinforcement must be consistent. The parents must reinforce the desired behavior each time that it occurs, and as soon as possible. It is hard to reinforce a child for taking out the trash when you just wrecked the car, the baby's diaper is wet, and you feel nauseous—but TRY! Try very hard, especially at first, to be quick and consistent with rewards. The child must be able to count on immediate reinforcers (a smile, ice cream, money, etc.) for the child to want to exhibit certain behaviors. If you simply cannot reinforce immediately, explain why and be sure that you follow through with a reward later.

The following is a good exercise for a group of parents. Send one of the participants out of the room. The rest of the group will decide on one thing, that is one behavior, that they want the absent person to do. Then ask the person to return to the room. Explain that you will clap when the person exhibits the behavior that the group has decided that they want the participant to do. Or, if the behavior is complex, tell the person that the group will clap when he or she exhibits a behavior that is close to what they want. When the exact behavior occurs, get the group to stand up and clap. The clapping is a positive reinforcer. Be sure to explain that. This exercise encourages parent participation and keeps them united as a group. Try it two to three times.

Another exercise for teams is conducted as follows. Divide the participants into pairs. Have one of the partners decide on a behavior that he or she wants the other partner to increase. Use M&M's or verbal praise as reinforcers for that behavior. In other words, one person gives the other one an M&M or verbal praise whenever the correct behavior is emitted. Give the individual the reward quickly and consistently after the behavior. Then, let the participant guess the behavior that you are trying to increase.

After you try these exercises, again reiterate how important consistency and immediacy of reinforcement can be to success. Spend a few minutes just talking with the group before you let them go. Ask about any problems or needed changes.

Session IV

Open the session as usual, talking about any substantial problems that have come up in the past week. Now is a good time to evaluate the learning that is taking place. Do this by asking the parents if they have noticed any changes that have happened at home. Next, review reinforcement. Ask for a definition from the group. Ask for an example of reinforcement. Check this definition and example with the rest of the group. Get as much input as you can. Then, ask for examples of reinforcements that could be used on these behaviors:

1. Good grades in school
2. Making beds
3. Quiet time after supper
4. Saying please and thank you
5. Reduced aggressive behavior

Remind the group that the reinforcement should increase these behaviors.

Next, the concept of shaping is introduced. For most behaviors, one cannot expect perfection at first. Just as one cannot expect a child to tie his or her shoes perfectly for the first time, one must learn to shape the behavior that one wants. If one expects perfection the first time, it serves to set oneself up for failure and frustration. If, for example, you want to teach a child to make the bed each morning, you may need to reinforce him or her for straightening the sheet first. Then, you may have to reinforce the child for folding the bedspread, and so on until the terminal goal is achieved. Explain all of this to the group. Ask for examples of behaviors that may need to be shaped. Discuss these behaviors. Then, ask the group to participate in this exercise. Start by picking one behavior. Give everyone a pencil and paper to write the behavior down in stepwise fashion. Write the behavior in as small, simple steps as possible. Then talk about the steps. Ask everyone to pick a separate behavior and do the same with it. Discuss the behaviors.

Now, quiz the group. Ask them to fill out the quiz in Table 1. If the clients cannot read, read the test to them aloud. Have them check the answers or tell you, the trainer, the answers. Discuss the quiz with the group. Compare answers. Accent positive points, right answers, and so forth. Correct wrong answers on the spot.

Table 1

Identify the reinforcer and the behavior that should increase.

1. Johnny goes to bed on time and he gets a nickel.
2. Susie does all of her homework and she gets to go shopping with mom.
3. For every time that John comes home sober, his wife will have sex with him.
4. Each day that Mary keeps the dishes washed, her husband marks it on the calendar. When she has five marks on the calendar, she gets to go out to dinner.
5. Each morning that Billy gets up with dry pants and dry sheets, he gets pancakes for breakfast.

What are two very important words to remember when you are reinforcing your child?

_____ and _____

What does reinforcement actually do?

Draw a diagram for this problem: John and his little sister, May, fight all the time. Their mother has about had it with them. Every time they spend one hour together without fighting, she gives them both a cookie.

What are some things that would be reinforcing to you?

1.
2.
3.
4.
5.

What are items that would be reinforcing to your child?

Session V

In this session the concept of negative reinforcement is introduced. Reinforcement does not always have to be positive or desirable. Although positive reinforcement is much preferred over negative reinforcement because it works faster and creates fewer hard feelings, negative reinforcement can be used to change behaviors. Negative reinforcement is more confusing, and may create hostile feelings and mistrust. The first thing to remember is that negative reinforcement increases behavior. It is still reinforcement. The difference is that negative reinforcement increases a behavior when it is taken away. In other words, the behavior increases when the reinforcement is taken away or stopped. The child behaves to avoid negative reinforcement. Explain this to your group and then present these exercises.

Little Johnny has a cat. He frequently forgets to change the kitty's litter box. So, the parents put the litter box in Johnny's room. If he doesn't change it, it smells. The smell is a negative reinforcement. The behavior that increases is changing the litter box. The boy behaves to avoid the bad smell.

Litter box smell .... changing the litter box
(negative reinforcement)   (increased behavior)

Another example of negative reinforcement is an alarm clock. When the alarm goes off in the morning, you push the button to stop it (to avoid the negative reinforcement). The alarm sound serves as a negative reinforcement. The behavior that increases is the turning off of the alarm. Diagram that situation on the board.

alarm sound .... punching the button
(negative reinforcement)   (increased behavior)

Give the class some examples of negative reinforcers and ask for the behaviors that could increase as a result of them. Examples include:

1. Getting wet on raining mornings (increased behavior of wearing a raincoat)
2. Burned finger on an iron (moving hand away from the iron)
3. Whining child (parent giving cookie to stop whining)
4. Pain from fingers slammed in door (moving fingers)
5. Weight gain (dieting)

Discuss these examples. Review the whole concept of negative reinforcement. Ask for examples from the group. Emphasize typical behaviors of whining and pestering and show how giving in to a child's demands is a dual rewarding process, one that serves as positive reinforcement for the child and negative reinforcement for the parent.

At this point, begin scheduling home visits with the group members.

Session VI

Review positive and negative reinforcement. Contrast and compare them verbally. What things are alike about the two procedures? What things are different? Ask for group input. This session is designed specifically for reviewing all of the principles presented thus far. It is up to the trainer to informally judge how well the trainees know these concepts. After talking about the differences and similarities of the types of reinforcement, list these examples on a board that everyone can see. Positive reinforcers include—candy, privileges, money, a smile, use of car. Ask the group for more examples. Write them down, too. Then write these examples of negative reinforcers: alarm clock ring, telephone ring, car horn. Ask for other examples relevant to home interactional situations.

Then, divide the large group into three or four smaller groups with at least three to a group. Give each group a piece of paper with a situation on it. Instruct them to decide on a positive or negative reinforcer that can be used to change the behavior. Describe how to do it, role play the situation in front of the group.

Next, call out situations listed below. Ask the group to write the negative or positive reinforcement used on a piece of paper. Discuss their responses. For each of the situations, talk about how one might shape the behavior.

Indicate to the participants that a quiz is upcoming. Plan an extra session or two here if groups need to review concepts.

Group Situations to Role Play

1. You want to increase the time your son spends on homework.
2. You want to increase the pleasant things that your daughter says.
3. You want to get your son up in the morning with little or no hassle.

Call Out Situations

1. You give your son a dime for every time he takes out the trash.
2. You agree to spend 30 minutes with your child playing ball every evening after he does his chores.
3. You take the phone off the hook to keep it from ringing.
4. Each time your spouse comes home sober you fix him or her a favorite meal.
5. Your son takes too long in the shower, so you turn off the hot water after 4 minutes.
6. You brush your teeth to get the onion taste out of your mouth.
7. You buy yourself a new dress when you lose 5 pounds.
8. You keep forgetting to take your umbrella to work and you get all wet.
9. Your hair gets itchy and greasy when it is dirty so you wash it every night.
10. You give your daughter a piece of gum every time she feeds the dog.
11. Your child yells and you give him what he wants.

Session VII

Written and/or oral quizzes. Discuss answers after the quiz.

Quiz

1. Reinforcement of any kind has what effect on behavior?

2. Explain the difference between positive and negative reinforcement.

3. Johnny is having a problem taking out the trash, his nightly or bi-weekly duty. How would you tackle that problem?

4. Your husband comes home at 11:30 pm three out of four nights a week . . . smashed on alcohol. How would you handle that?

5. You want to change one of your child's behaviors. You want little Johnny to stop being such a smart alec. First, narrow the problem to a manageable set of behaviors to work on. List them. Then state your strategy.

6. You are visiting a friend's house. Your child wants a piece of candy. Upon being refused, he or she throws him or herself on the floor, begins to cry and scream, kicks, etc. What do you do?

7. Your daughter is playing with older children that you do not approve of. What method of reinforcement could you use to change that?

8. Get with a partner and act out a situation calling for positive reinforcement, and then negative reinforcement.

9. Name three behaviors that your child does now that could be reduced by ignoring them. Name three that you think are pleasant and that you want to increase. State how you might go about shaping these behaviors.

10. What is shaping?

Session VIII

This session focuses on punishment. Sometimes punishment must be used, but it should be limited to certain circumstances and to specific types of punishment. Punishment is a negative reaction to a behavior. It can be a frown, a smack on the bottom, a loss of privileges, and so forth. Punishment reduces the chances that the behavior will occur again. For example, if you stay out late and you are grounded for it, the frequency of your being late usually decreases. The difficulty is that most persons over-use punishment and under-use positive reinforcement. There are times when punishment is appropriate, for example, for intolerable or dangerous behaviors. For instance, when a little tot reaches for a hot stove, he or she must be stopped quickly and forcefully. A smack on the hand is acceptable, *along with* an explanation. Tell the child why he or she is being punished. Punishment, as well as reinforcement, must be consistent. Emphasize this point. It should also be as immediate as possible to be effective with small children. One of the consistent mistakes that parents make in discipline is the "wait until Daddy gets home" approach. When Dad does get home, he is faced with disciplining a child for a behavior that happened a long time ago and that did not involve Dad himself. The key to successful parenting is to punish quickly, sparingly, adequately, and consistently.

There are many behaviors than can be dealt with by ignoring them (called *extinction*). By positive reinforcement of alternative prosocial behavior, the probability of nonsocial and/or antisocial behavior occurring is substantially reduced. Many children whine and cry in public places for treats or attention. For example, Joey may whine for a candy bar in a grocery store. Ignore him. He may cry; he may even cause a scene—but ignore him. It may be embarassing for you, but bear with it; it will pay off in the end. Do not give in. When you give in and buy the candy, the toy, whatever, you are teaching your child that his crying will eventually get him what he wants. When he exhibits *appropriate* behaviors in the store, use positive reinforcement extensively.

Conduct this exercise:
Circle the behaviors that must be treated through punishment and cross out behaviors

that can/should be ignored. List the appropriate behavior that positive reinforcement can increase.

running in the street	playing with matches
whining	refusing to eat
crying (due to no physical pain)	snapping fingers at you
hitting a smaller brother	smart alec remarks
stomping foot	telling tall tales
tantrums	touching a hot iron

Discuss the participants' answers.

Try this exercise with partners. Give one partner a list of six to seven behaviors to do at once. The list can include such behaviors as tapping fingers, licking lips, messing with hair, swinging a crossed leg, and coughing. Have one partner exhibit all of the behaviors, one right after the other, or intermingled. Have the other partner ignore the behaviors. Pick one particularly annoying behavior to punish. Decide on a punishment, a tasteful verbal remark, an ugly face, a pinch on the arm, and so forth. Engage in this interaction for 5 minutes. One person should be engaging in behaviors, and one should be ignoring and/or punishing behaviors. After 5 minutes, discuss the exercise. Talk about how the person exhibiting the behaviors felt when the punisher was ignoring/punishing the behavior. Did he or she feel like continuing the behavior? Was the punishment strong enough? Did it make any difference in the number of times the person engaged in the behavior?

Try role plays with the group in which participants ignore unattractive habits or behaviors. The idea here is that many people behave the way they do to get attention. Any attention, even gasping or staring at a person, may reinforce the behavior and it becomes likely that it will happen again. Be careful not to reinforce behaviors that you do not want to continue. Be strong and use consistent positive reinforcement for appropriate behavior.

Session IX

Review the concept of punishment. Ask for examples of behaviors for which punishment is appropriate. Get class input on how and why punishment is used.

One procedure that almost always must be utilized is time-out. Time-out is exactly what it sounds like, time-out from the situation. If nothing else works, remove either the child or yourself from the situation. Taking a child home when he or she is misbehaving in a grocery store is a good example of time-out. Sit the child in a quiet, separate place, until he or she calms down or stops the misbehavior. Do not send a child to his or her room if there are toys, puzzles, or TV to entertain. On the other hand, do not lock the child in a closet. Often, just having the child sit in a special chair or go to a separate room is enough. There are certain guidelines for time-out. Specify a time limit. An egg timer is great to help with time-out. Three to 5 minutes is usually adequate for a time-out. Do not let the child come back into the situation if he or she is still crying or misbehaving. For example, if he or she is cursing, send the child to the bedroom and set the timer for 3 to 5 minutes. This is usually adequate. If the child continues to curse, explain that the time will begin when cursing stops. Start the timer when the child is quiet. Be firm! Be consistent! Approach the implementation in a nonemotional manner maintaining such behaviors throughout the whole process. It will be tough at first, but hang on. It will pay off later.

If you cannot execute the time-out process in this manner, do not even attempt it. If you really feel frustrated and feel like you want to physically assault the child, *you* take a time out. *You* leave. Now, there are some limitations to your time out, too. Do not leave the children in a shopping center. Instead drop them off somewhere, at a relative's house or at a friend's. Call a neighbor. Call a crisis nursery. But you take a time-out. You get out of the environment. Take a walk, jog, have a glass of tea. When you cool off, come back and settle the situation. This can be done through either talking, ignoring, or punishment—but when you are in control of the situation.

Have all participants make a list of neighbors, friends, and relatives who could be used as time-out helpers. Have each pre-warn the friend, to facilitate the process. Encourage parents within the group to serve as back-up friends for time-out. They can certainly relate to the situation. Also, have all participants make lists of different time-out activities that they can engage in (walking, singing, jogging, and so forth). Role play a situation in which time-out would be appropriate. If needed, you, the trainer, take part in the role play. Then discuss it.

Next try this exercise. Below are some examples of misbehaviors. Circle the ones that are appropriate situations for time-out.

1. When Billy spits at his sister, lock him in the closet for 5 or 10 minutes.
2. When Suzanne smacks her brother, ask her to sit in her special chair for 5 minutes while the rest of the family plays games, eats, talks, and so forth.
3. When Lucy begins to cry and throw a tantrum at a neighbor's house, remove her from the situation, but let her come back after 5 minutes even though she is still crying.
4. After Joanie uses a stream of curse words, send her to her room where her TV, stereo, and phone are.
5. When Al cries and pounds his fists, sit him in a corner. Start timing when he stops crying and pounding. Have him sit quietly for 5 minutes in the corner. Explain the rationale to him.
6. After a long day, the kids are screaming, one child is sick, and you have had it. Throw up your hands and announce "I'm leaving!"
7. Your two boys have been fighting all day and you are ready to gag them and tie them up. Call a neighbor over for 20 minutes while you take a walk in the woods or down the street.
8. After a long day at work you come home and your wife starts nagging. You leave to go get drunk.

Review time-out and answer any questions that participants might have. Talk about the examples and exercises.

Session X

One very important part of behavior modification is listening. Everyone talks, but how many people ever really listen to their children, their spouses, their relatives? And, do these people listen to you? Many people sit and talk *at* each other. They never really listen to what the other person is saying. To really hear what your child is saying, you must actively listen.

This exercise will help you to learn to actively listen. Divide the group into pairs of people. Person 1 will state a problem. Person 2 must not interrupt or speak until Person 1 is finished. Then, the listener should repeat what Person 1 has just stated, almost word for word. It is good to start with a statement like, "what I hear you saying is . . ." or "I hear you saying that you need . . ." Explain that participants should do whatever is comfortable for them. Each person should send two or three messages for the other person to repeat. Then switch the listener to the teller.

After this exercise, ask participants how they felt about it. Then stress the following. This kind of repeating message does several things. It makes the listener *listen*. Because he or she will have to perform by repeating, the listener is more likely to listen to what is being said. It also clarifies the message. Often people do not hear the message clearly. The listener may have heard the problem wrong, or the teller may not be saying what he or she thinks. In any event, this direct feedback of problems will clear up the messages being sent between participants.

Now, role play this exercise in front of the group. The trainer is to whisper or state a problem to each trainee. The trainee must restate the problem to the trainer and the rest of the group. Just go quickly around the room with this one. See if anyone is hearing what you are saying. Also, see if everyone is listening to what is being said.

Next, try this exercise. State a problem to the whole class. Ask everyone to restate the problem, verbally or in writing. Check to see if the messages are being sent clearly, and heard clearly. Discuss any misconceptions in the exercise. Review the listening techniques. Talk about any problems that have come up in the last few sessions.

Session XI

The next, logical, reasonable question that your participants may have is "how do all of these wonderful principles affect me?" How do participants apply the techniques in order to get them to work for them? How do they apply them in specific situations? Create the expectation that the participants can use these techniques at home, and with good results.

The next step is to actually implement at home the reinforcement guides that the trainer has been elaborating on in the classroom. Indicate that they must follow them faithfully. If they, as parents, use them sometimes and forget them sometimes, the procedures will be ineffective. Children will just think that they are crazy and unpredictable. Be consistent. Listen to your children and to yourself, and follow the procedures as we have practiced them.

Select a problem. Ask parents to write down three real problems at home. Each parent should have a list. The first step is for each person to admit to the difficulty. Is it the child's problem or is it a problem of yours? What are things that you will have to change to help change the overall situation? Discuss the lists. Check to see if the spouse's list agrees. If not, be sure to discuss them.

Here is an example to use to get parents started:

Your husband does not come home right after work. Maybe it is because you:

1. Look like a truck hit you when he walks in the door
2. Have numerous children lined up for him to punish
3. Have not started dinner yet
4. Are always away from home
5. Or maybe it is not your fault at all.

In the majority of instances, it takes at least two people to have a problem. Mutual concessions have to be made for a problem to be solved. After discussing who owns the problems on everyone's list, tell each participant to pick one problem to work on. It can be one of their own problems, or their child's. Ask the parents to write the problem down. Now, everyone must define what that problem is. Defining a problem may be just a bit more complicated than it may seem. The problem must be broken down into observable, countable behaviors for this program to work. That can be very tricky and hard for rural individuals and will take patience and time.

Some good examples of behaviors to work on include cursing, spitting, not fixing dinner, and not picking up clothes off the floor.

Write this example on the board. "I want my husband to be nicer to me." What is nicer? What does nicer really mean? It is much too broad a word. Get everyone to list what they think nicer means. Read everyone's list aloud. Pick five definitions. Write them on the board. A list of things that nicer means might include:

Coming home after work
A kiss at the door
Spending 15 minutes with you before dinner
Talking together during those 15 minutes
Helping to wash dishes
Spending time with the children
Appropriate compliments for task accomplished

Break the problem or the statement into small, countable behaviors. This will help you to measure success and to be successful. After you break the problems into behaviors, decide how each person will reinforce the behavior, and what other techniques to use. Decide exactly how you define the behavior to be worked on, what amount and type of reinforcement you will use, and when you will reinforce.

Remember that consistency and immediacy is very important in this program. Moreover, remember that punishment is used as a last resort. An easy way to keep track of successes and failures is to keep a chart. In this session, everyone should practice setting up a chart for the specific behavior. Mark off each day, each behavior, and how many times the participant reinforced the behavior. The chart will help to get into the reinforcement routine, plus it will show you just how successful you are. You, the trainer, can make out a sample chart on the board to help your group understand, as illustrated in Table 2. Ask the class to fill in the missing information.

Table 2

Behavior	Times exhibited							Times reinforced						
	S	M	T	W	Th	F	S	S	M	T	W	Th	F	S
Picked up clothes														
Spitting														
Cursing														
Kiss at the door														
Washing dishes														
Spending time with the children														
Appropriate compliments for tasks accomplished														

Talk about the problem with your spouse or child. Discuss the types of rewards. Tell your child or husband the rules of the system. For parents with older children, behavior contracts may be in order. Discuss the contract with the child and write it up like a formal contract. Write in specific things to which you both agree. Make the expectations as specific as possible. Be sure that you both understand the terms of the contract and live up to them. For example:

I_____(the parent) agree to the following: I will pay $5.00 weekly for these chores to be done by my child_____ .
☐ Take the trash out daily
☐ Feed the dog after supper daily
☐ Pick up clothes daily
☐ Make the bed daily

In return, I_____(the child) agree to do these chores for the sum of $5.00 weekly, to be paid in cash to me on Friday at 5:00.

For an excellent discussion of the formulation of contracts see the text by W. DeRisi and G. Butz (1975) entitled *Writing Behavioral Contracts*.

Getting everyone to sign impresses upon them just how important this contract is. Review the idea of charts. Help everyone get a notion of a chart for their specific behavior problem. If possible, help them set up the chart during class. The starting date for the charts will be the day after this session. Tell participants that you will check the charts next week.

Sessions XII to XV

Discuss the charts and check them. Make charts for new behaviors to work on. Talk about the problems that are occurring at home. Praise good things that are going on at home. Review any unclear points about the techniques. Have the children come to one session during this time frame. Make videotape schedules for the group. On the child's nights have parents and children watch the videotape of the family. A group discussion on how to handle a certain type of problem at home is very beneficial. Weekly home visits should be continuing for 1 to 2 months after training. One additional point should be made about techniques of behavior change. Once a behavior is altered it is no longer necessary to reinforce it every time it occurs (Wodarski, 1980). Such a procedure ensures that the behaviors will continue as reinforcement becomes intermittent.

After these tasks are completed, the group can terminate, or it can continue as a parent support group.

Chapter 6

Rural Community Mental Health Program Evaluation

Beginning in 1963, with the advent of major federal legislation funding programs in community mental health, there was increasing demand for accountability, and this demand has grown substantially over the last several years (Coursey, 1977). Program evaluation is now a specific task to be accomplished by the social work field. It is mandated that agencies funded by public monies conduct program evaluation. Public Law 94–63, the Community Mental Health Centers Amendments of 1975, requires all Community Mental Health Centers (CMHCs) to conduct program evaluation on an annual basis. The program evaluation provisions in the Amendments (P.L. 94–63) which apply directly to Community Mental Health Centers are as follows:

1. Community mental health centers must establish "an ongoing quality assurance program (including utilization and peer review systems) respecting the center's services." [Section 201]
2. Grant applicants shall contain assurances that the center will provide:
   - an effective procedure for developing, compiling, evaluating, and reporting to the Secretary statistics and other information (which the Secretary shall publish and disseminate on a periodic basis and which the center shall disclose at least annually to the general public) relating to (I) the cost of the center's operation, (II) the availability, accessibility and acceptability of its services, (III) the impact of its services upon the mental health of the residents of its catchment area, and (IV) such other matters as the Secretary may require; [Section 206 (c) (I) (A) (ii)]
   - such community mental health centers will, in consultation with the residents of its catchment area, review its program of services and the statistics and the other pertinent information referred to (in the preceding paragraph) to assure that its services are responsive to the needs of the residents of the catchment area. [Section 206 (c) (I) (B)]

3. In each year, the "center shall obligate for a program of continuing evaluation of the effectiveness of its programs in serving the needs of the residents of its catchment area and for a review of the quality of the services provided by the center not less than an amount equal to 2 per centum of the amount obligated by the center in the preceding fiscal year for its operating expenses." [Section 206 (c) (4)]

Evaluation methods and activity have become topics of increasing importance. In a recent survey 65% of a sample of directors of CMHCs and state hospitals rated program evaluation as a critical issue in mental health service delivery (McIntyre, Attkisson, and Keller, 1977; Norris and Larsen, 1976). Extensive work has been done to help centers develop sufficient program evaluation capabilities to comply with the requirements of the law. The National Institute of Mental Health (NIMH) has prepared program evaluation guidelines for CMHCs to implement P.L. 94–63 (NIMH, 1977). The guidelines suggest an outline for the annual program evaluation report (See Appendix A). NIMH has also generated a number of publications providing technical advice on evaluation and on the dissemination of evaluation findings (Davidoff, Guttentag, and Offutt, 1977; Flaherty and Windle, 1981; Hagedorn et al., 1976; Hargreaves, Attkisson, and Sorensen, 1977; Landsberg et al., 1979). Topics include cost analysis, outcome evaluation, needs assessment, patterns of use, quality assurance, plus many other relevant materials.

Federal exhortation, advice, requirements, and technical assistance are evident. Despite this federal support and the specificity of the law concerning the topics to be evaluated, there is still a great deal of doubt as to whether a rural CMHC with limited resources can meet the federal guidelines for program evaluation (Hargreaves and DeLay, 1979). Gertz, Meider, and Pluckhan (1975) in their survey of rural mental health programs, found that there was a need to find comprehensive, measurable, and easy program evaluation systems that rural mental health centers with inadequate resources could perform. After a review of the general principles of program evaluation that includes the contents of the federal guidelines and program evaluation techniques, this chapter will propose a useful approach to program evaluation that is well within the means of a rural CMHC. The emphasis is on the evaluation of total programs; however, the majority of items are relevant to individual case evaluation. (For a presentation of the requisites of such evaluations, see John S. Wodarski, The Role of Research in Clinical Practice, 1981, Chapters 4, 5, 6, and 7).

GENERAL PRINCIPLES

What is Program Evaluation?

Program evaluation is a tool designed to assist in the process of decision making. It enables program directors, staff, and others to measure program effectiveness so as to determine the future of those programs. The benefits of program evaluation can be notable if properly carried out. Effective program management requires program evaluation (Stevenson and Longabaugh, 1980; Wholey et al., 1970).

Ideally, the benefits of program evaluations are: 1) it provides information about the outcome of a program in order for planners to determine if program goals are being met; 2) it provides information about efficiency, in terms of cost versus goal achievement or program impact; 3) it provides proof of a program's accomplishments and the staff's capabilities; and 4) it provides information about the needs within the agency such as more staff, specialization, extra funding, and/or new service techniques (Hagedorn et al., 1976; Landsberg et al., 1979; Wholey et al., 1970). Davis, Windle, and Sharfstein (1977), in their article on program evaluation in CMHCs, list three benefits of evaluation: 1) continued improvement of services to clients; 2) rewards to the providers of services in the form of tangible feedback on attainments; and 3) accountability to the multiple sources of sanctions and funds for the services provided" (p. 25).

Many definitions of program evaluation and descriptions of its benefits can be found in the literature. Most all seem to include key terms such as "effectiveness," "efficiency," and "impact."

Many definitions of program evaluation exist. The following definition is most appropriate here: "it assesses the effectiveness of an ongoing program in achieving its objectives" (Biggerstaff, 1977). With similar thoughts, Weiss (1972) describes the purpose of program evaluation as "to measure the effects of a program against the goals it set out to accomplish" (p. 4). More detailed definitions such as the following have also been proposed. Program evaluation is: "1) A process of making reasonable judgements about program effort, effectiveness, efficiency, and adequacy; 2) based on a systematic data collection and analysis; 3) designed for use in program management, external accountability, and future planning; 4) focuses especially on accessibility, acceptability, awareness, availability, comprehensiveness, continuity, integration, and cost of services" (Attkisson and Broskowski, 1978, p. 24).

It is valuable that such extensive literature exists to describe to CMHCs program evaluation and its purposes and benefits. However, this is not enough. Before CMHCs can be expected to perform effective program evaluations, the management and staff must know concete ways to perform an evaluation and how to adapt them to their local needs (such ways will be discussed in later sections).

Program evaluation is an essential means of providing effective services to rural areas. It takes time, effort, planning, and good management, however, to make it useful. The next section considers how to initiate effective evaluation.

Planning and Administrating Program Evaluation

For an evaluation to be successful, the cooperation of all, staff as well as management, must be elicited (Beigel and Levenson, 1978; Davis et al., 1977; Hagedorn et al., 1976). All individuals involved should made a commitment to do their best. This is a commitment that cannot be legislated (NIMH, 1977). The motivation for carrying out an effective evaluation has to come from within the center involved. The program evaluator or the management will be the key to eliciting everyone's cooperation. If this individual is not competent in the skills of program evaluation, it is probable that the evaluation will not prove useful. McIntyre et al. (1977) suggest that evaluators will be most effective when they are simultaneously program administrators, hence apparently guaranteeing evaluation in the service of vested interest.

Weiss (1972) points out five characteristics an evaluator should have. An evaluator "must have confidence in the professional skills of the evaluation staff, must be insulated from any possibility of biasing the data or its interpretation by a desire to make things look good, must possess an understanding of agency operations and services, must be in a position to make recommendations to the agency, and must be able to view the agency in a wide perspective and as a system of interrelated units" (pp. 20–21).

Thus, in order to effectively carry out an evaluation, one must have adequate interpersonal, administrative, and evaluative skills (Attkisson, Brown, and Hargreaves, 1978; Hagedorn et al., 1976). One must have a working knowledge of the skills involved in program evaluation and must know how to best use them to elicit staff cooperation in an effective way. But a problem exists. Very few of those with the responsibility of handling the evaluation have adequate training for the tasks inherent in evaluation (Beigel and Levenson, 1978). Many agency administrators in rural CMHCs in charge of program evaluation have clinical backgrounds both in training and work experience. Their interest lies in the area of clinical service. When faced with the responsibility of carrying out an evaluation, many reject the task. This usually means that either the task is dropped or an ineffective evaluation is done.

There is a solution to this lack of adequate training in the tasks of evaluation. Each agency could mandate that its administrators receive the necessary training in evaluation skills. Workshops on program evaluation skills could be arranged. This is a good idea if the time, resources, and workshop are available. Another solution, one that takes more effort on the part of the management or evaluators, involves evaluators making a commitment to do their best at all tasks, including evaluation tasks. If it means the evaluator has to study and learn new skills, then the professional must respond to the need. If the evaluator is unwilling to work at doing his or her best, it is unlikely that an effective evaluation will take place.

The management or evaluator alone cannot make program evaluation useful. This person will be the key but the cooperation of all staff involved is essential. Before beginning any part of an evaluation, the staff and their attitude toward the evaluation must be considered (Wodarski and Feldman, 1974). It is most beneficial to have positive attitudes about the evaluation throughout the center. In many instances, this is hard to accomplish. Many workers resent being made to spend their valuable time on something they feel will not help in any way (Davis et al., 1977; Hagedorn et al., 1976; Ward, 1977). Social workers are receiving two messages regarding evaluation that are putting them in a bind. "One message (is) demanding accountability, the other (is) arguing no benefit" (Piliavin and McDonald, 1977, p. 64). For many workers it is seen only as an obstacle diverting resources from direct services, and the results of the evaluation may not even be used at all. It is no wonder that social workers are reluctant to carry out evaluations.

The reluctance on the part of the workers to carry out the evaluations can be changed but it is up to the management to bring about the change. "A positive approach to program evaluation can be gained if center management comes to understand how evaluation can contribute to center management and the improvement of center operations" (Hagedorn et al., 1976, p. 9). It is then the job of the management to communicate to the staff the benefits of the evaluation. Management should also try to stimulate staff participation. Staff participation can be gained by continuously asking for input and assistance on all matters, keeping them well informed, and giving recognition and rewards for cooperative participation (Attkisson et al., 1978). Feedback is likely to enhance the staff's understanding of the usefulness of the evaluation and to encourage their cooperation in the evaluation process (Freid, 1977). The attitude and cooperation of everyone in an agency is of key importance in program evaluation. If management and staff can approach evaluation in a positive way, this will be the first step toward an effective evaluation. Next, management can move on to the actual process of evaluation.

Proper Evaluation Procedures

Planning and administering program evaluation is a substantial task. Unless proper procedures are followed, the evaluation will not produce useful results. Program management must make use of good evaluative procedures in order to obtain the appropriate information with which services can be improved. Ward (1977) summarizes it well by saying, "Successful management of the evaluation must be based on a clearly conceived plan. The plan must specify the type of evaluation needed, the roles and responsibilities of staff, the cost of conducting the evaluation, and a timetable for the delivery of evaluation products."

Despite the acknowledged need for a clearly conceived plan, data indicate practitioners continue to go about program evaluation in a haphazard way. It is generally agreed that many evaluators have no idea where to begin an evaluation and no idea of the methodology that must be used (Biggerstaff, 1977; Keenen, 1975). There are certain steps that an evaluator should follow in the development and execution of an evaluation. These steps can serve as guidelines for management and staff to follow to ascertain the achievement of a successful evaluation. The list of steps that follows is for management and staff to use in planning and conducting projects in program evaluation. It is in no way comprehensive but can help the evaluator begin the process of eliciting and clarifying the agency's needs and the issues the professional will face.

1. Choose program to evaluate.
2. Establish program goals.
3. Translate goals into measurable indicators of goal achievement (i.e., define adequate outcome criteria).
4. Design the evaluation project and commit resources needed to support the effort.
5. Implement the evaluation and collect data.
6. Analyze evaluation data.
7. Report on evaluation results.
8. Utilize results.

Step 1: Choose Program to Evaluate   A decision to evaluate should be based on the need or demand for that evaluation (Davis et al., 1977; Hagedorn et al., 1976; NIMH, 1977). Management should look at the primary concern of the agency, whether it be an administrative operation, a staff function, a need in the community, a specific service, or a specific therapeutic technique.

In selecting the area of an agency on which to focus evaluative time and efforts the input from all the staff is important. The workers see what goes on each day and take note of the needs of the agency. Management should always consult with staff members and listen to their opinions, thus providing a different view toward the evaluation and increasing the probability that relevant factors will be considered. Also, including the staff in choosing the area to evaluate can lower some of their resistance to having their activities evaluated (Wodarski, 1980).

Especially in the smaller rural CMHCs, it is a good idea for management and staff to work together. In many ways, these agencies are like a family (Freid, 1977). And, as in a family, all members should be included when important decisions are made. This facilitates the worker's commitment to the evaluation (Feldman and Wodarski, 1974; Wodarski, 1981).

Requisite items an agency needs to consider when choosing what to evaluate are: Will the evaluation accomplish anything? Is the information needed for the evaluation attainable? Will the results of the evaluation be used? Unless these questions can be answered "yes," the evaluator is not ready to move on with the next step of the evaluation.

Step 2: Establish Program Goals   "In planning the development of an evaluation project, the rock bottom starting point is a specification and delineation of the service program's objectives and goals" (Speer and Tapp, 1976). Predetermined goals establish criteria to assess performance. It would be impossible to evaluate a program without a statement of the goals against which success or failure can be measured. Specification of outcome criteria, however, is difficult in terms of time and energy.

The first step in establishing program goals is to develop broad general statements about what one is trying to accomplish. At this point, specific, measurable statements are not necessary. For example, a program goal could be something as broad as "adjustment in the community." These statements cannot be measured. For the next step in the evaluative process to proceed, general statements need to be translated into statements of goals that can be measured.

Step 3: Translate the Goals into Measurable Indicators of Goal Achievement (i.e., Define Adequate Outcome Criteria)   Translating the goal into a measurable indicator is often regarded as the key to successful evaluation (Coursey, 1977; Weiss, 1972). "Practical and relevant evaluation demands that the objectives of service programs be spelled out in terms as concrete and behavioral as possible" (Speer and Tapp, 1976). Terms such as *good, better, improvement, adequate,* and so forth should be defined in behaviorally observable terms. For instance, the goal of "adjustment in the community" could be translated into measurable terms, such as "for one year without rehospitalization, number of reports to law enforcement agents of such acts of violence, and so forth."

Brody and Krailo (1978) provide a guide for preparing statements of measurable objectives or goals. The statements should include the following elements:

1. Situation or condition to be attained
2. Target population
3. Quantity or amount of change to be attained
4. Time by which desired situation should exist.

An example of an objective containing these elements follows:

1. Improve personal adjustment (desired situation)
2. Of ex-mental hospital patients (target population)
3. To be measured by the number of the population remaining in the community without rehospitalization (75% of the cases served staying out of the hospital would be the target of performance)
4. Over a 1-year period (time frame).

After translating the goal into concrete measurable terms, the next step is to design the evaluation project.

Step 4: Design the Evaluation Project and Commit Resources Needed to Support the Effort   The program evaluator has an important job in this step. The professional is responsible for selecting, proposing, and developing the evaluation design. The evaluator must be willing to take initiative in making decisions and then be willing to stand by them; flexibility and openness to getting input from others is also important. The staff involved in the evaluation should always be kept well informed. It is the evaluator's job to clarify with everyone exactly what is occurring in each step of the evaluation.

It is generally agreed that one of the best ways to begin this design step is to have a staff brainstorming session, with the intent of generating new ideas and getting everyone involved. To get ideas on as many strategies as possible to accomplish the objectives is the purpose of this session. Leave no stone unturned. Strategies used by already successful programs or creative new strategies should be brought up for discussion.

After the group brainstorming session, the evaluator has the individual task of analyzing all the strategies and deciding which one is the most feasible. The first thing the professional can do to narrow down the list is to look at the resources needed to carry out each design and then to look at the available resources. Resources that must be considered are: money, personnel, equipment, time, facilities, knowledge, and skill. If adequate resources such as these are not available to carry out a design and cannot be acquired, then the design should be crossed off the list of possible alternatives and another, more feasible design should be chosen.

The second thing the evaluator can do to narrow down the list is to consider all possible things that might affect the outcome of the evaluation. The professional should weigh the positive and negative influences that can act on each design and then exclude the designs in which there are more negative than positive influences. Remember, the goal is to come up with the best possible design.

Next, the evaluator must make subjective comparisons among the designs from which the professional has left to choose. The evaluator must draw on knowledge, past experiences, and common sense in making a final decision on the evaluative design that will be used. When adequate research and thought have gone into selecting the design, the evaluator should be able to make a reasonable decision and then should stick behind it.

Finally, in a staff and management meeting, the evaluative design that has been selected should be presented and discussed. The evaluator should be explicit about the reasons for making the choice. Then the professional should present in detail what has to be done, by whom, how, and when. The evaluator should review the selection of measurement instruments and techniques to be used during the evaluation and should review the proper ways of gathering and documenting data. All of this information does not have to be presented in one staff meeting. It is a good idea to bring up the highlights of the evaluation project and to plan for later meetings to review the details. A detailed discussion of all the evaluation procedures before getting started helps to ensure a successful evaluation. Everyone involved should always know what is expected of them and how to do it. Such an involvement process will increase the participants' commitment to the evaluation.

Step 5. Implement the Evaluation and Collect Data   In this step, the program evaluator is responsible for activating the evaluation plans. Whether a decision has been made to implement a continuous or episodic evaluation project, the evaluator must coordinate the activities and see that the evaluation operates as planned.

The evaluation should run smoothly if adequately planned in the earlier stages. Every detail should already be specified in concrete, understandable terms. There should be no question in anyone's mind about what his or her responsibilities are. All loose ends must be tied up before implementing the evaluation and collecting data. The evaluator should keep abreast of everything that goes on. It is a good idea for the professional to periodically review the evaluation plans.

This will alert the professional to any problems that may arise and to any changes that should be made, and provides a check on all the details that must be executed.

As the evaluation gets under way, data collection will begin. The data collection process should be specifically spelled out in the design and understood by all. This process should be as simple and unobtrusive as possible. In the majority of instances, not only are staff not adequately trained to collect data, but no one wants to do it because it means extra paperwork. The easier it is to do, the easier it will be to gain staff cooperation. Staff cooperation in the data collection stage is essential. This is a step that has to be taken seriously by all.

In order to make the best decisions, the data must be reliable. Program evaluators must relay to their data collectors the importance of their jobs. Many biasing factors exist that can influence data collection, such as history, selection, maturation, and so forth. All these factors should be discussed prior to implementing the procedure. (For an extended discussion, see John S. Wodarski, *The Role of Research in Clinical Practice,* Chapter 6.)

Step 6: Analyze Evaluation Data   The agency management responsible for the evaluation plan will also play a major role in analyzing the collected data. It is their job to draw conclusions from the information gathered. "The simplest and most useful way to analyze data for evaluation is to relate program achievements to explicit goals of the program agreed upon by management. It is also helpful to include comparative information on other types of service programs" (NIMH, 1977). The CMHC profile pack provided by the NIMH Division of Biometry and Epidemiology is one source of comparative data.

As with every other step of the evaluation, it is useful to include the staff in all discussions. Especially in the analysis step, they can render valuable input. Interpretation of the data is made much easier when all who were involved in the evaluation generate personal ideas. Discussions of findings with the staff also help to further the staff's involvement in the evaluation. After discussions, the evaluator then should integrate the information and draw up a set of recommendations based on the staff's input and ideas.

Step 7: Report on Evaluation Findings   Evaluation findings can be presented informally and verbally or formally and in writing. The exact form of the evaluation depends on the audience addressed. Whatever type audience is addressed, the information should always be presented in a clear and concise manner to facilitate its acceptance. Weiss (1972) gives valuable hints for getting a positive response to the evaluation report.

1. Use existing channels of communication and decision making in the organization, both formal and informal. Having a leader sanction the report adds to its acceptability.
2. Build incentives and rewards for using the information.
3. Present useful comparisons.
4. Be nondefensive about the information. Share and explore the findings rather than give orders or advice.

5. Use simple and direct language. Many may resent a report that is complicated and full of professional jargon.
6. Use various media aids to present main ideas (i.e., charts, tables, graphs, and so forth).

In general, presenting findings in a positive way makes it easier for others to accept and respond.

Step 8: Utilize Findings   Based on the evaluation findings, make necessary decisions. Weiss (1972) lists several decisions that can be made: ''1) to continue or discontinue a program; 2) to improve its practices or procedures; 3) to add or drop specific program strategies or techniques; 4) to institute similar programs elsewhere; 5) to allocate resources among competing programs; and 6) to accept or reject a program approach or theory'' (p. 16).

Annual Evaluation Report

This introduction and general discussion has highlighted a number of central issues in the evaluation of mental health programs. It is timely to take a more in-depth look at the contents of the required annual evaluation report. First, there are nine topic areas that should provide the focus for an evaluation. These correspond roughly to the areas required in CMHC program evaluation under the Community Mental Health Center Amendments of 1975. The nine areas are as follows:

1. Cost of operation
2. Use of services
3. Availability
4. Accessibility
5. Acceptability
6. Awareness
7. Impact of services on residents of the catchment area
8. Impact of consultation and education services
9. Impact of inappropriate institutionalization

Each of these areas is important and should not be overlooked. Literature and research is available covering all nine topics. Other content sections of the annual evaluation report include: peer review and utilization studies, citizen reviews, center goals, and next year's evaluation plan.

The law is very specific as to the content for program evaluation. NIMH has prepared guidelines for program evaluation that simplify the description of this required content and suggest an outline for the annual program evaluation report (See Appendix A). Even with the guidelines and the flexibility they provide, many CMHC personnel believe it will be difficult for centers to satisfy the requirements of the law (Davis et al., 1977). This would hold true especially for rural centers—given the limited staff time, resources, and prior experience in program evaluation.

Considering the difficulty that centers may face in complying with the law, every effort should be made to develop relatively simple standard methods to deal with common evaluation issues. Additional guidance in preparing an annual program evaluation report is needed, especially at centers with limited resources and trained personnel. The following reviews the contents required by the guidelines and offers additional guidance on preparing the annual report.

Contents   The annual report should include evaluative information on the topics specified by the law and elaborated in the guidelines. For each topic, the report should briefly describe the program concerns, the method to study the concerns, the results, the actions taken, and the rationale for such actions. Emphasis on these topics can vary depending on their importance to the center. Centers are expected to focus on those evaluative studies most important to improving their own operations and the populations they serve (Davis et al., 1977). Ideas to consider in evaluating and reporting each of the topics follow.

Cost of Operation   Under the guidelines for program evaluation, CMHCs are asked to report the estimated cost of the center's operation. Furthermore, to be meaningful and to avoid misinterpretation, careful definitions of the units of service, the clients, and the nature and results of the service should accompany the cost estimates (NIMH, 1977). Realizing the structural, developmental, and financial limitations centers face, they are allowed to calculate only what their conditions permit.

Estimates of cost alone are not usually thought of as evaluative but they can be meaningful when merged with outcome measures. ''When costs are merged with outcomes, cost analysis becomes possible and when cost outcomes are compared, cost-effectiveness analysis emerges'' (Sorensen and Binner, 1979). By comparing the cost and outcomes for two or more service interventions, the more cost-effective program or technique can be determined.

Sorensen and Grove (1978) summarize the steps for a cost-effectiveness analysis:

1. Identification of the service goals to be achieved for specific target groups (i.e., children, adolescents, the aged, and so forth).
2. Random assignment or other approaches for comparing equivalent groups of clients who are provided alternative service strategies designed to achieve these same service goals.
3. Use of accrual accounting, operating statistics, and cost finding to determine the cost per episode for each client.
4. Preintervention versus postintervention assessment of clients to determine the service outcomes within the groups of clients provided each service strategy.
5. Statistical analysis to determine the average cost per episode and average outcome in each service strategy, and to determine what cost and outcome differences can be detected with confidence.
6. Presentation of cost and outcome summaries in cost-outcome and cost-effectiveness matrices for decision consideration.

7. In ambiguous situations, it may be necessary to make further judgments about the relative utilities of unobserved outcomes in relation to observed outcomes.

Sorensen and Grove (1978) note that this approach is "neither easy nor obvious when extended in realistic program decision making and accountability." There is the need for such comprehensive approaches like the one above, however, especially in attempting to meet demands of accountability and for improved program management.

Patterns of Use of Services Patterns of use studies are basically descriptions. They describe "the numbers and rates of catchment area residents' use of the center's services, by element of service (e.g., inpatient care and outpatient care) and client age, sex, family income, race and geographic subarea including 'subareas of poverty,' if applicable" (NIMH, 1977). These descriptive studies are "the most frequent type of mental health program evaluation activity" (Windle and Voldman, 1973) and can provide evaluative information.

There are many different ways to determine patterns of service use. The simplest way is to determine who is receiving services and what services they are receiving or to determine the utilization rates of different services by clients (Roth, Lecklitner, and Landsberg, 1979).

Utilization rates are expressed as the number of clients served per 1,000 catchment area residents (NIMH, 1977). They are simple to develop and valuable when they can be interpreted. Utilization rates can be compared to various norms or other measures, including: 1) what are the sex, age, and ethnic characteristics of catchment area residents; 2) what is the estimated incidence of mental illness in the catchment area; 3) what subpopulations in the catchment area are not receiving center services; 4) what needs for mental health services in the catchment area can be ascertained; and 5) what subpopulations can be shown to be at high risk in the catchment area (Hagedorn et al, 1976). Comparisons can be made among programs, from an earlier to a later time period, with other CMHCs, or with other kinds of service delivery programs.

Availability, Accessibility, Acceptability and Awareness Overcoming barriers to service delivery is a topic of key importance in the CMHC Amendments of 1975 and in the NIMH guidelines. This is reflected in their requirement that centers evaluate their programs on four topics related to service delivery. These topics are the "Availability," "Accessibility," "Acceptibility," and "Awareness," of mental health services. The first three topics deal with how well a program reaches people who need services.

Availability of services, defined as the amount of various types of services the center can provide at any given time to given client groups (NIMH, 1977).

To evaluate availability, Windle (1979) suggests each type of service should be described and compared with estimates of total community need. What other services are available for the catchment area through other agencies should also be considered.

Hagedorn et al. (1976) suggest more specific techniques for assessing the availability of services.

Service ratios should be calculated of staff days available in various types of services and beds in all facilities and private practice practitioners serving the catchment area, per thousand catchment area population. The portions of the population eligible for each of these services must be noted in order that availability can be determined for various segments of the population.

Types of services offered should be related to catchment area needs. This will require a key informant survey, including other community caretakers to determine whether or not they believe adequate mental health services of the various types are available in the community.

Accessibility of services, defined as the ease of reaching a center and obtaining its services. Accessibility usually includes the following dimensions ... Temporal ... Geographic ... Financial ... Psychological and Sociocultural (NIMH, 1977).

Techniques for assessing accessibility of services are as follows: *Temporal accessibility* can be measured by the hours that the center is open for various types of services and the speed with which requests for services can be met (Windle, 1979). A simple technique is to measure the scheduling for appointments (time lapse; ability to meet clients' first, second, or third preference for appointments; time required to make the appointment by telephone or face to face) (Hagedorn et al., 1976; Windle, 1979). Waiting time measures can also provide information (Hagedorn et al., 1976). An actual sample of waiting times can easily be collected, and people's attitudes toward the waiting period ascertained.

Geographic accessibility is the difficulty catchment area residents experience in getting to the center for services. It can be measured by noting the steps the center has taken to make services readily available, such as establishing satellites or making home visits, measuring the amount of travel time required to go to center offices from various parts of the catchment area, assessing the various transportation means available to catchment area residents, and by obtaining the evaluative judgments by clients or others of the inconvenience in getting to the center (Hagedorn et al., 1976; Windle, 1979).

Financial accessibility relates to fees for services in relation to clients' ability to pay and the rules for eligibility (Hagedorn et al., 1976; Windle, 1979). The clients' attitudes toward cost of services can aid in measuring financial accessibility.

Psychological and Sociocultural accessibility refer to conditions which affect persons' attitudes in ways which deter their getting services. These conditions may be characteristics of the center that frighten, humiliate, or alienate clients. Measures of these conditions may come from client satisfaction surveys; surveys assessing the attractiveness or forbidding qualities of the facility, staff, and administrative procedures; or judgments of experts concerning the center's reputation, physical arrangements, provisions to accompany specific populations, and appointment scheduling procedures (Hagedorn et al., 1976; Windle, 1979).

Information about problems in accessibility may also be obtained from differences in utilization rates not in accord with need.

Accessibility of services, defined as a predilection by clients, community residents and caretakers to use and to continue to use a center (NIMH, 1977).

Windle (1979) suggests that acceptability can be measured by client satisfaction studies, complaint systems, frequency of threats of malpractice suits, and limited queries of citizens and other caregivers. Other techniques for assessing acceptability of services include: a community forum approach, which is like an open town meeting; a psychological attitudinal questionnaire of current CMHC clients to determine their awareness of service alternatives, their views of alternatives, their feelings about alternatives, their feelings about the convenience, pleasantness, and ease of using center services as well as their understanding of what services are available; and a survey of other caregivers' and community leaders' attitudes in terms of their willingness to refer and receive CMHC clients and their desire to participate in CMHC-sponsored activities (Hagedorn et al., 1976).

The fourth topic, Awareness, has been added as a specific requirement by the NIMH guidelines because it seemed a logical part of the conditions which determine centers' utilization.

Awareness of services, defined as knowledge by the local population and community caretakers about the existence of a center, the services it offers and the conditions for which these services are appropriate (NIMH, 1977).

Techniques for assessing awareness of services are to survey relevant caretakers in the community and community leaders to determine their awareness of the existence, nature, and procedures to obtain CMHC services (Hagedorn et al., 1976; Windle, 1979). Other techniques that can be of use are a survey of the catchment area residents, chosen subpopulations, or small samples of high risk groups.

Impact of Services on Residents in the Catchment Area   As the demand for program evaluation in CMHCs increases, more emphasis is being placed on the effectiveness of treatment services. The key word, effectiveness, delineates a most important category of evaluation. To measure "the extent to which a center's services help the people it serves directly" is a central concern of program evaluation (NIMH, 1977). Client outcome evaluations are the means available for measuring the impact or effectiveness of treatment services. Speer and Tapp (1976) specifically state "outcome of services are the only ultimate criteria of program effectiveness."

Assessing program effectiveness can be costly and technologically sophisticated (Hagedorn et al., 1976; Landsberg et al., 1979). Also, it requires the availability of knowledgeable people in the area of mental health program evaluation. Because of such factors—cost, technological sophistications, and knowledgeable staff—outcome evaluations are not being conducted to the extent that they should be in rural mental health centers. Regular, effective use of outcome studies is an advanced stage in the maturation of program evaluation capability (Attkisson et al., 1978; McIntyre et al., 1977).

Although never extensively used, many outcome measurement instruments have been developed over the years. The following will review a variety of instruments which appear to have the best track record in terms of their usefulness, reliability, validity, and their cost of administration and implementation in terms of time and energy (Hagedorn et al., 1976; Wodarski and Buckholdt, 1975).

1. *Goal Attainment Scaling* (Kiresuk and Sherman, 1968). A measure of the attainment of specific treatment goals from the vantage points of the client and the therapists, or of the client and an independent evaluator.
2. *The SCL-90:* Symptom Checklist (Derogatis, Lipman, and Covi, 1973; Derogatis et al., 1974). A measure of the client's symptoms from the vantage point of the client himself.
3. *The Katz Adjustment Scale* (Katz and Lyerly, 1963); The *Personal Adjustment and Role Skills Scale* (Ellsworth et al., 1968); The *Adams County Mental Health Center C.O.C.E. Adult Interview* (1975); and *The Denver County Community Mental Questionnaire* (Ciarlo and Reihman, 1974); These techniques measure the client's personal, social, and community adjustment from a variety of vantage points.
4. *The Global Assessment Scale* (Spitzer, Gibbon, and Endicott, 1973). A measure of the client's overall level of functioning from the vantage point of the therapist.
5. *Client Satisfaction Questionnaire: Salt Lake CMHC Consumer Satisfaction Inventory; Client Satisfaction Questionnaire* (Larsen, Attkisson, and Hargreaves, 1978); and *Hennepin County CMHC "Tell-It-Like-It-Was" Questionnaire* (Tillman, 1976).

Other instruments that are appropriate (see Hargreaves et al., 1977) are: the Psychiatric Status Schedule; the Brief Psychiatric Rating Scale; the Periodic Evaluation Record; the Social Adjustment Scale; the Client Episode Outcome Summary; Progress Evaluation Scales (see Ihilevich et al., 1981); and Assessment of Social Functioning (MacNair, Wodarski, and Giordano, in press).

Impact—Consultation and Education   The impact of a center's consultation and education services is another service focus centers must address, but not necessarily annually. Program evaluation guidelines require that a center consider the impact of its indirect consultation and education services in attaining program goals (NIMH, 1977). Windle and Flaherty (1979) suggest that indirect services can benefit from program evaluation in two ways: such evaluations may reveal the benefits of the indirect service, and evaluation may suggest ways to improve the effectiveness or efficiency of indirect services.

Unfortunately, indirect services have been unable to achieve these benefits.

The difficulty and complexity of evaluating indirect services has resulted in the lack of relatively complete evaluation systems for consultation and education (Hagedorn et al., 1976).

Program evaluation guidelines suggest that at a minimum CMHCs obtain the judgments of the agencies and persons receiving these services about the results of the services, using procedures to encourage candor and accuracy, and making comparisons between the relative efficiency of direct and indirect services in achieving program goals.

Windle (1979) and Windle and Flaherty (1979) suggest another approach often employed in the evaluation of direct services, and found to be useful for indirect services. The strategy is goal attainment scaling, most practical when used in conjunction with ongoing program and client satisfaction studies.

Impact on Inappropriate Institutionalization This topic refers to a center's effectiveness in reducing inappropriate institutionalization by: 1) assisting courts and other public agencies in screening and arranging alternative treatment for potential referrals to state mental health inpatient facilities; 2) providing follow-up care to catchment area residents discharged from a mental health facility; 3) encouraging community placement of state hospital patients with center follow-up and support (NIMH, 1977).

Other requirements listed in the annual evaluation report are as follows:

Peer Review and Utilization Studies The statistical results of the center's peer review and utilization studies should be described. This report should give numbers of cases reviewed, numbers and types of inadequacies, and remedial actions taken, but should not reveal the identity of individual patients or clinicians (NIMH, 1977).

Citizens Review The purpose of the review is to assure that the center's services are known to, understood by, and desired by the community and to ensure center accountability to the citizens. This section should include the following specific types of information.

1. The procedures used to provide copies and summaries of the last evaluation report reviewed by citizens (if not the present report, the plans for citizen review of this report)
2. The procedures used to publicize the availability of the last evaluation report (and/or the plans for the present report)
3. The procedures used for the last citizens review (and/or planned for the next one)
4. A summary of the suggestions from citizens during and after their review of the last (or present) annual report and the center's responses
5. The involvement of the center's governing board in reviewing the last or present evaluation report (NIMH, 1977)

Center Goals A statement of the main objectives sought by management in the last year and data on how well and under what conditions these were attained (NIMH, 1977; Windle, 1979).

Plans for Next Year's Center Evaluation A brief description of the major issues to be studied (including how the evaluation plan responds to citizen review suggestions), expected program implications of these evaluations, methods to be used, and proposed changes in citizen review procedures (NIMH, 1977; Windle, 1979).

A COMPREHENSIVE EVALUATION PLAN FOR RURAL CMHCs

Despite the pressures to rapidly develop a program evaluation capability, a center must take its time and proceed realistically. "Growth in evaluative capacity must proceed in harmony with the organization's present level of systematic maturity, the kinds of information tools needed for current and future tasks, and the multiple functions evaluation must perform in relation to program leadership and other staff" (Attkisson, Brown, and Hargreaves, 1978).

It is understandable that new programs with limited evaluative experiences and resources will require much developmental work. P.L. 94–63 supports the gradual development of program evaluation capability, maximizing incentives for the usefulness of results. Davis et al. (1977) suggest that CMHCs choose from various available evaluation possibilities those most appropriate to improving their own operations. Existing evaluation possibilities vary in the amount of resources they require and their degree of sophistication. Many strategies require a developed, high level of evaluative capability, and adequate resources must be available in order to carry out a successful project.

Before planning an evaluation, each center should review its capabilities and inventory its resources. In the absence of adequate fiscal and staffing resources, simple, cost-effective evaluations are most feasible to use (Kivens and Bolin, 1976). This reasoning is especially relevant for rural CMHCs as these most likely operate on a tight budget and very seldom have any extra monies available to spend for costly evaluations. As stated before, evaluations require resources—money, time, staff, and equipment. When an agency is not adequately staffed and equipped, as is frequently the case in rural areas, the monies they have to spend go toward purchasing the essentials. Direct service delivery expenses are given top priority over such things as program evaluation expenses. A common attitude rural CMHC staff may take is that the little money the center has might better be used to hire extra staff or to purchase needed equipment than spent on a costly evaluation. If all centers, including rural ones, were adequately staffed and equipped, then they may feel better about spending their time and money on evaluations. As it stands now, many CMHCs, especially the rural ones try to meet program evaluation requirements by using as few of their resources as possible.

Furthermore, many rural CMHCs do not have the staff trained to do mental health evaluations or to use sophisticated instruments (Gertz et al., 1975). A 1977 survey showed that "rural centers had significantly fewer mental health trainees in three of the major mental health disciplines (psychiatry, psychology, and social work) and fewer affiliations with training institutions, factors that contribute to the maldistribution of mental health professions in rural areas'' (Pearls, Winslow, and Pathak, 1980). Unless trained staff are made available, rural CMHCs cannot be expected to carry out the same level of evaluation as urban or semi-urban centers that have the "know-how" staff available.

For rural CMHCs with relatively low levels of program evaluation capability, it is best if they focus their evaluation efforts on tasks that parallel their present ability level. McIntyre, Attkisson, and Keller (1977) present a conceptual model centers can use in planning and structuring a useful evaluation that corresponds to their capability level. This model outlines three essential dimensions of internal evaluation: 1) evolving levels of evaluative activity, 2) information capability, and 3) functional roles of the evaluator. These dimensions describe the minimal framework necessary to produce the kind of information that can make evaluation an effective support system for program administration.

The central dimension consists of four levels of evaluation activity: systems resource management; client utilization; outcome of intervention; and community impact. The four levels of activity are described as "evolving levels . . . because they are naturally ordered on a hierarchy which reflects current practice, levels of measurement difficulty, and relationship to the range of program goals" (McIntyre et al., 1977, p. 79). The other two dimensions, information capability and functional role of the evaluator, determine the quality and utility of evaluation activity within a human service organization.

Attkisson and Hargreaves (1977) propose that there are typical management tasks and evaluation functions at each level of evaluation activity. These are presented in Table 3. New evaluation efforts may focus only on the first level, but as conditions become optimal will progressively address all four levels.

In designing an evaluation plan tailored to the resources and needs of a rural CMHC, this chapter suggests that rural centers are operating at a low level of evaluation capability and, therefore, should focus only on evaluation strategies that parallel their capabilities.

There is little detailed literature describing program evaluation plans, either existing or possible, for small, rural CMHCs. Efforts to assist centers to develop useful program evaluations are largely urban influenced and oriented, often requiring multiple specialized techniques ill suited to a rural area (Flax et al., 1979). With only a few evaluation studies of rural programs, how does a rural center approach all mandated evaluation requirements? Can a rural CMHC go beyond basic accountability requirements and perform evaluations documenting the need for more staff, specialization, extra funding, and/or new services? Hargreaves and DeLay (1979) have presented one conceptual program evaluation work plan adaptable to a rural setting. The following discussion proposes another fairly comprehensive approach to evaluation developed in the context of the limitations inherent in the rural setting. This work plan was designed to meet the requirements specified in the Federal Guidelines for Program Evaluation and to meet them in ways that would be most useful to rural centers. The plan suggests study methods or evaluation strategies for each topic specified in the law and guidelines previously discussed (See Appendix A).

Cost Analysis Of the annual "cost per unit service" indices for major treatment modalities, there are two that are most commonly used for evaluation purposes. These are total cost per encounter and total cost per hour of professional service (Hagedorn et al., 1976).

1. Total cost per encounter—total expenses are divided by the number of transactions to give a cost per transaction, as in the following example: outpatient service—total expenses $195,843: number of transactions, 19,584; cost per transaction, $10.
2. Total cost per hour of professional service—total expenses are divided by the number of hours of professional service to give total cost per professional hour of service.

These figures can be computed for various services: outpatient, inpatient, adult day treatment, emergency, alcohol and drug, child and adolescent, geriatric, and consultation and education.

After cost per unit service is figured, it is useful to make comparisons with other CMHCs. Every center should have available to it the NIMH profile package, including the cost norms generated from the biometry inventory data.

Patterns of Use Important evaluation information may be found in the demographic characteristics of clients served by the center. There must be developed a report on the active caseload—the aproximate number of clients and a demographic breakdown of the caseload (race, sex, age, annual household income, and education level).

The active caseload for a center can be compared with data for other CMHCs. Such comparisons are made possible by the Biometry Office, NIMH.

Availability The center being evaluated can be assessed by comparing a center to others on several indexes for which comparable regional and national data are available. Information should be collected on the scheduled weekly staff hours per 1,000 catchment area residents and inpatient beds per 1,000 residents. Again, comparisons are made possible by the CMHC profiles for 1975 provided by the Biometry Office, NIMH.

Acceptability Client satisfaction surveys and surveys of citizens and other caregiving agencies can be used to measure acceptability. Information should be gathered on the predilection by clients, community residents, and caretakers to use and to continue to use a center. One survey can be incorporated to assess several topics at the same time. Examples of surveys to use can be found in the appendix (see Appendices B and C).

Accessibility Indicators relevant to the ease of obtaining needed services are outlined below.

Temporal Accessibility Information on a center's "open hours" should be compared with other CMHCs. A survey can be used to question if appointment

Table 3. Typical management tasks and evaluation activities at four progressively evolving levels of evaluation activity

Level of evaluation activity	Typical management tasks	Typical evaluation activities
1. Systems resource management	Clarify organizational objectives Develop program plan and budget Establish lines of management responsibility Obtain and maintain financial support Allocate fiscal resources and staff effort Coordinate personnel supervision Establish new services and phase out existing services Relate to community advisory groups Meet external reporting requirements and program standards Monitor income and expenditures Establish fees and billings rates	Review objectives and formulate indicators of attainment Meet external reporting requirements Clarify roles of evaluator and integrate with management tasks Develop improved information capability and integrate data collection systems Review mandated services or documented needs Establish evaluation liaison with community advisory groups and evaluators from other organizational levels Monitor staff effort and development of human, fiscal, and physical resources Collaborate in establishment of a cost-finding system and determine unit costs of services Provide effort feedback to management and service staff
2. Client utilization	Make workload projections Maintain efficiency of service delivery Assure equity of service access Assure appropriate client screening and treatment assignment Assure adequate treatment planning	Monitor unduplicated counts of clients served Analyze caseloads and client flow Compare client demographics to census data and high risk-need populations Analyze reasons for premature dropout and under-utilization of services
2. Client utilization (continued)	Assure appropriate service utilization and integration with other community services at the individual client level	Assist in installation of problem-oriented client record and monitor service needs of clients Provide technical support for utilization review

			and other quality assurance activities Analyze continuity of care Analyze costs per episode of care within specific client groups or service settings
3.	Outcome of intervention	Assure continuity of care Establish quality assurance program	Provide services acceptable to clients and referral sources Detect and correct grossly ineffective service activities Assure that services are generally effective Improve cost-effectiveness of services Reallocate resources to support and enhance most cost-effective services Communicate service effectiveness to funding sources and advisory groups	Routinely monitor client status Study client and referral source satisfaction Study posttreatment outcomes Compare program outcomes to outcome norms Undertake comparative outcome experiments Do systems simulation and optimization studies Compare cost-outcomes of different approaches to service needs and establish cost-effectiveness of services Find cost-outcome per duration of problem or illness within specific client groups and/or service settings
4.	Community Impact		Participate in regional health assessment Develop joint interagency services and administrative support systems Provide effective primary prevention and indirect services Collaborate in integration of services for multi-problems clients and stimulate effective interagency referral system	Assess community needs Undertake incidence and prevalence studies Test primary prevention strategies Evaluate consultation and education services Participate in systematic regional need assessment Facilitate and provide technical assistance to citizen and consumer input to need assessment, program planning, and evaluation

Source: Attkisson and Hargreaves (1977).

times are convenient for clients and if the waiting time from date of application to the first appointment time is suitable to clients (see Appendix C). Again, comparison with other centers is useful.

Geographic Accessibility   A map showing the location of service elements will demonstrate geographic accessibility. Provisions of transportation options for clients who cannot walk, drive, or pay for transportation to the center should be reported. And the number of home visits (if any) should be reported.

Financial Accessibility   The percentage of new cases with weekly family incomes under $100 should be assessed and compared with the national percentage. Also, the average fee per visit for clients who pay can be assessed and compared with national statistics.

Psychological and Sociocultural Accessibility   Assess services to major ethnic minorities in catchment areas and assess services for different age groups. These asessments show whether or not "underserved" populations are using center services. Client satisfaction surveys used for other topics can also provide useful information for psychological accessibility.

Awareness   is evaluated through a survey of the local population and community professionals of the existence of a center, the services it offers, and the conditions for which these services are appropriate will demonstrate awareness (See Appendix B).

Impact of Consultation and Education Services   Data should be kept on the professional staff time spent delivering consultation and education services, for example, the number of hours. This information can be compared with national statistics.

Impact on Inappropriate Institutionalization   A center should report area admission and residency rates to State hospitals per 1,000 of the population. Rates should be compared with the rates from past years in order to determine if there is an increase or decrease in admission and residence in State hospitals.

Impact on Catchment Area Residents   Demonstrating program impact is the most difficult topic to evaluate but one of the most important. A variety of evaluation strategies exist for centers' use. These strategies focus on different criteria for measuring treatment outcome from different vantage points (Hagedorn et al., 1976). Limiting an evaluation to the use of one type outcome measure from one vantage point may cause the evaluation results to be invalid and unreliable, and may miss relevant information needed to assess the center's functioning. On the other hand, using several outcome measures assessed from multiple vantage points may yield more accurate, reliable results.

Three kinds of outcome evaluations are useful and relevant for mental health evaluations. They are: routine monitoring of a program or activity, evaluation aimed at demonstrating program effectiveness, and evaluation to aid administrative decision making. Each kind of evaluation yields valuable information. Therefore, an approach integrating these three types into a balanced outcome strategy is desired. The following outlines a balanced outcome strategy making use of several outcome measures, several vantage points, and both routine and episodic studies.

The initial step of this evaluation strategy involves establishing a routine system to monitor outcome. This will provide a basic measure of client outcome. An economical approach must be used because this step entails ongoing monitoring of every client. Only easily collected and inexpensive outcome indicators are practical for day-to-day monitoring of service in rural areas (Attkisson et al., 1978). The techniques chosen on the basis of these criteria are:

1. The Global Assessment Scale: A measure of the client's overall level of functioning from the vantage point of the therapist (See Appendix D).
2. The SCL-90-R Symptom Checklist: A measure of the client's symptoms from the vantage point of the client himself (See Appendix E).
3. Client Satisfaction Questionnaire: A measure of the client's satisfaction with the outcome of clinical and nonclinical processes of treatment (See Appendices F and G).

The use of a routine monitoring strategy is a reasonable first step to take in evaluating program effectiveness and client outcome. When used alone to serve as the entire evaluation, it is adequate. There must be at least one other approach involved in an effective outcome evaluation strategy. It should be an efficient, valid approach and should be capable of demonstating the effectiveness of individual programs with precision. One such approach that is well studied and relevant in clinical settings is Goal Attainment Scaling (GAS). GAS is a measure of the attainment of specific treatment goals from the vantage point of the client and the therapist. It does require more than minimal staff investment, thus it is not feasible to administer on a continuous basis. A time-limited study using samples of clients must therefore be employed. It is left up to each agency to review its resources and to design its own strategy. Smaller, rural agencies should probably aim toward short-term studies lasting only a few months. For more information, see Kiresuk and Sherman, 1968.

Peer Review and Utilization Studies Activities   Describe the process the agency carried out to meet this requirement. This will be somewhat different for each agency. Describe the guidelines that have been set up to monitor patient records and drug use profiles in accordance with Federal requirements.

Citizens Review   Describe all procedures used to involve citizens in reviewing the Annual Evaluation Report.

Center Goals   Review last year's centerwide annual report and note the goals that were identified. Next discuss and report on the progress made to date toward meeting these goals.

Next Year's Plan   Describe the major issues to be studied. Elucidate program implications of these evaluations, methods to be used, and proposed changes in citizen review procedures, if any.

SUMMARY

In program evaluation, the end is but the beginning—a time to start implementing changes and to begin the continued process of planning and evaluation. This continual process must exist and it is up to the program management to establish "active feedback loops." Hagedorn et al. (1976) suggest a feedback loop through which evaluation results should flow:

1. Program
2. Program information
3. Information gathering and analysis
4. Results of evaluation
5. Management, including program management

To ensure that an agency's evaluation results are used effectively, program evaluation and administrative decision making must be integrated activities. "We shall continue to see poorly administered programs and disregarded evaluation findings until the self-evaluating organization becomes a reality and there is a day-to-day working integration of administration and evaluation fully using the organization's evaluative capability" (Attkisson et al., 1978, p. 83).

Ronald Havelock (cited in Attkisson et al., 1978) outlines seven principles that are relevant requisites for use in integrating evaluation with administrative decision making: linkage methods, program structure, openness, capacity, reward, proximity, and synergy.

Linkage Methods   Evaluation and administration should be linked together at all levels of an organization. "Linkage" is determined by the degree to which two systems collaborate or work together. The more linkages there are, the better. With linkages, communication is made easier and the impact each system can make increases.

Program Structure   Programs must have effectively organized structural framework in order for evaluative information to be successfully incorporated into administrative decision making.

Openness   Program management must be willing to give and receive information. All must be open to change. They must accept that change is necessary.

Capacity   In order for program evaluation findings to be utilized, agencies must have adequate resources and competence to perform effectively. Adequate administrative and evaluative capacities are the basis for both good programs and effective evaluations.

Reward   The use of positive reinforcement with staff and management makes for more effective evaluations. Rewards build incentives for participation in the evaluation process.

Proximity   A close "proximity" between staff and management increases the likelihood of effective linkages between them. This means greater utilization of evaluative information.

Synergy   Evaluation information is better received, absorbed, and utilized the more times it is reviewed and discussed. Redundant communication of the evaluative findings makes for better understanding and utilization.

These seven principles facilitate integration of evaluation and administration. Agencies having established this integration will be well on their way toward becoming a self-evaluating organization.

To become a self-evaluating organization is a goal to aim toward. Wildavsky (cited in Attkisson et al., 1978) proposed the concept of a self-evaluating organization and holds that it is an ideal stage. A self-evaluating organization continuously monitors and evaluates its activities. Then, evaluation findings are utilized for the purpose of program development, change, and improvement.

In the future, all agencies need to work toward becoming more like Wildavsky's self-evaluating organization. This would make for the development of more relevant and effective community mental health agencies in rural areas.

REFERENCES

Adams County Mental Health Center C.O.C.E. Adult Interview. 1975. In W. Hargreaves, C. Attkisson, L. Siegel, M. McIntyre, and J. Sorenson (eds.), Resource Materials for Community Mental Health Evaluation (Park IV), DHEW Publication No. (ADM) 75–222, U.S. Government Printing Office, Washington D.C.

Attkisson, C. C., and Broskowski, A. 1978. Evaluation and the emerging human service concept. In Attkisson et al. (eds.) 1977. Evaluation of Human Service Programs. Academic Press, New York.

Attkisson, C. C., Brown, T. R., and Hargreaves, W. A. 1978. Roles and functions of evaluation in human service programs. In Attkisson et al. (eds.), Evaluation of Human Service Programs. Academic Press, New York.

Attkisson, C. C., and Hargreaves, W. A. 1977. A conceptual model for program evaluation in health organizations. In H. C. Shulberg and F. Baker (eds.), Program Evaluation in the Health Fields (Vol. II). Behavioral Publications, New York.

Beigel, A., and Levenson, A. 1978. Program evaluation on a shoestring budget. In Attkisson et al. (eds.), Evaluating of Human Service Programs. New York: Academic Press.

Biggerstaff, M. A. 1977. The administrator and social agency evaluation. Admin. Soc. Work 1:71–78.

Brody, R., and Krailo, H. 1978. An approach to reviewing the effectiveness of programs. Soc. Work 5:226–232.

Ciarlo, J. A., and Reihman, J. 1974. The Denver Community Mental Health Questionnaire: Development of multidimensional program evaluation instrument. Unpublished report. Available from the Mental Health Systems Evaluation Project, 70 W. Sixth Avenue, Denver, Colorado, 80204.

Coursey, R. D. 1977. Basic questions and tasks. In R. D. Coursey et al. (eds.), Program Evaluation for Mental Health. Grune & Stratton, New York.

Davis, H. R., Windle, C., and Sharfstein, S. S. 1977. Developing guidelines for program evaluation capability in community mental health centers. Evaluation 4:25–29.

Davidoff, I., Guttentag, M., and Offutt, J. (eds.). 1977. Evaluating Community Mental Health Services. DHEW Publication No. (ADM) 77–465, U.S. Government Printing Office, Washington, D.C.

Derogatis, L. R., Lipman, R. F., and Covi, L. 1973 SCL–90: An outpatient psychiatric rating scale. Psychopharmacol. Bull. 9:13–28.

Derogatis, L. R., Lipman, R. S., Rickels, K., Uhlenhuth, E. H., and Covi, L. 1974. The Hopkins Symptom Checklist (HSCL): A self-report symptom inventory. Behav. Sci. 19:1–15.

Ellsworth, R. B., Foster, L., Childers, B., Arthur, G., and Krocker, D. 1968. Hospital and community adjustments as perceived by psychiatric patients, their families, and staff. J. Counsult. Clin. Psychol. Monogr. 32:Part 2, 41.

Feldman, R., and Wodarski, J. S. 1974. Bureaucratic constraints and methodological adaptations in community-based research. Am. J. Community Psychol. 2:211–224.

Flaherty, E. W., and Windle, C. 1981. Mandated evaluation in community mental health centers: Framework for a new policy. Eval. Rev. J. Appl. Soc. Res. 5:620–638.

Flax, J. W., Wagenfeld, M. O., Ivens, R. E., and Weiss, R. J. 1979. Mental Health and Rural America: An Overview and Annotated Bibliography. DHEW Publication No. (ADM) 78–753. U.S. Government Printing Office, Washington, D.C.

Freid, J. B. 1977. Evaluation as a cooperative effort in a mental health clinic: A family affair. Evaluation 4:208–210.

Gertz, B., Meider, J., and Pluckhan, M. L. 1975. A survey of rural community mental health needs and resources.Hosp. Community Psych. 26:816–819.

Hagedorn, H. J., Beck, K. J., Neubert, S. F., and Werlin, S. H. 1976. A Working Manual of Simple Program Evaluation Techniques for Community Mental Health Centers. DHEW Publication No. (ADM) 76–404. U.S. Government Printing Office, Washington, D.C.

Hargreaves, W. A., Attkisson, C. C., and Ochberg, F. M. 1975. Outcome studies in mental health program evaluation. In W. A. Hargreaves, C. C. Attkisson, L. M. Siegel, M. H. McIntyre, and J. E. Sorensen (eds.), Resource Materials for Community Mental Health Evaluation Part IV, DHEW Publication No. (ADM) 75–222, U.S. Government Printing Office, Washington, D.C.

Hargreaves, W. A., Attkisson, C. C., and Sorensen, J. E. (eds.). 1977. Resource Materials for Community Mental Health Centers Evaluation. DHEW Publication No. (ADM) 77–328. U.S. Government Printing Office, Washington, D.C.

Hargreaves, W. A., and DeLay, E. A. 1979. Program evaluation in a rural community mental health center. Community Ment. Health J. 15:104–119.

Ihilevich, D., Gleser, G., Gritter, G., Kroman, L., and Watson, A. 1981. Measuring program outcome: The progress evaluation scales. Eval. Rev. 5:451–477.

Katz, M. M., and Lyerly, S. B. 1963. Methods for measuring adjustment and social behavior in the community: I. Rationale description discriminative validity and scale development. Psychol. Rep. 13:503–535.

Keenen, M. A. 1975. Essentials of methodology for mental health evaluations. Hosp. Community Psych. 26:730–733.

Kiresuk, T. J., and Sherman, R. E. 1968. Goal attainment scaling: A general method for evaluating comprehensive community mental health programs. Community Ment. Health J. 4:443–453.

Kivens, L., and Bolin, D. C. 1976. Evaluation in community mental health center: Hillsborough CMHC, Tampa, Florida. Evaluations 3:98–105.

Landsberg, G., Neigher, W. D., Hammer, R. J., Windle, C., and Woy, J. F. (eds.). 1979. Evaluation in Practice. DHEW Publications No. (ADM) 78–763, U.S. Government Printing Office, Washington, D.C.

Larsen, D. L., Attkisson, C., and Hargreaves, W. 1978. Salt Lake CMHC consumer satisfaction inventory. In Attkisson et al. (eds.), Evaluation of Human Service Programs. Academic Press, New York.

McIntyre, M. H., Attkisson, C. C., and Keller, T. W. 1977. Components of program evaluation capability in community mental health centers. In Hargreaves et al. (eds.),

Resource Materials for Community Mental Health Program Evaluation. DHEW Publication (ADM) No. 77–328, U.S. Government Printing Office, Washington, D.C.

MacNair, R., Wodarski, J. S., and Giordano, J. Social instrumentation: The implications for delivery of human resources. In press.

National Institute of Mental Health. 1977. Guidelines for Program Evaluation. Working Draft.

Norris, E. L., and Larsen, J. K. 1976. Critical issues in mental health service delivery: What are the priorities? Hosp. Community Psych. 27:561–566.

Pearls, S. R., Winslow, W. W., and Pathak, D. R. 1980. Staffing patterns in community mental health centers. Hosp. Community Psych. 31:119–121.

Piliavin, I., and McDonald, T. 1977. On the fruits of evaluative research for the social services. Admin. Soc. Work 1:63–70.

Roth, D., Lecklitner, G., and Landsberg, G. 1979. Overview. In Landsberg et al. (eds.), Evaluation in Practice. DHEW Publication No. (ADM) 78–763, U.S. Government Printing Office, Washington, D.C.

Sorensen, J. E., and Binner, P. R. 1979. Overview. In Landsberg et al. (eds.), Evaluation in Practice, DHEW Publication No. (ADM) 78–763, U.S. Government Printing Office, Washington, D.C.

Sorensen, J. E., and Grove, H. D. 1978. Using cost-outcome and cost-effectiveness analyses for improved program management and accountability. In Attkisson et al. (eds.), Evaluation of Human Service Programs. Academic Press, New York.

Speer, D. C., and Tapp, J. C. 1976. Evaluation of mental health service effectiveness. Am. J. Orthopsych. 46:217–227.

Spitzer, R. L., Gibbon, M., and Endicott, J. 1973. Global Assessment Scale (GAS), Unpublished report.

Stevenson, J. F., and Longabaugh, R. H. 1980. The role of evaluation in mental health. Eval. Rev. 4:461–480.

Tillman, H. 1976. Hennepin County CMHC. "Telling-it-like-it-was" questionnaire. In H. Hagedorn, K. Beck, S. Neubert, and S. Werlin (eds.), A Working Manual of Simple Program Evaluation Techniques for Community Mental Health Centers. DHEW Publicaion No. (ADM) 76–404. U.S. Government Printing Office, Washington, D.C.

Ward, J. H. 1977. An approach to measuring effectiveness of social services: Problems and resolutions, Admin. Soc. Work 1:409–419.

Weiss, C. H. 1972. Evaluation Research: Methods of Assessing Program Effectiveness. Prentice-Hall, Inc., Englewood Cliffs, N.J.

Wholey, J. S., Scanlon, J. W., Duffy, H. G., Fukumoto, J. S., and Vogt, L. M. 1970. Federal Evaluation Policy: Analysis of Effects of Public Programs. The Urban Institute, Washington, D.C.

Windle, C. (ed.). 1979. Reporting Program Evaluations: Two Sample Community Mental Health Center Annual Evaluation Reports. DHEW Publications No. (ADM) 79–607. U.S. Government Printing Office, Washington, D.C.

Windle, C., and Flaherty, E. W. 1979. Overview. In Landsberg et al. (eds.), Evaluation in Practice. PHEW Publication No. (ADM) 78–763, U.S. Government Printing Office, Washington, D.C.

Windle, C., and Voldman, E. M. 1973. Evaluation in the centers programs. Evaluation 1:69–70.

Wodarski, J. S. 1980. Requisites for the establishment and implementation of competency-based agency practice. Arete 6:17–28.

Wodarski, J. S. 1981. Role of Research in Clinical Practice. University Park Press, Baltimore.

Wodarski, J. S., and Buckholdt, D. 1975. Behavioral instruction in college classrooms: A review of methodological procedures. In J. M. Johnston (ed.), Behavior Research and Technology in Higher Education. Charles C Thomas, Springfield Ill.

Wodarski, J. S., and Feldman, R. A. 1974. Practical aspects of field research. Clin. Soc. Work J. 2:182–193.

APPENDIX A: SUGGESTED OUTLINE FOR ANNUAL EVALUATION REPORT

A one-page summary for each heading is desired.

A. The study purposes, methods, empirical data, and evaluation results from the past year.
    1. Cost of operation
    2. Use of services
    3. Availability, accessibility, and acceptability
    4. Impact
    5. Other matters
        a. Consultation and education
        b. Awareness of services
        c. Reduction of inappropriate institutionalization
B. The results from peer and utilization reviews and clinical care evaluation studies done as part of quality assurance. (This report should give numbers of cases reviewed, numbers and types of inadequacies and remedial actions taken, but not reveal the identity of individual patients or clinicians).
C. Procedures used to publicize the last evaluation report.
D. The procedures used to provide copies and summaries of the last evaluation report.
E. The amount and types of citizen review and consultation and resulting citizen suggestions, together with an indication of the extent to which the center board has been involved in the preparation and approval of the center's program evaluation report.
F. The plan for the next year's evaluation of center services, taking into account center program priorities and problems and results of past evaluations.
G. Conclusions reached on the basis of the review of evaluation information, decisions reached, consequent action on policy and practice changes, and management rationale for not taking actions suggested by evaluative information.
H. A summary of extent to which center's goals are being met.

APPENDIX B: AGENCY AWARENESS AND
SATISFACTION QUESTIONNAIRE

Agency _____

Contact person _____

Position _____

Length of employment _____

1. What percentages of your time are spent in each of the following duties?
    _____ % administrative
    _____ % ongoing services delivery or counseling with clients
    _____ % community liaison work
    _____ % consultation with other agencies
    _____ % other (specify)

2. Which of the services offered by _____ CMHC are you aware of?
    Which services have you referred clients to in the past 6 months? (Check off as
    the person names them)

    Aware of   Referred

_____	_____	Outpatient
_____	_____	Inpatient
_____	_____	Emergency Walk-In
_____	_____	Day Care (Adult Day Treatment)
_____	_____	Children's Services
_____	_____	Aging Program
_____	_____	Consultation and Education
_____	_____	Aftercare
_____	_____	Alcohol Services
_____	_____	Halfway House
_____	_____	Diagnostic Screening for Courts

3. How many clients would you estimate you referred to _____ CMHC in
    the past 6 months?
    _____ None (If none, go to 3 A and B).
    _____ 1–2
    _____ 3–4
    _____ 5–7
    _____ 8 or more

3A. Reasons for not referring patients to _____ CMHC:
    _____ not appropriate
    _____ not aware of services
    _____ other (specify)

3B. Are you aware of the procedures required for referring clients to _____
    CMHC?
    _____ yes
    _____ no

4. Have you received any referrals from ＿＿＿＿＿＿ CMHC in the past 6 months?

＿＿＿＿＿ yes

＿＿＿＿＿ no

Were they appropriate?

＿＿＿＿＿ yes

＿＿＿＿＿ no

For questions 5 to 10, please select the response choice which you feel most accurately describes your feelings about the statement. Your choices will be strongly agree, agree, disagree, strongly disagree. (Read all four choices after each question).

	Strongly agree	Agree	Disagree	Strongly disagree
5. When I have contacted the center's secretarial staff, they have been cooperative and helpful.				
6. There is usually prompt reporting to me from ＿＿ CMHC concerning the clients I have referred.				
7. Most clients report they have a good feeling about the treatment they receive at the center.				
8. When I refer a client to the center, he/she is seen by a counselor within a short time.				
9. The staff at the center have usually shown interest in my clients.				
10. I will continue to refer appropriate clients to ＿＿＿＿＿＿ CMHC.				

11. How generally satisfied are you with the services your clients are receiving at the ＿＿＿＿ CMHC?

＿＿＿＿＿ Satisfied

＿＿＿＿＿ Somewhat satisfied

＿＿＿＿＿ Somewhat dissatisfied

＿＿＿＿＿ Dissatisfied

12. In your opinion, what can the ＿＿＿＿＿＿＿ CMHC do to improve the staff, facilities, programs, and services it is now providing to your referred clients?

Source: Hennepin County CMHC

APPENDIX C: CONSUMER SATISFACTION/FOLLOW-UP QUESTIONNAIRE

1. How many times have you been here?
    a. 1
    b. 2
    c. 3
    d. 4
    e. 5 or more (specify)
2. What type of service(s) are you receiving?
    a. Individual
    b. Group/Family
    c. Aftercare
    d. Children's services
    e. Evaluation
    f. Other, specify medication
3. How generally satisfied are you with services you receive here?

1	2	3	4	5
satisfied	somewhat satisfied	no opinion	somewhat dissatisfied	dissatisfied

4. In general, was it easy to be seen here?
    _____ Yes
    _____ No
5. Was the appointment scheduled at a time that was convenient for you?
    _____ Yes
    _____ No
    _____ Sometimes
6. After you arrived here today, how soon were you seen?
    a. Immediately
    b. 5 minutes
    c. 15 minutes
    d. 30 minutes
    e. One hour
    f. Longer than one hour
7. Was there a goal(s) set in your therapy?
    _____ Yes
    _____ No
    _____ Don't know
8. What are your service goals?
9. How much progress do you feel you are making toward reaching this/these goal(s)?
    a. A great deal of progress
    b. Some progress
    c. No progress

10. Were you ever in the hospital for psychiatric reasons?
   _____ Yes   _____ VA
   _____ No   _____ State
                                  _____ Local
                                  _____ Private

11. Are you working now?
   _____ Yes
   _____ No

12. Were you working before you came here?
   _____ Yes
   _____ No (If no, ask why)
   _____ Not working since working would be inappropriate (e.g., fully disabled, dependent spouse, etc.)
   _____ Not working since either was in the hospital or had just gotten out of the hospital
   _____ Other, specify unemployed, child, student, etc.

13. Is there anything at the center you did not like?
   _____ Yes
   _____ No
   Specify community not aware of services, vending machines, doctors hard to understand, don't see doctor much or easily, no psychiatric care—just medication, receptionist oblivious to goings on, therapy should be more behaviorist/goal oriented, etc.

14. If you feel that any part of the service at the center was especially good, briefly explain what it was.

15. Are you coming back?
   _____ Yes
   _____ No
   _____ Don't know
   If yes, are you clear on whom you will be seeing for your next visit?
   _____ Yes
   _____ No

16. As a result of your treatment here, do you feel you understand yourself/your child better?
   _____ Yes
   _____ No
   _____ Don't know

Source: Hennepin County CMHC

APPENDIX D: GLOBAL ASSESSMENT SCALE

Rate the subject's lowest level of functioning in the last week by selecting the lowest range which describes his functioning on a hypothethetical continuum of mental health-illness. For example, a subject whose "behavior is considerably influenced by delusions" (range 21–30) should be given a rating in that range even though he/she has "major impairment in several areas" (range 31–40). Use intermediary levels when appropriate (e.g., 35, 58, 63). Rate actual functioning independent of whether or not client is receiving and may be helped by medication or some other form of treatment.

91–100   No symptoms, superior functioning in a wide range of activities, life's problems never seem to get out of hand, is sought out by others because of his or her warmth and integrity.

81–90   Transient symptoms may occur, but good functioning in all areas, interested and involved in a wide range of activities, socially effective, generally satisfied with life, "everyday" worries that only occasionally get out of hand.

71–80   Minimal symptoms may be present but no more than slight impairment in functioning, varying degrees of "everyday" worries and problems that sometimes get out of hand.

61–70   Some mild symptoms (e.g., depressive mood and mild insomnia) *or* some difficulty in several areas of functioning, but generally functioning pretty well, has some meaningful interpersonal relationships and most untrained people would not consider him or her "sick."

51–60   Moderate symptoms or generally functioning with some difficulty (e.g., few friends and flat affect, depressed mood and pathological self-doubt, euphoric mood and pressure of speech, moderately severe antisocial behavior).

41–50   Any serious symptomatology or impairment in functioning that most clinicians would think obviously requires treatment or attention (e.g., suicidal preoccupation or gesture, severe obsessional rituals, frequent anxiety attacks, serious antisocial behavior, compulsive drinking).

31–40   Major impairment in several areas such as work, family relations, judgment, thinking, or mood (e.g., depressed woman avoids friends, neglects family, unable to do housework), *or* some impairment in reality testing or communication (e.g., speech is at times obscure, illogical or irrelevant), *or* single serious suicidal attempt.

21–30   Unable to function in almost all areas (e.g., stays in bed all day), *or* behavior is considerably influenced by either delusions or hallucinations, *or* serious impairment in communication (e.g., sometimes incoherent or unresponsive) or judgment (e.g., acts grossly inappropriately).

11-20   Needs some supervision to prevent hurting self or others or to maintain minimal personal hygiene (e.g., repeated suicide attempts, frequently violent, manic excitement, smears feces), *or* gross impairment in communication (e.g., largely incoherent or mute).

1-10   Needs constant supervision for several days to prevent hurting self or others or makes no attempt to maintain minimal personal hygiene (e.g., requires an intensive care unit with special observations by staff).

Source: Robert L. Spitzer, M.D.; Miriam Gibbon, M.S.W.; Jean Endicott, Ph.D. (cited in Hagedorn et al., 1976, p. 207)

APPENDIX E: SCL-90-R

NAME: _____

LOCATION: _____DATE: _____

RATER:_____ TECH:_____ S.NO _____

REMARKS: _____

DO NOT MARK IN SHADED AREA BELOW

	:0: :1: :2: :3: :4:		:5: :6: :7: :8: :9:
	:0: :1: :2: :3: :4:	PATIENT	:5: :6: :7: :8: :9:
	:0: :1: :2: :3: :4:		:5: :6: :7: :8: :9:
	:0: :1: :2: :3: :4:	VISIT	:5: :6: :7: :8: :9:
	:0: :1: :2: :3: :4:		:5: :6: :7: :8: :9:
	:0: :1: :2: :3: :4:	RATER	:5: :6: :7: :8: :9:
	:0: :1: :2: :3: :4:		:5: :6: :7: :8: :9:
	▬▬	P. NO.	

INSTRUCTIONS

Below is a list of problems and complaints that people some-times have. Please read each one carefully. After you have done so, please fill in one of the numbered spaces to the right that best describes HOW MUCH THAT PROBLEM HAS BOTHERED OR DISTRESSED YOU DURING THE PAST INCLUDING TODAY. Mark only one numbered space for each problem and do not skip any items. Make your marks carefully using a No. 2 pencil. DO NOT USE A BALLPOINT PEN. If you change your mind, erase your first mark completely. Please do not make any extra marks on the sheet. Please read the example before beginning.

PLEASE CONTINUE ON THE FOLLOWING PAGE

APPENDIX E: SCL-90-R (continued)

	EXAMPLE					
		NOT AT ALL	A LITTLE BIT	MODERATELY	QUITE A BIT	EXTREMELY
HOW MUCH WERE YOU BOTHERED BY:						
1.	Backaches	⁼0⁼	■■■	⁼2⁼	⁼3⁼	⁼4⁼

	HOW MUCH WERE YOU BOTHERED BY:	NOT AT ALL	A LITTLE BIT	MODERATELY	QUITE A BIT	EXTREMELY
1.	Nervousness or shakiness inside	⁼0⁼	⁼1⁼	⁼2⁼	⁼3⁼	⁼4⁼
2.	Unwanted thoughts, words, or ideas that won't leave your mind	⁼0⁼	⁼1⁼	⁼2⁼	⁼3⁼	⁼4⁼
3.	Hearing voices that other people do not hear	⁼0⁼	⁼1⁼	⁼2⁼	⁼3⁼	⁼4⁼
4.	Crying easily	⁼0⁼	⁼1⁼	⁼2⁼	⁼3⁼	⁼4⁼
5.	Feeling that people are unfriendly or dislike you	⁼0⁼	⁼1⁼	⁼2⁼	⁼3⁼	⁼4⁼
6.	Feeling that you are watched or talked about by others	⁼0⁼	⁼1⁼	⁼2⁼	⁼3⁼	⁼4⁼
7.	Having urges to break or smash things	⁼0⁼	⁼1⁼	⁼2⁼	⁼3⁼	⁼4⁼
8.	Feelings of worthlessness	⁼0⁼	⁼1⁼	⁼2⁼	⁼3⁼	⁼4⁼
9.	The idea that something is wrong with your mind	⁼0⁼	⁼1⁼	⁼2⁼	⁼3⁼	⁼4⁼

The nine items are reproduced here with the permission of the author of the SCL-90-R, Leonard R. Derogatis, Ph.D., Director, Division of Medical Psychology, The Johns Hopkins University School of Medicine, Baltimore. This is intended as a sample only, and conveys the comprehensiveness of the scale itself. The SCL-90-R is copyrighted and is distributed by Clinical Psychometric Research in Baltimore.

APPENDIX F: CLIENT SATISFACTION QUESTIONNAIRE

Please help us improve our program by answering some questions about the services you have received at the _____ . We are interested in your honest opinions, whether they are positive or negative. Please answer all of the questions. We also welcome your comments and suggestions. Thank you very much, we appreciate your help!

CIRCLE YOUR ANSWER

1. How would you rate the quality of service you received?

4	3	2	1
Excellent	Good	Fair	Poor

2. Did you get the kind of service you wanted?

1	2	3	4
No, definitely not	No, not really	Yes, generally	Yes, definitely

3. To what extent has our program met your needs?

4	3	2	1
Almost all of my needs have been met	Most of my needs have been met	Only a few of my needs have been met	None of my needs have been met

4. If a friend were in need of similar help, would you recommend your program to him/her?

1	2	3	4
No, definitely not	No, I don't think so	Yes, I think so	Yes, definitely

5. How satisfied are you with the amount of help you received?

1	2	3	4
Quite dissatisfied	Indifferent or mildly dissatisfied	Mostly satisfied	Very satisfied

6. Have the services you received helped you to deal more effectively with your problems?

4	3	2	1
Yes, they helped a great deal	Yes, they helped somewhat	No, they really didn't help	No, they seemed to make things worse

7. In an overall, general sense, how satisfied are you with the services you received?

4	3	2	1
Very satisfied	Mostly satisfied	Indifferent or mildly dissatisfied	Quite dissatisfied

8.   If you were to seek help again, would you come back to our program?

1	2	3	4
No,	No, I don't	Yes,	Yes,
definitely not	think so	I think so	definitely

Write comments below:

Source: D. L. Larsen, C. C. Attkisson, and W. A. Hargreaves (cited in Attkisson et al., 1978, p. 309).

APPENDIX G: TELL-IT-LIKE-IT-WAS

For each question listed below, please circle the appropriate answer.

A. How do you feel about the location of this agency in getting there for services?
   1. very satisfied
   2. not satisfied
   3. no particular feelings one way or the other
   4. satisfactory
   5. very satisfactory
   If you have circled 1 or 2, please make comments here.

B. How were you personally treated by the receptionists and clerks?
   1. very satisfactorily
   2. not satisfactorily
   3. no particular feeling one way or the other
   4. satisfactorily
   5. very satisfactorily
   If you circled 1 or 2, please make comments here.

C. How do you feel about the length of time before our agency dealt with your particular situation/problem(s) after you first contacted? (Be sure you consider the urgency of your concerns).
   1. very unsatisfied
   2. not satisfied
   3. no particular feelings one way or the other
   4. satisfied
   5. very satisfied
   If you have circled 1 or 2, please make comments here.

D. How do you feel your situation/problem(s) has changed since you have become involved with this agency?
   1. become much worse
   2. become somewhat worse
   3. better in some ways but worse in others
   4. become somewhat better
   5. become much better
   If you have circled 1 or 2, please make comments here.

E. How do you feel about the helpfulness of the primary staff who dealt with your situation/problem(s)?
   1. very satisfied
   2. not satisfied
   3. no particular feelings one way or the other
   4. satisfied
   5. very satisfied
   If you have circled 1 or 2, please make comments here.

F. If a friend asked, would you recommend the service of this agency?
   1. never
   2. hardly ever recommend
   3. usually recommend
   4. almost always recommend
   5. always recommend
   If you have circled 1 or 2, please make comments here.

G. If needed, would you come back or contact us again?
   1. never come back or contact
   2. hardly ever come back or contact
   3. usually come back or contact
   4. almost always come back or contact
   5. always come back or contact
   If you have circled 1 or 2, please make comments here.

H. In general, what do you think of the overall service that you received?
   1. very unsatisfied
   2. not satisfied
   3. no particular feelings one way or the other
   4. satisfied
   5. very satisfied
   If you have circled 1 or 2, please make comments here.

I. Who filled out this questionnaire?
   1. male consumer
   2. female consumer
   3. male and female consumers (couple)
   4. parent of consumer
   5. other than parents of consumer

Source: Harvey Tillman (cited in Hagedorn et al., 1976, pp. 238–240)

Chapter 7

Competencies for Effective Rural Practice

Formal community mental health services are relatively new to rural America. There are early indications that services that are planned and executed in urban settings are often difficult to duplicate in the rural area. Likewise, roles and functions of social workers in the cities are likely in need of modification and/or expansion to be workable in the rural setting.

A look at life in rural America and the community mental health program that is possible there shed considerable light on competencies needed by rural mental community health practitioners in general, and bachelor level and graduate level social workers, in particular. The competencies are conceptualized on a continuum, that is, basic, intermediate, and advanced. These competencies point to curriculum changes and additions that are needed to prepare social workers for rural practice.

PROFILE OF THE RURAL COMMUNITY MENTAL HEALTH CENTER

Rural mental health services are primarily those provided through the community mental health centers. Although hospital services are extended to rural clients, a study published in 1973 revealed that comparable rates of psychiatric admissions in the four most rural states were 1/10 that of the four most urban (Wagenfield and Robin, 1976). Because hospital services are underutilized for rural areas, and private services are most likely not available, the community mental health program has emerged as a powerful resource to fill a substantial service void.

The study conducted by Wagenfield and Robin (1976) on the emerging role of community mental health workers yielded information on the rural community mental health center activities and the staff involved in this programming. At the time of this survey, only 11% of all CMHCs in operation were designated as serving an all rural catchment area, that which is outside a standard metropolitan statistical area and consists only of counties in which more than 50% of the 1970 population live in communities of 2,500 or less. Moreover, these rural centers tended to be those most recently established.

Rural CMHCs depend heavily on various government agencies for funding, with only 13% of the revenue coming from receipts for services. This is opposed to 25% for nonrural centers. Only 40% of rural staff members work full time as opposed to 66% in nonrural centers, and there are less than half the proportion of psychiatrists. Proportions of social workers, psychologists, and nurses, however, are roughly comparable.

Another significant staffing characteristic is the high proportion of para-professionals. Because most of these persons are indigenous to the area, they assist in putting the community emphasis in the CMHC and offer the element of trust necessary for clients in rural areas (Jeffrey and Reeve, 1978). On the other hand, many times these workers are not well-trained and, therefore, have limited utility.

> In one sense rural CMHCs are an innovative vanguard; on the other hand, their heavy reliance on nonprofessional staff may be another index of the professional resources deficit that characterizes many rural human services programs (Wagenfield and Robin, 1976, p. 71).

GENERAL COMPETENCIES NEEDED FOR
RURAL COMMUNITY MENTAL HEALTH WORK

A worker within the rural mental health setting may be described as the proverbial jack-of-all-trades. Unlike the urban counterpart who sees clients on a regular basis in a comfortable office, the rural worker may spend a good deal of work time away from the office interviewing a potentially suicidal person at the jail, visiting a home-bound elderly client who needs a medication evaluation, or making contact with a worker at the welfare services concerning a shared client. The rural worker may be in one part of the catchment area one day a week and many miles away serving the center's clients the next. Because catchment areas are determined on the basis of population (75,000 to 200,000) and rural areas are sparsely populated, distance creates a particularly difficult problem in the delivery of rural mental health services (Wagenfield and Robin, 1976). In many instances, the automobile is the worker's office.

In an area in which there are few social services available for clients, there is a demand for rural workers to be capable of autonomous work. The rural worker must be a self-starter because there is less likelihood of receiving supervision or team backup than for the urban counterpart. The rural worker must be able to develop personal guidelines and standards and adhere to these with little support (Ginsberg, 1969; Jankovic and Anderson, 1979). Imagination may be one of the worker's most useful tools to secure needed (Snyder, Kane, and Conover, 1978).

It is generally agreed that a major requisite for the rural worker is to be self-motivated in terms of professional growth and stimulation (Ginsberg, 1969;

Horejsi and Deaton, 1977). The practitioner does not have access to the professional contacts and stimulation that occur naturally during coffee breaks in large organizations. It is up to individual workers then to expand their contacts and skills through attending workshops largely available in urban areas, reading the current literature, and seeking out the limited number of professionals in a rural area.

The rural worker must know how to create and use social services that are not, in the traditional sense, viewed as social services. The worker must know how to identify the network of services that are hidden. It is the role of the rural worker to assess the strength of the network and to assist it in improving, rather than viewing it as nonprofessional and disregarding it (Ginsberg, 1969). For example, the local sheriff may be the county's answer to Traveler's Aid by housing transients in jail overnight.

In the rural setting, it is important for the worker to be able to establish trust. Personal trust supercedes issues of competence, and a person can function as a useful worker only if he or she can be seen as a trustworthy individual. It may be of more benefit to have coffee with the director of the welfare system locally or to exchange fish stories during this trust-building time than to introduce imaginative programs (Jeffrey and Reeve, 1978). This time spent may be more cost-effective than first meets the eye since the rural art of doing business is a person-to-person one.

The rural worker must have the capacity for quickly building relationships with all types of people in all types of roles (i.e., other workers, ministers, political and business figures). Although the rural worker may have the opportunity to develop long-term relationships with many clients, the number of contacts will be irregular, due to the wide areas served by rural agencies. It is important that this person be able to make the occasional contact count. The practitioner must be able to work with the client in such a way that the work continues under the auspices of existing organizations that fill the roles of social agencies (Ginsberg, 1969).

Another important trait that the rural mental health worker must possess in order to survive in the setting is the ability to set realistic goals in accordance with the needs of the client group being served. The clinician will have more than a fair share of unmotivated clients and those with multiple needs exacerbated by the scarcity of services. If a goal of "personality reorganization" is set for these clients, the worker will rapidly become discouraged with inappropriateness and subsequent lack of success. The rural worker needs to define success for a client in small increments such as helping a female client see that being beaten by a husband is not a normal part of everyone's life and supporting her appropriate anger. This step alone may not improve her situation but may be the first in her discovery of alternatives to her situation and her own strengths in pursuing such alternatives (Jeffrey and Reeve, 1978).

To work effectively in the rural setting, Fenby (1978), Kiesler (1969), and Tranel (1970) indicate that the rural worker must become identified with the area by becoming a resident.

Not only our personal attributes but also our interests, our life styles, our drinking habits, our marriages, our children, our religious practices, our politics, and our positions on various issues of current concern had to be catalogued before we could become personally predictable enough to be trusted with more than technical professional questions. Only when professionals have lived in rural areas long enough to emerge as citizens with as much personal stake in the future of the community as anyone else can their community begin to make full use of their capabilities ... (Kiesler, 1969).

In all cases possible, students in the rural community mental health project described herein were strongly encouraged to live in the rural area where they practiced.

The rural worker confronts the accompanying element of high visibility, the loss of personal privacy and the ability to exercise control over social contacts (Horejsi and Deaton, 1977; Riggs and Kugel, 1976; Snyder, Kane, and Conover, 1978). This leads to role-juggling. When an acquaintance of the mental health worker calls on him or her, it may not be clear as to whether the person comes as client, friend, or member of a committee on which both of them serve. During a single encounter the practitioner may have to adapt to all three situations (Bachrach, 1977; Cummings, 1978).

The worker must be able to assess the norms of the rural community to avoid violating those norms and offending people, particularly those in the power structure. Anonymity is almost impossible in the rural area, and separation of one's private self from one's work is nearly as impossible. Overt violation of local norms can lead to painful confrontations. There is nowhere to hide for the rural worker in violation (Ginsberg, 1969; Horejsi and Deaton, 1977).

In 1974 Gertz, Meider, and Pluckhan conducted a survey of 215 rural community mental health centers across the United States. Part of the survey had to do with the qualities and skills needed by rural workers. From the 92 responses, skills were categorized as academic preparation, personal qualities, general abilities, and those requirements unique to the rural setting.

In terms of academic preparation, the disciplines of training mentioned were the usual ones of psychology, social work, and psychiatry, with the addition of anthropology. Specific skills mentioned were in the areas of individual, group, and family counseling. Knowledge of community resources was considered beneficial. The three most often mentioned personal qualities were good communication skills, the ability to function autonomously, and the ability to make and maintain good interpersonal relationships. One more ability noted is that of tolerating isolation while still remaining visible to the community. General abilities listed were those skills in teaching, consultation, public relations, management, and problem-solving. Assessment skills in recognizing the social network of the area, social planning skills, and those having to do with community organization were also indicated as requisites.

In looking at the uniqueness of the rural setting and preparation for it, the questionnaire's respondents noted that a knowledge of rural politics and power structures and the ability to develop informal patterns of communication with leaders in the community was necessary for effective functioning of staff. The ability to recognize informal pressure groups that exert control in the area was essential. Other requisite skills listed which have special importance for the rural worker are "familiarity and empathy with the particular cultures, socioeconomic levels, values, and mores of rural residents" (Gertz, Meider, and Pluckhan, 1975). Additional staff attributes noted were acceptance of the conservative rural ethic and a grasp of the demographic characteristics of the area.

In summary, the research indicates that the practitioner in rural community mental health needs the basic skills of working with clients in a helping fashion, in assessing and working with the local power structure, communicating effectively in a rural culture, and working autonomously, often in an innovative fashion. The literature also indicates that the way to gain acceptance for mental health programs within the rural setting is through an informal network of getting things done.

PRACTICE IN THE PUBLIC SECTOR—WHAT BSWs AND MSWs DO

A review of the literature and data from the rural community mental health project indicate that bachelor's level social workers tend to provide direct service to clients. This is in line with the goals of the majority of undergraduate social work programs; that is, to prepare students for these service line positions (H. H. Jarrett, personal communication; Loewenberg, 1972; Wodarski, Giordano, and Bagarozzi, 1981). In the Georgia state merit system, these positions are classified as human services technicians and caseworkers. There is the occasional BSW who is drafted into an administratively oriented position, usually in a rural area, but due to the educational criteria for a number of administrative positions, this is the rare exception.

A substantial number of master's-level programs offer students either a direct practice tract or an administrative tract, and numbers indicate that within the University of Georgia and a number of other institutions the vast majority of students opt for the clinical tract. A 1976 survey of its MSW graduates conducted by the School of Social Work at the University of Texas at Austin revealed that 64% of the graduates had majored in the Interpersonal Helping (IH) tract, whereas 36% majored in the Social Planning and Program Development (SPPD) tract. The study also indicated that within an average of 3 years, 91% of SPPD individuals moved into positions compatible with their training. IH majors, on the other hand, appeared to be moving out of their direct service emphasis in substantial numbers (Sherwood and Daley, 1979). Teare (1979), reporting on a 1977 Job Analysis Survey conducted within a state public welfare agency employing 4,000 workers in the southeastern United States, revealed that only 27% of those with graduate degrees were classified in the provision of direct services. The majority were supervisors, administrators, or shared administrative and supervisory roles. Abramczyk (1980) supports this trend in human services, noting that it is not unusual for social workers to go directly from graduate school into supervisory positions or to be quickly promoted into such, often within 18 months.

In an article reviewing the job tasks and job perceptions of various practitioners from disciplines of social work, psychiatry, and psychology in an evening mental health clinic, House, Miller, and Schlachter (1978) reported interesting discrepancies. The MSW social workers interviewed perceived themselves as spending 51% of their time in direct practice. In actuality, they were spending 27% of their time in the clinical area. Perhaps this distortion assists the clinically oriented and trained MSWs in finding their increasingly administrative positions palatable.

The dream of the MSW providing the bulk of front-line direct service to clients has never been realized, and due to economic conditions of the foreseeable future, will not be a reality in rural areas. Sherwood and Daley (1979) suggest that from a professional view, this dream should not come to pass. Their suggestion is that it is better that many direct service jobs, especially those at lower salary levels and those in public agencies, should be filled by BSWs. Due to the lack of a career ladder in direct service, an MSW must move into administration for additional salary, power to effect change, and to have professional status, which the majority of graduates desire.

COMPETENCIES FOR BSWs AND MSWs IN RURAL MENTAL HEALTH

One of the debatable principles of social work in rural mental health and rural social work in general is that the practitioner needs to be a generalist (Fenby, 1978; Ginsberg, 1969, 1971, 1976; Horejsi and Deaton, 1977). Although Specht (1979) and Teare (1979) are not focusing on social workers in the rural area in particular, they take issue with generalist preparation. They consider the expectations of the generalist model, that practitioners be equally well versed in dealing with direct and indirect service tasks, to demand too much of a practitioner. The concern here is that the social worker will not receive knowledge specific enough to handle these tasks.

From the experiences of 18 MSW students in rural field placements under the auspices of the rural training grant in mental health (Wodarski, Giordano, and Bagarozzi, 1981) and those in a rural VA Hospital placement (Synder, Kane, and Conover, 1978), there is additional support for the generalist model. There is not the luxury of specialized focus in a rural area of diversity and few mental health workers. The rural mental health social worker may see children as well as aging clients, do crisis intervention work, present a community workshop on drug education and abuse, and confer with another agency worker about a cooperative programming effort, all in a single day. For this, the rural social worker needs a variety of skills that are applicable to the particular practice situation. The task comes in teasing out the competencies which a BSW needs to master as opposed to the MSW.

In talking about competencies, reference is directed toward the person's ability to do (i.e., the performance of specified skills). During the last decade, competency-based education has been heralded as the way of the future. It is an approach that includes carefully defined learning objectives that both students and instructors are aware of, a definite plan of assessment in which each student is judged in terms of her or his attainment of objectives, individualized instruction, and a variety of experiences and instruction modules that build competence (Jarrett, 1974).

BSW Competencies

There is substantial agreement in the literature that front line clinical work is nearly always in the realm of the BSW social worker. The provision of services to individuals, families, and groups is the focus.

An excellent source of defining BSW competencies for rural community mental health practice is found in a programmed self study prepared by the undergraduate social work faculty of the University of Georgia (1981). The most obvious competency heading the list is that of interpersonal communication. Without the underlying skill of communication, the practitioner cannot effectively work with clients or community resource persons. This competency can be broken down to include skills in verbal and nonverbal attending behavior; the communication of empathy, respect, genuineness, and warmth; and an accurate communication of understanding of the verbal and nonverbal content and feelings being expressed. This is the basic competency upon which all other practice endeavors are built.

A requisite competency for the rural BSW is becoming aware of his or her own biases and prejudices and controlling for them. With a mastery of this competency, the worker will be seeing persons as individuals with unique problems and strengths and will be clear about the client's area of concern. Likewise, the worker can prevent personal bias from distorting the service process.

Conducting oneself in a professional manner with clients and community persons is a primary competency. This includes adhering to confidentiality which may at times be difficult in the rural setting in which everyone may know everyone else's family members. A major facet of this professionalism involves meeting the standards of acceptable work for one's agency. In line with the Social Work Code of Ethics (1979) developed by the National Association of Social Workers, the BSW would identify, develop, and utilize knowledge of professional practice.

A prerequisite practice competency is one of assessment. The BSW needs to be able to work with the client system to identify and assess the factors impinging on a problem. Analogous to this competency, the BSW practitioner should be able to work with the client to formulate a plan of intervention and to assess the outcome of this plan. This presupposes that the worker has theoretical models that provide the rationale for the intervention, can make the choice of the appropriate change agent, and has the skills to apply the knowledge through interventions. Models that seem to be most appropriate in rural practice are those of short-term intervention dealing with concrete problems (Wodarski, 1981; Wodarski, Giordano, and Bagarozzi, 1981).

One observation has been that a practice competency of great value to the rural BSW is the ability to link clients with desired or needed resources. This is particularly important in rural areas where there are few formal services. This demands that the BSW have a knowledge of civic and church groups and concerned citizens who serve as the informal helping network that fill this void. Moreover, it also requires that the BSW be able to inform and assist the client in taking advantage of these resources.

The BSW practitioner must be able to analyze the organizational workings of his or her own agency and the way that the agency interfaces with the community, both of which subsequently affect practice endeavors. Services and programs are influenced by the social context, and the BSW, in order to work effectively, must have an understanding of the impact on practice endeavors of the rural community and values placed on these services. This involves the BSW identifying and working within the power structure of the rural community.

An essential competency for the BSW is the ability to understand cultural diversity. It is imperative for an identification of the existing subcultures and their value systems for the determination of how they will affect practice interventions. The worker will need to be aware of the value structure of the rural majority and how this differs from the subgroups within the community. This competency involves complex skills in both being able to assess subgroup behavior and being able to identify individual characteristics and needs. Moreover, the BSW must have a working knowledge of social welfare policies and programs and research as they relate to the effective delivery of services in rural areas.

A practical competency, suggested by those in rural field placements (Wodarski, Giordano, and Bagarozzi, 1981), is that the rural BSW must be familiar with psychotropic medications and their expected and problematic side effects. The BSW must be able to describe behavioral symptoms that will assist the psychiatrist, often in touch only by telephone, to identify the need for and to prescribe medication for clients where warranted.

MSW Competencies

General   Identified competencies at the graduate level at this time are much more ambiguous for rural community mental health practice. Loewenberg (1972, p. 20) says that "the specific goal of social work education at the master's degree level is to prepare students for a level of competence necessary for responsible professional practice and sufficient to serve as a creative and productive professional career." That "specific goal" is a substantial broad mandate and certainly not defined as to the components that go into forming this professional preparation. This ambiguity is reflected in graduate school curricula in which the focus differs with the school. Competencies for the MSW are often so generally stated because graduate educators cannot agree about the work for which they need to be trained (Wodarski, 1979).

In conjunction with the lack of agreement on competencies needed, there is a dearth of students clamoring for rural training. In many cases, the MSW who practices in rural areas is not there because of planned career choices but may have moved there because of a spouse's job or family connections (R. J. Anderson, personal communication).

Having MSW practitioners in rural areas is a relatively recent phenomenon. A National Association of Social Workers (NASW) survey of members conducted by Stamm in 1969 revealed that only 4% of MSWs worked in rural areas of less than 10,000 (Ginsberg, 1971). Although this number may have expanded somewhat, in a 1978 article, Fenby describes as a usual phenomenon the autonomous, lone-ranger rural MSW in mental health work. If the MSW is not a single-person agency, then she or he is one of only a handful of workers and usually the program's administrator.

Competencies thought to be necessary for the MSW build on requisites for BSW practitioners and specifically include advanced practice technologies (including work with individuals, families, and groups), and enabling skills in administration, community organization, social planning, and public relations (Ginsberg, 1976).

R. J. Anderson (personal communication) and Hollister (1976) suggest a reassessment of services provided in rural community mental health and thus of the competencies required. The model of service provided is dependent upon whether one is *treating* mental illness in the rural catchment area or *supporting* good community mental health by contributing to family, neighborhood, and community problem-solving.

> A rural mental health program strategy that defines and responds to each presenting individual need as a clinical problem to be dealt with by clinical resources, results very quickly in overwhelming the scarce clinical (staff) available. All too soon there is a waiting list of persons who have been classified by staff as "patients to be seen." A high clinical commitment leaves no time to deal with the host of people with psychological disabilities, some severe and some mild, that do not directly present themselves for care to a mental health unit. (Hollister, 1976)

Gottlieb and Schroter (1978), Hollister (1976), Magel and Price (1979), Seibert (1979) and an article published in *Human Services in the Rural Environment* (Informal Helping Systems for the Child Welfare Workers, 1980) all strongly support the MSW's competency in utilizing informal helping systems and offering consultation rather than direct services. Data from the project described here, however, indicate it will take time to establish the contents of practice functions because social work endeavors in many rural communities are relatively new phenomena.

MSWs are operating within a national mental health system, with all the mandates and constraints imposed. It appears that the rural MSW must be able to do some of everything. Rural MSWs must offer advanced direct services to those individuals who come to the clinic, particularly those deinstitutionalized persons who have returned to the community. They must also master more indirect prevention and consultative skills to serve the rural population not seeking direct treatment. Simultaneously, they must act as administrators. This model is appropriate if the agency has workers trained at different levels of practice.

Specific First and foremost, the MSW must have interpersonal competencies to deliver advanced clinical services as set forth in the section on competencies needed by the BSW. Many rural MSWs do not have the luxury of working as a supervisor, administrator, clinician, *or* program specialist in consultation and education. They must do it all, and these firing line clinical skills are essential. They must have skills in working with individuals, families, and groups that present a variety of problems. Where possible, the MSW should supervise the bachelor's-level practitioner in the provision of these services. Thus, MSW practitioners must attain advanced practice skills through graduate education to be prepared to offer such supervision.

Moreover, MSWs must have the requisite competencies in administration and management. In many instances, the MSW in the rural mental health agency is the only professional employed and, thus, must be skillful in using supportive personnel effectively, in preparing and evaluating a budget, in administering personnel effectively, in setting up linkages with other agencies and key individuals in the community, and in hiring and firing staff. It is the MSW who must have competence in program development. He or she must be able to create and follow through with a program, which may involve organizing and delegating roles, fund raising, finding volunteers, and evaluating whether objectives were attained.

An indispensable competency for the MSW practitioner who has at least one other employee is that of supervision. The MSW will be orienting the employee, offering on-the-job training, offering case consultation, setting limits, providing feedback on position performance, supporting the isolated worker, and providing continuing education.

Another critical competency that MSWs in rural community mental health need is in the area of social policy planning. The MSWs should be skilled in making the view from rural areas known to these larger planning groups by providing rationales based on data. In many instances, this takes energy and time beyond agency hours. If the preventive approach is to be implemented, then these macro-level skills will be essential.

Rural MSWs must possess intermediate research skills. Adequate programs that serve the population in which they work require data on population trends, social problems, and community attitudes. Such skills should increase the ability to delineate a problem, to build an intervention plan based on behavioral science, and to conduct subsequent evaluation through predetermined outcome criteria to determine the effectiveness of the intervention (Wodarski, 1981).

A key competency lies in the area of consultation and education. In order to survive in an area with many needs and few services, MSWs must be able to support professionals already in existence. This includes case consultation with another agency's staff, program consultation, and community education as well as inservice education for community helpers.

Ginsberg (1976) sums up the expectations of the rural MSW by saying that this person does not need to be a super social worker with the high degree of skill in every area that the urban MSW has in one, but the rural MSW does need an adequate skill in everything. This is a rather overwhelming but apparently accurate assessment of the MSW in rural mental health.

Implications for Curriculum Development

In looking at ways of more effectively designing a curriculum to meet the practice needs of social workers in rural mental health, Feldman (1978) suggests that "services are significantly modified by the nature of the setting in which they are provided and, to be effective, training must reflect the needs of these settings." The most obvious reflection of need is that the BSW must continue to be trained as the direct service worker, one who can function with autonomy and creativity. The MSW needs a wide range of advanced competencies in direct service, administration, supervision, consultation and education, social policy planning, and research. Moreover, graduate-level preparation as an advanced generalist seems imperative along with the development of the abilities to apply the advanced competencies in a variety of practice contexts.

Arkava and Brennan (1975) enumerate those competencies that they believe should be attained and support the use of an oral or written examination for an assessment of practice skills for the bachelor level social worker. They are as follows: knowledge of the agency, knowledge of community resources, understanding of what social work is as it relates to the BSW's own work, skill in information gathering, ability to design and implement a plan of intervention, communication skills, and skill in assessing intervention processes and results. Subsequent tests should also be developed for the graduate social worker before he or she enters in practice to assess whether a differentiation of competencies is occurring at the various levels of social work education.

A must in the preparation of rural practitioners is that the field placement experience be in a rural mental health center. Field placements in cities cannot offer models of how to get things done in the rural environment.

> For many students, the rural field placement is an altogether different work from what they have previously experienced. Exposure to rural poverty, isolated living conditions, lack of transportation, and scarcity of other resources may bring about value and attitude changes. Students may commute to out-lying (even more rural) counties for clinics, day treatment centers, home visits, or other services. The contacts made with a wide variety of settings, agencies, and staff and then shared among students are rewarding and beneficial in the education and resocialization process (Jarrett and Kilpatrick, 1978, p. 18).

There should be an intensive module of training designed for BSW and MSW students preparing themselves for rural practice. The curriculum should include a cross-cultural learning emphasis that would assist the student in the learning of new, appropriate habits and unlearning old ones, careful preparation for entry into rural work, and the recognition that learning to live and work in a rural area takes time. Supportive materials concerning rural social problems, policies, and community behavior would be helpful (Ginsberg, 1976). Local experts (residents) from the area to which the students are going for field placement could be brought in to offer basic how-to's for work in the area. The key points to be stressed include defining the rural culture and different groups that are part of it, assessing the area as to formal and informal service providers, alliances and conflictual relationships, and power structure (formal and informal), and becoming aware of what local residents find annoying about newcomers (M. Reul, personal communication). The local experts could also give pointers for establishing credibility and learning the ropes in a rural area which include finding a mentor, making community contacts, and utilizing local ideas in programming efforts (B. Foster, personal communication).

There is also a need to prepare these rural practitioners for independent, minimally supervised, professionally isolated, and often lonely practice. Information on burn-out and on ways of finding support for oneself and one's work in the rural sphere are essential.

CONCLUSIONS

If social workers in rural mental health are to practice effectively, they must be aware of the rural environment and the impact it has on mental health services. They must come into the rural area with skills that are in line with the demands of rural practice. Curricula in undergraduate and graduate social work programs must build those skills needed for competent rural mental health practice.

Suggestions have been made as to what competencies are needed by BSWs and MSWs working in rural mental health. Further research is needed here to expand and more finely tune these suggested competencies.

Enumerating the competencies does little if curricula are not developed to teach and measure performance of them. Despite much interest in competency-based education in the literature (Arkava and Brennan, 1975; Duehn and Mayadas, 1977; Jarrett, 1974, 1979; Jarrett and Clark, 1978; Jarrett, Kilpatrick, and Pollane, 1977; Peterson, 1976), there are few well developed and evaluative training programs for rural social work practitioners in community mental health.

It is posited that competencies rest on continuing with bachelor's-level practitioners providing direct services and the master's-level practitioner providing advanced services in terms of advanced direct practice, administration and management, supervision, social policy and planning, research and consultation, and education.

REFERENCES

Abramczyk, L. W. 1980. The new M.S.W. supervisor: Problems of role transition. Soc. Casework 61:83–89.

Arkava, M. L., and Brennan, C. C. 1975. Toward a competency examination for the baccalaureate social worker. J. Educ. Soc. Work 11:22–29.

Bachrach, L. L. 1977. Deinstitutionalization of mental health services in rural areas. Hosp. Community Psych. 28:669–672.

Cummings, D. 1978. What a rural FNP needs to know. Am. J. Nurs. 78:1332–1333.

Duehn, W., and Mayadas, N. S. 1977. Entrance and exit requirements of professional social work education. J. Educ. Soc. Work, 13:22–29.

Feldman, S. 1978. Promises, promises or community mental health services and training: Ships that pass in the night. Commun. Ment. Health J. 14:83–91.

Fenby, B. L. 1978. Social work in a rural setting. Soc. Work 23:162–163.

Gertz, B., Meider, J., and Pluckhan, M. 1975. A survey of rural community mental health needs and resources. Hosp. Commun. Psych. 26:816–819.

Ginsberg, L. H. 1969. Education for social work in rural settings. Soc. Work Educ. Rep. 17:28–32, 60–61.

Ginsberg, L. H. 1971. Rural social work. Encycl. Soc. Work 2:1138–1144.

Ginsberg, L. H. 1976. An overview of social work education for rural areas. In L. H. Ginsberg (ed.), Social Work in Rural Communities: A Book of Readings, Council on Social Work Education, Inc., New York.

Gottlieb, B. H., and Schroter, C. 1978. Collaboration and resource exchange between professionals and natural support systems. Prof. Psychol. 9:614–622.

Hollister, W. G. 1976. Experiences in rural mental health. In L. H. Ginsberg (ed.), Social Work in Rural Communities: A Book of Readings. Council on Social Work Education, Inc., New York.

Horejsi, C. R., and Deaton, R. L. 1977. The cracker-barrel classroom: Rural programming for continuing education. J. Educ. Soc. Work, 13:37–43.

House, W. C., Miller, S. I., and Schlachter, R. H. 1978. Role definitions among mental health professionals. Compr. Psych. 19:469–476.

Informal helping systems for child welfare workers 1980. Hum. Serv. Rural Envir. 5:29–30.

Jankovic, J., and Anderson, R. J. 1979. Professional education for rural practice. Soc. Work Educ. 1:5–14.

Jarrett, H. H. 1974. Competency-based education in the liberal arts. Unpublished doctoral dissertation, University of Georgia.

Jarrett, H. H. 1979. Operationalizing educational outcomes in the curriculum. In B. L. Baer and R. C. Federico (eds.), Educating the Baccalaureate Social Worker. Ballinger Publishing Company, Cambridge, Mass.

Jarrett, H. H., and Clark, F. W. 1978. Variety in competency-based education: A program comparison. Alt. Higher Educ. 3:104–113.

Jarrett, H. H., and Kilpatrick, A. C. 1978. Country roads . . . rural field instruction. Hum. Serv. Rural Envir. 3:13–21.

Jarrett, H. H., Kilpatrick, A. C., and Pollane, L. P. 1977. Operationalizing competency-based B.S.W. field experience. Paper presented at the Annual Program Meeting of the Council on Social Work Educational Innovations Exchange, February, Phoenix, Ariz.

Jeffrey, M., and Reeve, R. 1978. Community mental health services in rural areas: Some practical issues. Commun. Ment. Health J. 14:54–62.

Kiesler, F. 1969. More than psychiatry: A rural program. In M. F. Shore and F. V. Mannino (eds.), Mental Health and the Community: Problems, Programs, and Strategies. Behavioral Publications, New York.

Loewenberg, F. M. 1972. Time and Quality in Graduate Social Work Education. Council on Social Work Education, Inc., New York.

Magel, D., and Price, C. 1979. Innovations in rural service delivery. Hum. Serv. Rural Envir. 4:20–28.

National Association of Social Workers. 1979. Code of Ethics. National Association of Social Workers, Washington, D.C.

Peterson, G. W. 1976. A strategy for instituting competency-based education in large colleges and universities: A pilot program. Educ. Technol. 16:30–34.

Riggs, R. T., and Kugel, L. F. 1976. Transition from urban to rural mental health practice. Soc. Casework 57:562–567.

Seibert, M. 1979. Developing self-help groups for a rural mental health center. Hum. Serv. Rural Envir. 4:33–34.

Sherwood, D. A., and Daley, M. R. 1979. Curriculum directions for an upgraded M.S.W.: Administration for everyone? J. Educ. Soc. Work 15:65–71.

Snyder, G. W., Kane, R. A., and Conover, C. G. 1978. Block placements in rural veteran administration hospitals: A consortium approach. Soc. Work Health Care 3:331–343.

Specht, H. 1979. Generalist and specialist approaches to practice and a new educational model. In F. W. Clark, M. L. Arkava, and Associates (eds.), The Pursuit of Competence in Social Work. Jossey-Bass Publishers, San Francisco.

Teare, R. J. 1979. A task analysis for public welfare practice and educational implications. In F. W. Clark, M. L. Arkava, and Associates (eds.), The Pursuit of Competence in Social Work. Jossey-Bass Publishers, San Francisco.

Tranel, N. 1970. Rural program development. In H. Grunebaum (ed.), The Practice of Community Mental Health. Little Brown & Company, Boston.

University of Georgia School of Social Work. 1981. B.S.W. program for self study. Vol. 2. Athens, Ga.

Wagenfield, M. O., and Robin, S. S. 1976. The social worker in the rural community mental health center. In L. H. Ginsberg (ed.), Social Work in Rural Communities: A Book of Readings. Council on Social Work Education, Inc., New York.

Wodarski, J. S. 1979. Critical issues in social work education, J. Educ. Soc. Work 15:5–13.

Wodarski, J. S. 1981. Role of Research in Clinical Practice. University Park Press, Baltimore.

Wodarski, J. S., Giordano, J., and Bagarozzi, D. A. 1981. Training for competent community mental health practice: Implications for rural social work. Paper presented at the annual meeting of the Council on Social Work Education, March, Louisville, Kentucky.

Chapter 8

Practicum

An Elucidation of the
Educational Process and Objectives

Practicum provides the major training experience for students who intend to practice in rural community mental health. Academic courses can provide an overview of the requisites of rural practice. Only the practicum, however, can reveal to the student the different organizational contexts for rural practice and the variety of skills necessary to execute the multitude of professional tasks. For the faculty member responsible for practicum instruction, the lack of appropriate supervision for students in rural areas creates a major training challenge, and the amount of travel for both students and faculty is substantial. This chapter presents the rationale for requisite practice instruction and an elucidation of its components.

KNOWING THE COMMUNITY

Rural areas may be defined as agricultural or remote from the larger society, or characterized as sparsely populated and nonindustrial. Edward Buxton (1973) defines rural as " . . . an area which lags behind in population per square mile, in education, in variety of experience and finally, in the power to control its own destiny . . . ." The problems faced by a social worker in a rural area are vastly different from those faced by his or her urban counterpart (Millar, 1977). Thus, one essential aspect of the practicum is to help a student understand their context of practice.

Differences between rural clients and those of other areas become particularly important in preparing social work students for rural field placements. In the community mental health training project it has been observed that many students have had no prior experience in rural areas. Moreover, they may be from a distant part of the country and have little knowledge of the school's geographic region. In order to be effective in a rural area, the student must have an understanding of the peculiarities of the clients with whom he or she will be working and the culture in which they live (Mermelstein and Sundet, 1977). The social worker entering into a rural area is set apart from the residents in many areas: education, dress, age, speech, mannerisms, even the type of car he or she drives. Workers must be aware of existing differences between themselves and their clients and must seek to understand the community in which they are practicing in order to find their "place" in that community (Buxton, 1973).

Community mental health practitioners going into rural areas face distinctly different problems with clients and service delivery than do their urban counterparts (Riggs and Kugel, 1976). "Rural clients are generally more reserved, concrete thinking, and traditional . . ." than middle class, white, urban clients (Nooe, 1977, p. 347). The isolation of rural clients affects their perceptions of themselves, outsiders, and the appropriateness of seeking help from them. Outside help—professionals and other authority figures—tends to be rejected and help is sought from traditional helpers in the community—preachers, teachers, doctors, older family members, and so forth (Bates, 1980; Nooe, 1977). Use of groups to provide support for clients tends to reduce the threat of "outsiders." Moreover, group procedures have been found to be especially effective with persons from deprived backgrounds. In the group setting, "individuals with similar problems and attitudes are brought together for educational, recreational, or counseling experiences where they gain confidence from each other" (Reul, 1974, p. 579).

The clinical model for the rural area should take into account the client's orientation toward concreteness, lack of regard for "expert opinion," and desire for immediate service effect. Services should be clearly defined and the method for obtaining them as obstacle-free as possible. The rural poor lack self-confidence and have little past experience in successful interaction with agencies (Nooe, 1977; Reul, 1974). Because of the need for nontraditional services and the scarcity of social services in the geographic area, the rural social worker must be able to perform a wide range of tasks. Workers trained in a variety of specialized skills can more easily adapt to different kinds of problem situations and the context in which they occur (Millar, 1977; Ramage, 1971). Thus, it is necessary to alter traditional clinical methods for use in rural mental health centers (Nooe, 1977).

Many rural mental health programs have failed to meet the needs of the people they were intended to serve. This is frequently due to failure to consult with potential clients to determine their perceptions of their own needs. Workers must understand how the people they will be serving define mental health problems (Fink, 1977). The milieu of the client—family, social organizations, and community—determine what is considered to be mental health or illness (Ramage, 1971). In an area such as the rural Appalachians, the socialization system is different from that of urban industrialized areas. In order to render effective intervention, the worker must have first hand, not theoretical, knowledge of the family structure and the dynamics of the client's social system (Aquizap and Vargas, 1970). The student social worker should learn the community in which he or she is to practice. A community immersion experience, therefore, is necessary to facilitate the student's appreciation of the environment in which the client functions (Mermelstein and Sundet, 1977).

Participant Observation

The anthropological tool of participant observation is one of the most feasible ways of obtaining needed information about communities to be served (Fink, 1977). The use of anthropological techniques to gather data about or to assess certain characteristics of a particular social group is one essential facet of applied anthropology. The anthropologist sees people "in the course of their daily lives, not in an artificial setting." This acquaints the anthropologist with "normal" behavioral interactional patterns of the persons under observation (Barnouw, 1973). Although not in itself a means of changing a group or culture, applied anthropology can be used to assess and predict behaviors. The applied anthropologist's function is to use the results of the analysis to state what a situation is, and if certain results are desired, what methods should be followed to obtain the desirable outcomes (Firth, 1971). Thus, through their ethnological study of a community, applied anthropologists are able to advise policy makers on the formulation of policy and change strategy for that community (Neville, 1978).

The objective of participant observation is "to develop a picture of the culture under review" (Barnouw, 1973). The anthropologist seeks to fit into a community of an alien culture and learn of that culture from the people who possess it. He or she "respects them, learns from them, and puts his/her knowledge of the outside world at their disposal" (Tax, 1977). The participant observer records observations of people in day-to-day interactions. The observer uses "informants," that is, members of the culture willing to answer their questions, to obtain information on the history of the group, social behavior not readily observable, and beliefs and attitudes in terms of mores and folkways commonly held by the group. Folktales, common jokes, and local sayings are collected and recorded (Barnouw, 1973). Thus, the observer becomes familiar with the language, including class variations and slang, of the group. Knowledge of the group will include both information it knows about itself and observations that only an objective outsider can make.

Skills of Participant Observation

The features of a group are as varied as the life histories of each of its individual members. By observation of the members, however, it is possible to make generalizations about the group's behavior and values. This is the personality of a culture.

It is essential that the participant observer live in or near the community under study in order to be able to participate in its life. The student practitioner must have easy access to people of the community; he or she must be able to interact with them in their day-to-day life. The student's goal is more than just to observe the community; the student must become a part of it. Students in the training program described here were strongly encouraged to live in rural areas where they practiced. Students who did indicated that their learning experiences were more valuable, as did their faculty supervisors.

By participating in the life of a community, students learn what it is like to be a member of that community. They are subjected to the same geographical and climatological conditions as the natives. The economic, political, and social conditions of the area are assessed and evaluated. They become familiar with the same magnificent old houses and rustic farms that the townspeople know and frequently use as landmarks. Such knowledge can be used to break the ice in essential interactions with clients and significant other community members. If the area is impoverished and businesses are closing down, the student may experience the same lack of availability of goods and services that the residents suffer. The abundance or absence of recreation or entertainment activities will be shared by community members and the participant observer. In this way, the student comes to understand some of the external presses that community members, including his or her clients, experience.

Possession of a common environment can serve to enhance the establishment of empathy between the practitioner and client. As the practitioner comes to understand circumstances that affect all members of the community, he or she can better assess clients' coping efforts. For example, by knowing that the county being served is low in business expansion and high in unemployment, the student practitioner can identify a client's inability to obtain employment as not unusual for that area and not necessarily indicative of a lack of desire or ability to work. The more the student understands of factors that affect the community as a whole, the more rapidly he or she can delineate the total gestalt of factors impinging on the client.

Indeed, as the student practitioner comes to understand problems of the whole community, he or she may come to believe that macro-system, and not only individual, changes are needed in order to ameliorate clients' problems. That macro-system change is needed may first come to students' attention through their own experiences. However, students cannot expect to make changes in the community unless local residents also define the problem and want to work to change it. An exception to this is the condition of local circumstances being at variance with state or federal laws, for example, failure to comply with mandatory desegregation of schools. The practitioner in such a case might face a dilemma between taking action against what is not tolerated elsewhere and maintaining trust and good relations with the community.

By being seen around the community, the student practitioner becomes familiar to local residents. If students do not live in the community it is likely that their only interactions would be with their clients and members of other social service agencies. By becoming familiar to a wider range of community members, the student has a better chance of gaining the trust of people who can provide information about relevant aspects of community life and of obtaining the data to assess the natural helping network of an area.

Long-time local residents who are willing to talk to the participant observer about the area and its history are of great value. They can rapidly provide information that the student might otherwise have to track down in newspapers or deduce from conversations with many different people. The student can simply ask the resident about people in power and how they achieved that power; responses may differ from one person to another, but the worker will soon get an idea of the true power structure of the community. One must be careful, however, to elicit relevant information and bits of "local color," and not mere gossip. Historical information about how the community was founded and got its name, what areas of the county were first settled, where the settlers were from, and/or the significance of certain landmarks can be quite helpful. A knowledge of local "hangouts" and their locations can help the practitioner when his or her clients make reference to them in interviews. An awareness of attitudes toward change, growth, and "outsiders coming in" can be used as an indicator of how the student, and other mental health staff, are viewed by residents. Local informants can explain to the participant observer the significance of current events such as court trials, county elections, or the formation of a union in a local factory.

As practitioners learn about a community they will recognize that there are cultural elements of which the community members themselves are unaware. To acquaint themselves with these behaviors practitioners will need to carefully observe interactions between community members. Through this observation workers will be able to generalize a set of rules about people in authority and how they are to be respected, individuals who are devalued and how they are treated, and appropriate social courtesies toward community members of all ages. Thus, through observation, the worker can assess the behavioral expectations of significant groups of the culture.

One important set of behaviors to observe is a culture's hidden rules in nonverbal communication. This is a complex set of behaviors including affect and mannerisms while talking, that is, eye contact, facial expressions, tone of voice, and so forth; proper distancing from other people; proper ways of entering rooms and joining groups; the accepted way of arranging office furniture; and other social rituals. The student practitioner in a rural area will be affected by these behaviors and will be taught what is or is not appropriate by the approval or disapproval of the local residents. It is more expedient for the student to be trained to recognize these behaviors and to learn the rules without violating them than to risk social disapproval. For example, a group's rules for distancing are readily observable by an outsider and may be used to determine how best to interact with them. Distances can be classified as intimate, personal, social, and public (Hall, 1969). After observing many interactions with people of differing ages and social status, the student can determine what distance must be kept for the dignity and comfort of the persons with whom the student communicates. Violations of the rules for distancing could indicate disrespect, hostility, an attempt to dominate, or a cold and withdrawn attitude. Different members of a group may be approached at varying distances, depending both on the rules of the group and individual idiosyncracies.

Knowledge of the rules of the group will help the social worker determine whether an individual's behavior is in keeping with those rules or not.

Eye contact is another important nonverbal communication. Before the student practitioner can judge whether the client's eye contact is appropriate he or she should assess what is typical for various social groups in that area. As a participant observer, the student should be attentive to eye contact in exchanges. Also, when watching an interaction of local residents, attention should be paid to the eye contact they have with each other (Hall, 1973).

Techniques of careful observation used to generalize rules by which a group interacts can be useful practice aids, for example, when working with groups as small as a family. It is quite possible that an entire family's behavior might differ from that of the larger community, especially if the family has moved in from another area. In such a case, the student practitioner would hardly be able to understand and subsequently to help the family without a working knowledge of the mores of the community.

While students are observing and learning from the community they are also becoming functioning members of it. In addition to the professional services student workers provide, they may be involved in a church, volunteer organizations, or local clubs. Through their involvement they may provide new ideas to a group or may be able to use their specialized knowledge of social service organizations to help community members better deal with agencies they may not understand. This kind of interaction not only promotes trust, but builds a link between the worker and community members and provides a tangible benefit to the community.

An essential element of social work intervention is "starting where the client is." For the student first encountering clients in a rural setting, the attributes of "location" may be difficult to assess. The techniques of participant observation serve to help students relate to clients in terms of their own community, the first requisite of effective practice.

ASSESSMENT OF PRACTICE COMPETENCIES

Development of student practice competencies is conceptualized along a continuum from beginning, intermediate, to advanced. Three general areas of competency should be assessed: interpersonal skills, theoretical knowledge, and practice skills.

Interpersonal Skills

Mechanisms must be provided for assessing three critical interpersonal skills— empathy, unconditional positive regard, and genuineness—characteristics that empirical research shows are necessary ingredients for therapeutic change, regardless of the therapeutic approach being utilized by the social worker. Empathy is generally defined as the worker's ability to understand the world according to each client's unique perspective. Workers who are empathetic can accurately feel and experience the world as the client does. Unconditional positive regard is usually defined as the ability to provide clients with a nonthreatening, safe, and secure atmosphere in which to express themselves. Genuineness is defined as the therapist's ability to establish genuine and nonexploitive relationships with clients. Additional research is showing that attending behaviors, accurate reflection, and summary of feelings may be other relative characteristics pertinent to inducing therapeutic change (Wodarski, 1979). These therapist traits can be readily measured within current agency practice because good measurement devices are available and are easily administered in terms of time and financial considerations and thus cause minimal disruption of the agency's regular mode of operation (Carkhuff, 1977).

Theoretical Knowledge

To assess the student practitioner's theoretical accuracy, an objective exam or assessment battery can be given, for example, on task-centered casework, family therapy, and behavioral social work. Once they achieve acceptable criterion levels on these assessment batteries, they can then move on to implementing interventions based on the theoretical framework.

Practice Skills

To determine practice skill levels, students might be asked to review a tape of a client interview or read a contrived case, make a diagnosis, design a corresponding intervention plan, and specify how they will evaluate the success of the plan to the satisfaction of practicing clinicians who have demonstrated their competencies. Once these tasks are successfully mastered, students are considered prepared for their initial contacts with clients.

Inventories such as the Barrett-Lennard, which measure the quality of the relationship between client and worker from the client's perspective, can be administered to clients to obtain consumer assessment of worker endeavors (Barrett-Lennard, 1962). This consumer aspect of the evaluation process is seldom addressed but is a requisite for a comprehensive evaluation and the provision of appropriate feedback to students (Wodarski et al., 1979).

SPECIFIC PRACTICE SKILLS

Specific practice skills have not been reviewed thus far. Necessary skills for rural community mental health practice are categorized into seven areas of competency, attainment of which can occur through case vignettes, simulation exercises, audio and visual taping, training exercises, and so forth. No distinction is made in training for micro- or macro-level practice because practicum sites require students to exhibit skills at both levels throughout their placements. Specific mechanisms for the assessment of these skills are reviewed in Chapter 9.

1. Skills involved in human relationship formation, maintenance and determination, such as verbal and non-verbal communication, that is, association

and clustering of words, duration of utterances, interpretative statements, verbal congruence, content relevance, and the length of silent periods; and such nonverbal details as posture, gestures, eye contact, hand touching, ability to reinforce others, indications of interest, concern and respect, encouragement, and model provisions.

2. Interviewing skills that facilitate securing information necessary to help clients change, and subsequent competencies in micro intervention techniques with individuals, families, and small groups. Emphasis needs to be on short-term social functioning oriented treatment, task-centered casework, crisis intervention counseling, reality therapy, and behavioral techniques (Berg, 1975).

3. Abilities to define the target of change, that is, should it be an individual, a group, community, and/or institution, and the definitions of behaviors to be changed in terms of observable referents for various groups such as the elderly, youth, retarded individuals, and so forth.

4. Competence in the assessment of the level on which the change strategy should be delivered, that is, individual, group, organizational, and/or societal. This includes decision-making and problem-solving skills relevant for rural areas and macro-skills in gaining community support for intervention and resource identification and development.

5. Skills in choosing the appropriate change agent, that is, associate-, bachelor's-, and/or master's-level worker who possesses such characteristics as unconditional positive regard, empathy, verbal congruence, verbal ability, physical attractiveness, warmth, self-adjustment, and so forth that facilitate behavioral changes; in choosing the length of treatment; in determining the criteria of success; and in preparing for the termination of treatment through such processes as substitution of "naturally occurring" reinforcers, training relatives or other individuals in the client's environment, gradually removing or fading the contingencies, varying the conditions of training, using different schedules of reinforcement, using delayed reinforcement and assuring that behaviors acquired in treatment are maintained (Anthony and Carkhuff, 1977; Carkhuff, 1969, 1971; Carkhuff and Berenson, 1967; Vitalo, 1975; Wells and Miller, 1973).

6. Skills in determining where treatment should be provided, that is, understanding how the organizational aspects of the treatment context will affect the service; how to establish and implement a program; and how staff should be trained. These considerations are emphasized in recent research investigations that provide data to suggest that many treatment contexts are inappropriate mechanisms for the performance of services (Caplinger, Feldman, and Wodarski, 1978; Feldman and Wodarski, 1974; Feldman et al., 1973; Wodarski, Feldman, and Pedi, 1976a, b; Wodarski and Pedi, 1977).

7. Ability to specify the requisites for the evaluation of treatment programs involving specific items, such as securement of an adequate pretreatment

baseline of behaviors, specification of client behaviors to be changed, specification of worker's behaviors in terms of relationship formation and intervention, monitoring of treatment to ensure that the quality of treatment is maintained over time, use of appropriate design and statistics, follow-up, and so forth.

Practice Techniques That Can Be Evaluated

There are numerous concrete items that can be easily assessed, regardless of the rural practice context. Contracts executed between client and workers can be checked for the inclusion of the following: purpose of the interaction; targeted problems and areas of difficulties to be worked on; various goals and objectives that might be accomplished; client and therapist duties; delineation of administrative procedures or constraints; techniques that will be used; duration of contracts and criteria for decisions for termination; and renegotiation procedures (Wodarski and Bagarozzi, 1979).

Agencies can use goal-setting forms that specify the type of client difficulty, plans for therapy, short- and long-term goals, plans for termination, follow-up procedures, and so forth. Such documentation should facilitate the evaluation of progress that is made toward treatment goals. Additionally, a summary form could be used to specify the overall treatment plan including termination and follow-up procedures.

Other means of evaluation might entail checking to see if practice notes summarizing the major events of the client's last visit are recorded within a reasonable time frame, such as 72 hours after each session, and determining if the following are executed and placed in the client's record within a reasonable time period: letter to referral professional (if necessary) regarding treatment plans and diagnosis, summary termination notes including follow-up procedures, and if necessary, a letter to the referring professional or family doctor regarding the termination of services within 1 week of said termination. In all instances, the energy and the time necessary to execute the forms should be kept at a minimum (Rinn and Vernon, 1975).

USE OF EVALUATION DATA TO IMPROVE PRACTICE

Adequate baseline data on practice competencies will provide the information necessary to facilitate the development of a competency-based student practicum. After collection of baseline data, steps may be taken to develop specific competencies. Supervision should be provided in such a manner as to help the worker alter dysfunctional service behaviors. This process should include:

1. Pinpointing behaviors that must be altered
2. Measuring the frequency of such behaviors
3. Developing a program to alter behavior
4. Providing feedback on targeted behaviors.

Videotaping client and practitioner interactions should facilitate isolation of those behaviors that need to be altered and likewise provide the opportunity for supervisors to reinforce the student's favorable practice behaviors.

The student practitioner should possess basic interpersonal skills to deliver any practice intervention. The intervention plan should be based on the best available theoretical rationale, and outcome criteria must be adequately specified. Practice episodes at the micro- and macro-level are subsequently evaluated on the criteria set forth.

ORIENTATION TO TRAINING FOR RURAL MENTAL HEALTH WORKERS

The training package set forth here provides basic instruction for all rural mental health workers. It represents an intensive experience to prepare students for initial contacts with clients and thus ensures their readiness for beginning practice endeavors. The training enhances placement and facilitates the learning experience in the rural area. The "crash" course is designed to be delivered in 3 weeks. Such an approach has been successful in training behavior specialists who are taught to do counseling with military personnel and their dependents (Peters and Rank, 1972).

Communication Skills

Whether the rural mental health practitioner is working directly with a client, a staff member, or a member of the community power structure, communication skills are a basic prerequisite to effective practice. The model used for training communication skills is Ivey's micro-counseling approach. The Ivey (1971) model teaches the individual skills of helping, utilizing videotaping, step-by-step training manuals, feedback from others, and self-observation. Several other models for training interpersonal skills are available. The Ivey model is chosen, however, due to its ease of implementation in terms of time, required resources, and clarity. The sequential steps of the approach are as follows:

1. Each trainee completes an initial (baseline) interview of 5 minutes with a volunteer client using a real or role-played concern.
2. The training process begins.
   a. The trainee studies a manual describing the single skill to be learned.
   b. The trainee views video models that illustrate the specific skill. The trainer discusses the single skill with rationale specified.
   c. The trainee views the original baseline interview, comparing his or her own performance with that of the models.
   d. The trainer maintains a warm supportive relationship with the trainee, pointing out positive aspects of the trainee's performance while focusing on the single skill being taught.
   e. A reinterview by the trainee is videotaped. The trainer gives special emphasis to the single skill being learned. The tape is then reviewed with the trainer with the trainer providing feedback (Ivey, 1971; Ivey and Authier, 1978).

The benefits of this approach are that the trainee has a simple and direct task—that of learning one skill at a time—and that the student is not overwhelmed with the complex task of learning how to communicate more effectively. Through this method, the practitioner gradually develops a repertoire of communication competencies.

The skills to be taught in this way include attending skills of open and closed questions, focusing and following, minimal encouragers, paraphrasing, reflection of feeling and content, and summarization. Influencing skills encompass directions, expressions of content and feeling, confrontation, self-disclosure, structuring, summary, and interpretation (Evans et al., 1979).

For attaining the next level of communication skills, Kagan's Interpersonal Process Recall (IPM) is employed (Ivey and Authier, 1978). Role plays are videotaped and then reviewed by a supervisor or instructor. During this review, the emphasis is on the trainee focusing on his or her subjective feelings rather than on specific skills. Discussion between trainee and supervisor centers on how the trainee might deal with these feelings when they arise in future sessions.

Techniques of Interviewing

Building upon the communication skills, there are a number of techniques that can be employed by the rural mental health worker to secure an adequate amount of information to be an effective facilitator with the person seeking mental health services. The training in communication skills will have provided basic information and a foundation for this set of skills. Now the rural worker is ready to learn the techniques of opening an interview, focusing in on the presenting problem, getting the needed information, and appropriately terminating the interview. Using a programmed text, the student traces an interview with a rural client. The trainee goes at his or her own pace through the text and chooses the most appropriate answers, modifying choices as suggested by the text (Augelli et al., 1980; Gazda et al., 1977). Following the completion of the programmed text, a class led by an instructor/facilitator is held to reiterate the main points of the interviewing process. The trainees then choose partners to do videotaped interviews in which one trainee role plays the client and the other the practitioner. The trainees then shift roles. After the filming, a trainer/facilitator meets with each dyad to discuss and critique their tapes. If necessary, the process can be repeated.

Exposure to a Classification of Psychiatric Disorders

In the rural setting workers must be clearly aware of psychiatric disorders because they most often will have to rely on their own recognition skills rather than on supervision from a highly trained clinician or psychiatrist. A programmed text prepared by the Academy of Health Sciences, U.S. Army Behavioral Sciences Division (Peters and Rank, 1972) offers an exposure to such disorders. The rural trainee can complete such a text in an hour.

After the initial textbook exposure, the trainee views a series of prepared videotapes illustrating symptoms typically encountered by the worker in rural practice. Trainees view these tapes in groups with an instructor/facilitator, and there is a question and answer period to discuss what the tapes illustrated (Research and Educational Association, 1981).

Counseling Strategies

There is a wide variety of theoretical models from which to choose in setting up a training program for rural mental health workers. The most important things to consider when making this choice are: Is the model appropriate? Will it help a particular client achieve service objectives? Is it culturally sensitive?

In choosing a treatment service model for rural mental health clients, the reasons for contact with a mental health worker must be assessed. To be placed in proper perspective, it is advisable to review the rural versus the urban conception of the help-seeking process. In the urban setting, clients usually contact a mental health worker because of a growth issue, that is, a life span developmental task. Such is not the case in rural America where mental health help is sought only if one is "sick." In order to be viewed as "sick" in the rural setting, one must be sick in an identifiable way, that is, the client exhibits behaviors the community does not approve of and an appropriate label is assigned. The work ethic dominates the definition of health in rural areas. In rural areas one is sick only if one cannot function in one's job. For males, employment outside the home is the prime focus; for females, taking care of the home is the major job. Interpersonal stresses may be present, but as long as one can work one certainly does not need any help. Tranel (1970) captures the picture as follows:

> Symptoms of mental illness in a rural situation which reach the professional mental health worker are frequently much more gross and would usually be considered much more severe than those observed in a more highly sophisticated social unit. This is so because of the prevalent attitude that people living in a rural condition must be very, very "crazy" before they can receive attention from the network of interpersonal attendants surrounding them (p. 420).

A model that is useful and relevant in the rural setting is one that supports the work ethic, one that focuses on returning individuals as quickly as possible to their employment environments.

There are several models that meet these criteria for the rural worker: the crisis intervention model (Aguilera, Messick, and Farrell, 1970); the problem-solving model (Perlman, 1957); and the task-centered model (Reid, 1978). All three methods maintain the basic assumption that a person is capable of problem-solving and can move from crisis to resolution. The mental health worker's role is that of facilitation of this process.

Training in the Crisis Intervention Model

The initial practice model for the rural worker is that of crisis intervention. The worker is taught to define a crisis, the facing of "an obstacle to important life goals that is, for a time, insurmountable through the utilization of customary methods of problem solving. The problem solving cycle involves a period of disorganization, a period of distress, during which many abortive attempts at solution are made'' (Aguilera, Messick, and Farrell, 1970, p. 5). The minimum goal of this model is the psychological resolution of the person's immediate crisis, restoring the client to at least the level of functioning that existed before the period of crisis. A maximum therapeutic goal is improvement in functioning above that of the precrisis level.

Crisis is viewed as time limited, lasting from 4 to 6 weeks. During this time the client is both psychologically vulnerable and open to new ways of solving problems. The outcome of the crisis may depend heavily on appropriate help. The duration of treatment under this model is from 4 to 6 weeks, with the median being 4 weeks (Aguilera, Messick, and Farrell, 1970). The pace of therapy is much faster and demands a goal-oriented focus of commitment from both client and therapist. Training in the model consists of:

1. Training in assessment of the individual and his or her problem: This utilizes the worker's communication skills that center on isolating precipitating events and the resulting crisis that brought the individual into treatment. Judgment must be made as to suicidal and homicidal risks. If the individual is a high risk, referral must be made for psychiatric evaluation for possible hospitalization.
2. Training in planning therapeutic intervention: In this step the trainee continues assessment as to how much the crisis has disrupted the client's life and the effects of this disruption on others in his or her environment. The trainee elicits information on the client's coping skills he or she may have used in the past and what people in the environment may serve as supports for the client. Search is made for alternative methods of coping not being employed at this time.
3. Training in intervention: The nature of the intervention makes use of the worker's preexisting skills, creativity, and flexibility. The four major components of this part of the crisis intervention process include:
    a. Helping the individual to gain an intellectual understanding of the crisis.
    b. Helping the individual to deal openly with present feelings which he or she may be ignoring or denying.
    c. Exploring alternative ways of coping.
    d. Reopening the individual's social world.
4. Training in crisis resolution and anticipatory planning procedures (Aguilera, Messick, and Farrell, 1970).

Using these components of crisis intervention, the trainee repeats the same format used for the communication skills. The trainer/facilitator first gives the trainee a written manual describing the components of the crisis intervention process. Videotapes of role plays among the trainees to both assess and improve their skills are then employed. Videotapes of successful interventions are viewed and discussed with the trainers/facilitators with the provision of appropriate feedback (Wodarski, 1980). In this training the trainer/facilitator (field instructor) is called upon to be a role model of the skills being presented, to be supportive and positive with the trainees, and to focus on the skills being learned.

Training in the Task-Centered Model

The second model that the rural community mental health practitioner must be prepared to implement is the task-centered model of casework. There are a number of reasons for developing skills in this model. Empirical foundations for this model consist largely of the outcomes of studies comparing short- and long-term casework, counseling, and psychotherapy. Generalizations derived from these studies include:

1. Recipients of brief, time-limited treatment show as much durable improvement as those in long-term, open-ended treatment.
2. Most of the improvement associated with long-term treatment occurs relatively soon after the beginning of treatment.
3. Regardless of their intended length, most courses of treatment turn out to be relatively brief (Reid, 1978).

Rural clients accept services that are more time-limited and concrete. In the rural area, where people seek services only when they are hurting enough to appear ''sick,'' the rural mental health worker usually has a limited number of sessions to assist them in changing. Data indicate that clients are very unlikely to remain for long periods of therapy. Also, in an area in which transportation is a problem, a worker needs to assist in fast problem-solving. The person may not be able to return for a number of future visits.

The task-centered approach focuses on these basic assumptions: 1) The problems to be worked on are ones acknowledged by the client. This means that the client can state the problem. 2) Clients can work on these problems outside the treatment session through homework assignments.

The role of the rural worker is to assist clients in alleviating or improving problems that concern them and to aid clients in having a constructive problem-solving experience that will enhance their capabilities to repeat such a process in the future. The relationship between the worker and client, as in every clinical encounter, must be one in which the client feels accepted, respected, liked, and understood. This relationship provides a means of stimulating and promoting problem-solving action. In this model, the ''practitioner expects the client to work on agreed-upon problems and tasks and communicates these expectations to the client both explicitly and implicitly. While the practitioner respects the client's decision to reject services, the worker also holds the client accountable for following through once a contract has been established'' (Reid, 1978, p. 89).

The training of the worker in this area consists of training in collecting basic data, identifying problems, problem assessment and planning, contracting, setting tasks, problem review, and post treatment planning and disposition.

The training model for this follows the other skill building training mentioned in this chapter. With the teacher/facilitator as a guide, the trainee reads a manual section for each process skill the practitioner is developing. The worker then practices with videotaped role plays and views exemplary tapes illustrating the particular skill they are learning. With the feedback from the trainer, the trainee makes another tape and views this with the trainer for critique.

Counseling Strategies for Work with the Chronic Client

The observation in the rural community mental health project has been that the rural worker frequently sees the deinstitutionalized patient with a history of chronic mental hospitalization. This individual may be seen by the worker as infrequently as once a month for medication monitoring. This contact may differ from state to state, but Medicaid mandates that once monthly is the minimal contact.

The chronic, long-term client will offer a different challenge to the rural worker. The primary goal for this client may be to maintain him or her at the current level of functioning. Other goals may be referral for supportive services such as an alternative living arrangement, food stamps or other welfare services, or structuring of the client's time during the day through participation in a day treatment program. There will be fewer of these support services in rural areas, and the worker may have to be innovative in getting any such service for the client.

This type of client is most likely taking psychotropic medication prescribed through the psychiatrist under contract to the rural clinic or through a local physician. It is important for the rural worker to be acquainted with the various medications, their attributes and side effects. Unlike the urban worker who may be within arm's reach of the staff psychiatrist, the rural worker may be many miles and several telephone calls away. The rural worker will have to be keenly aware of whether the client's medications are appropriate, whether the client's condition remains stable, or whether the client needs to be evaluated by the psychiatrist for medication change or possible hospitalization.

In working with chronic clients, skills training should be in medication monitoring and in developing advocacy and referral skills. Certainly communication skills will be employed and goal-oriented casework strategies are also useful, but this group of clients, who may be within a state mental health system for years, requires the worker to focus on the therapeutic services rather than therapy per se.

Training in medication monitoring is provided rural trainees in a programmed learning fashion. Audio tapes that explain the different drugs used, their properties, doses, and possible side effects, are assigned to each trainee. Trainees have a programmed text to accompany the tape, and they proceed at their own pace through the material. To supplement this programmed material, trainees also view video productions illustrating clinicians working with clients who are taking various medications. Side effects and the red flag behaviors resulting from improper medication schedules are illustrated. After exposure to the training packet, trainees are tested on their information about medications and their own observations of drug problems and courses of action to take with clients. The testing consists of objective paper and pencil tests and verbal reactions to video vignettes of clients displaying various drug reactions. Trainees report their observations and recommend courses of action, such as referral to a medical advisor, to the trainer for critique.

Training in advocacy and referral skills is accomplished through a course in resource discovery. The trainee becomes a part of a small group of five or six who are to investigate the services offered in the area in which they are housed for this training. They are presented with several problem situations of client needs by the trainer. Their tasks are to locate services and advocacy assistance for a client in this position. Trainees are encouraged to call upon agencies and individuals in the community for assistance. The various task groups make presentations to the entire training group. Trainers and trainees critique the presentations and offer any additional approaches that may be possible.

Training in Advanced Interpersonal Practice Technologies

Students should not only be trained in crisis intervention, the task-centered model, and counseling strategies for work with the chronic client, but should have the opportunity for training in advanced interpersonal treatment technologies. These consist of behavioral approaches to the solution of interpersonal problems. Numerous data-based behavioral technologies are available for workers to use in helping clients acquire necessary behaviors to operate in their environments. Every year more data support the successful history of behavior modification practice with children classified as: hyperactive (Hamblin, et al., 1971; Patterson, 1973; Patterson et al.; 1965); autistic (Browning and Stover, 1971; Hamblin et al., 1971; Graziano, 1971, 1975; Lovaas and Koegel, 1973; Margolies, 1977; O'Leary and Wilson, 1975); delinquent (Braukmann and Fixsen, 1975; Cohen, 1973; Graziano, 1975; O'Leary and Wilson, 1975; Patterson, 1973); and retarded (Bijou, 1973; Graziano, 1975; O'Leary and Wilson, 1975; Tavormina, 1975), and adults classified as: antisocial (Cohen and Filipczak, 1971; O'Leary and Wilson, 1975; Yates, 1970); retarded (Forehand and Baumeister, 1976; O'Leary and Wilson, 1975; Yates, 1970); neurotic (Marks, 1975; O'Leary and Wilson, 1975; Wolpe, 1973; Yates, 1970); and psychotic (Allyon and Azrin, 1968; Kazdin, 1975a, b; Lewinsohn, 1975; O'Leary and Wilson, 1975; Yates, 1970).

The following is a categorization of the areas of possible application of behavioral technology in social work practice. Each application has substantial empirical support. A further elaboration of theory, research, and illustrations of the application of the techniques is available in *Behavioral Social Work* (Wodarski and Bagarozzi, 1979).

Children and Adolescents

Foster Care   Development of behavioral management programs and appropriate parenting skills for both natural and foster parents. Training parents of children to use contingency contracts, stimulus control, and time-out procedures to facilitate their development of social skills needed for effective adult functioning.

Schools   Helping decrease absenteeism; increasing appropriate academic behavior, such as reading comprehension, vocabulary development, and computational skills; increasing interpersonal skills, such as the ability to share and cooperate with other children and adults; and decreasing disruptive behavior.

Juvenile Courts   Helping decrease deviant behavior and increase prosocial behavior by contingency contracting, programming significant adults to provide reinforcement for prosocial behavior, developing programs for training children in those behavioral skills that will allow them to experience satisfaction and to gain desired reinforcements through socially acceptable means.

Community Centers   Helping children develop appropriate social skills, such as working together, participating in decision making, making and discussing plans, and successfully carrying plans through.

Outpatient Clinics   Helping clients reduce anxiety, eliminate disturbing behavioral problems, define goals in terms of career and lifestyle, increase self-esteem, gain employment, solve problems (both concrete and interpersonal), develop satisfying life styles, and learn skills necessary for successful adult functioning in society.

Adults

Family Service   Helping in the development of marital interactional skills for effective problem-solving and goal-setting behaviors, development of better parenting behaviors, and development of clearer communication structures to facilitate interaction among family members.

Community Mental Health Centers   Helping individuals reduce anxieties through relaxation techniques. Teaching self-control to enable clients to alter certain problem-causing behaviors. Offering assertiveness training as one means of having personal needs met. Helping in the acquisition of behaviors to facilitate interaction with family, friends, and co-workers.

Psychiatric Hospitals   Using token economies to help clients acquire necessary prosocial behaviors for their effective reintegration into society. Structuring clients' environments through provision, by significant others, of reinforcement for the maintenance of appropriate social behaviors, such as self-care, employment, and social interactional skills. Analogous emphasis is indicated for working with the retarded in institutions.

Public Welfare   Helping clients achieve self-sufficiency, learn effective child management and financial management procedures, and develop social behaviors, skills and competencies needed to gain employment.

Corrections   Using token economies to increase prosocial behaviors, to learn new job skills, and to develop self-control and problem-solving strategies that are not antisocial.

Cross-Cultural Learning: Approaching Living and Working in a Rural Area

This aspect of training will be of utmost importance to the rural trainee who is not indigenous to the area in which he or she will practice. The training module is based on the one developed for Peace Corps volunteers by Vittilow et al. (1980).

A successful move to working in rural community mental health depends upon the learning of new, appropriate habits and unlearning old ones, and the recognition that learning to live and work in the rural area takes time.

Training for the rural worker is designed so that the student works in groups of five or six trainees using a workbook with basic didactic material and a number of exercises. A facilitator is assigned to each group to help in expanding and interpreting the exercises during discussion periods. Ideally, the facilitator is a person from the rural area in which the trainees will practice.

The layout of the workbook is as follows:

1. Historical encounters of people of different cultures, positive and negative
2. Learned attitudes from childhood about strangers and individuals who are different
3. Past experience in one culture, personal needs, and the tasks of satisfying old needs in new ways
4. Development of a problem list
5. Response to a new culture through cultural shock, feedback, and over identification
6. Development of a plan for action (Vittilow et al., 1980)

Following this cultural sensitization training, rural "experts" from the area in which the trainees are going are brought in to offer basic how-to's for work in the area. Key points stressed are:

1. How to define the rural culture and differing groups who are a part of it
2. How to assess the area as to where people go for services, alliances and conflictual relationships, power structures (formal and informal)
3. What is annoying about newcomers (M. R. Reul, personal communication)
4. Looking at the rural area in terms of family dynamics:
   a. Seeing the area as a large family with certain alliances, rivalries and roles
   b. Interdependence on other agencies and groups in that area
   c. Censoring of criticism (Everyone is related by marriage, work situation, etc.)
   d. Identification with rural area versus the larger metropolitan or academic community
5. How to establish credibility and learn the ropes:
   a. Finding a mentor
   b. Making community contacts

c. Utilizing local ideas in programming efforts (M. Daniels, personal communication)

THE RURAL MENTAL HEALTH WORKER
AS AN AGENT OF SOCIAL CHANGE

"The intent of the community mental health program to alter the existing balance of social forces requires that mental health workers act as agents of social change, a role outside their traditional repertoire" (Jones, Robin, and Wagenfield, 1974, p. 78). Ginsberg (1969) supports this in suggesting that a rural worker who knows how to get things done is extremely valuable to his or her community. His definition of getting things done includes helping to build and mobilize a constituency, securing legislation in the State or the United States Congress, and helping local institutions become more powerful in the administrative and regulatory affairs of the State and Federal governments.

In training rural workers for this community development role, there should be basic understanding of the necessary conditions for change, the process involved in implementing change, and the most important aspect, the effects of change on individuals, families, and communities involved in the process (Reul, 1972).

One model for community development has been suggested by Reul (1972). In using this model the rural worker in his or her social planning role can look at the various alternatives of conditions remaining as they are, closing the gaps in present human needs, and at the growth toward human and natural resource potential.

In training rural workers to evaluate their efforts in social planning, Reul (personal communication) suggests that the worker not only appreciate the rural culture but strive to preserve it. The 1960s initiated the age of sameness as rural residents began watching the same television shows, building the same types of shopping centers featuring the same brand of products, getting the same movies, living in the same ranch style houses, and having the same conversations on the same subjects as their urban counterparts who saw the same television news broadcast at the same time. Rural workers must evaluate their own interests in the rural area maintaining its uniqueness and not just being unwittingly stamped into sameness.

Rural social planners have a formidable task. It is their job to be aware not only of the mental health of the individual but of the community as a whole (Jones, Wagenfield, and Robin, 1976). In the rural community mental health training project students defined a service need, designed a system to meet that need, and secured the requisite political and financial support.

SUMMARY

This chapter reviews the practicum experience in terms of getting to know the rural community and appropriate training exercises to help prepare for rural community mental health practice. Topics center on the worker practicing autonomously, maintaining a great deal of flexibility, recognizing and working within the rural power structure, becoming established as a trustworthy person, quickly building relationships, role-juggling, and working with clients in a helping fashion—all of which demand innovation on the part of the worker.

A training program has been set forth that can be tailored to meet the needs of those who are in graduate social work programs. The skills providing the focus for the program are communication skills, techniques of interviewing, recognition of psychiatric disorders, counseling strategies, advanced training in interpersonal treatment technologies, medication monitoring, cultural sensitivity, and evaluation of one's role in social change.

The specified program can assist in the preparation of the practitioner for rural mental health practice. It can best assist the person who enters into training with a desire to work in the rural setting, who meets people easily, and who is flexible. Appendix A contains the syllabi for the three practicum courses which include course objectives, outlines of topics covered, simulation exercises, performance criteria, and suggested readings.

REFERENCES

Aguilera, D. C., Messick, J. M., and Farrell, M. S. 1970. Crisis Intervention: Theory and Methodology. C. V. Mosby Co., St. Louis.

Anthony, W. A., and Carkhuff, R. R. 1977. The functional professional therapeutic agent. In A. S. Gurman and A. M. Razin (eds.), Effective Psychotherapy. Pergamon, New York.

Aquizap, R. B., and Vargas, E. 1970. Technology, power, and socialization in Appalachia. Soc. Casework 51:131–139.

Augelli, A. R., Danish, S. J., Hauer, A. L., and Conter, J. J. 1980. Helping Skills: A Basic Training Program. 2nd Ed. Sciences Press, New York.

Ayllon, T., and Azrin, N. 1968. The Token Economy. Appleton-Century-Crofts, New York.

Barnouw, V. 1973. Culture and Personality. The Dorsey Press, Homewood, Ill.

Barrett-Lennard, G. T. 1962. Dimensions of therapist response as causal factors in therapeutic change. Psychol. Monogr. 43:Whole No. 562.

Bates, V. E. 1980. Developing a comprehensive community helping system in a rural boom town: A potential for informal helping. Paper presented at the Council on Social Work Education Annual Program Meeting, March, Los Angeles.

Berg, L. 1975. Knowledge, skills and values essential to social work practice in community mental health. In Community Mental Health in Social Work Education, Southern Regional Educational Board, Atlanta, Ga.

Bijou, S. W. 1973. Behavior modification in teaching the retarded child. In C. E. Thoreson (ed.), Behavior Modification in Education. The University of Chicago Press, Chicago.

Braukmann, C. J., and Fixsen, D. L. 1975. Behavior modification with delinquents. In M Herson, R. M. Eisler, and P. M. Miller (eds.), Progress in Behavior Modification Vol. 1. Academic Press, New York.

Browning, R., and Stover, D. O. 1971. Behavior Modification and Child Treatment. Aldine-Atherton, Chicago.

Buxton, E. B. 1973. Delivering social services in rural areas. Public Welfare, 31:15–20.

Caplinger, T. E., Feldman, R. A., and Wodarski, J. S. 1978. Agents of Social Control:

Pro-social and Anti-social Peer Groups. Paper presented at 9th World Congress of Sociology, August, Uppsala, Sweden.

Carkhuff, R. R. 1969. Helping and Human Relations. Holt, Rinehart and Winston, New York.

Carkhuff, R. R. 1971. Training as a preferred mode of treatment. J. Counsel. Psychol. 18:123–131.

Carkhuff, R. R. 1977. The functional professional therapeutic agent. In A. S. Gurman and A. M. Razin (eds.), Effective Psychotherapy. Pergamon, New York.

Carkhuff, R. R., and Berenson, B. G. 1967. Beyond Counseling and Therapy. Holt, Rinehart and Winston, New York.

Cohen, H. L. 1973. Behavior modification and socially deviant youth. In C. E. Thoreson (ed.), Behavior Modification in Education. The University of Chicago Press, Chicago.

Cohen, H. L., and Filipczak, J. 1971. A New Learning Environment. Jossey-Bass. San Francisco.

Evans, D. R., Hearn, M. T., Uhlemann, M. R., and Ivey, A. E. 1979. Essential Interviewing. Wadsworth Inc. Belmont, Calif.

Feldman, R. A., and Wodarski, J. S. 1974. Bureaucratic constraints and methodological adaptations in community-based research. Am. J. Commun. Psychol. 2:211–224.

Feldman, R. A., Wodarski, J. S., Goodman, M., and Flax, N. 1973. Pro-social and anti-social boys together. Soc. Work 18:26–37.

Fink, R. L. 1977. The role of mental health programs in rural areas. In R. K. Green and S. A. Webster (eds.), Social Work in Rural Areas. University of Tennessee School of Social Work, Knoxville, Tenn.

Firth, R. 1971. Applied anthropology. In L. D. Holmes (ed.), Readings in General Anthropology. Ronald Press Co., New York.

Forehand, R., and Baumeister, A. A. 1976. Deceleration of aberrant behavior among retarded individuals. In M. Hersen, R. M. Eisler, and P. M. Miller (eds.), Progress in Behavior Modification, Vol. 1. Academic Press, New York.

Gazda, G. M., Asbury, F. R., Balzer, F. J., Childers, W. C., and Walters, R. P. 1977. Human Relations Development: A Manual for Educators. 2nd Ed. Allyn and Bacon, Boston.

Ginsberg, L. H. 1969. Education for social work in rural settings. Soc. Work Educ. Rep. 9:28–32.

Graziano, A. M. (ed.). 1971. Behavior Therapy with Children. Aldine, Chicago.

Graziano, A. M. (ed.). 1975. Behavior Therapy with Children. Vol. 2. Aldine, Chicago.

Hall, E. T. 1969. The Hidden Dimension. Anchor Books, Garden City, N.Y.

Hall, E. T. 1973. The Silent Language. Anchor Books, Garden City, N.Y.

Hamblin, R. L., Buckholdt, D., Ferritor, D., Kozloff, M., and Blackwell, L. 1971. Humanization Process. John Wiley, New York.

Ivey, A. E. 1971. Microcounseling: Innovations in Interview Training. Charles C Thomas, Springfield, Ill.

Ivey, A. E., and Authier, J. 1978. Microcounseling: Innovations in Interviewing, Counseling, Psychotherapy, and Psychoeducation. Charles C Thomas, Springfield, Ill.

Jones, J. D., Robin, S. S., and Wagenfield, M. O. 1974. Rural mental health centers: Are they different? Commun. Ment. Health J. 14:77–92.

Jones, J. D., Wagenfield, M. O., and Robin, S. S. 1976. A profile of the rural community mental health center. Commun. Ment. Health J. 12:176–181.

Kazdin, A. E. 1975a. Behavior Modification in Applied Settings. The Dorsey Press, Homewood, Ill.

Kazdin, A. E. 1975b. Recent advances in token economy research. In M. Hersen, R. M. Eisler, and P. M. Miller (eds.), Progress in Behavior Modification, Vol. 1. Academic Press, New York.

Lewinsohn, P. M. 1975. The behavioral study and treatment of depression. In M. Hersen, R. M. Eisler, and P. M. Miller (eds..), Progress in Behavior Modification, Vol. 1. Academic Press, New York.

Lovaas, O. I., and Koegel, R. I. 1973. Behavior therapy with autistic children. In C. E. Thoreson (ed.), Behavior Modification in Education, Vol. 1. Academic Press, New York.

Margolies, P. J. 1977. Behavioral approaches to the treatment of early infantile autism: A review. Psychol. Bull. 84:249–264.

Marks, I. 1975. Behavioral treatments of phobia and obsessive-compulsive disorders: A critical appraisal. In M. Hersen, R. M. Eisler, and P. M. Miller (eds.), Progress in Behavior Modification, Vol. 1. Academic Press, New York.

Mermelstein, J., and Sundet, P. 1977. A teaching model for rural field instruction. In R. K. Green and S. A. Webster (eds.), Social Work in Rural Areas. University of Tennessee School of Social Work, Knoxville, Tenn.

Millar, K. 1977. Canadian rural social work. In R. K. Green and S. A. Webster (eds.), Social Work in Rural Areas. University of Tennessee School of Social Work, Knoxville, Tenn.

Neville, G. K. 1978. Marginal communicant: The anthropologist in religious groups and agencies. In E. M. Eddy and W. L. Partridge (eds.), Applied Anthropology in America. Columbia University Press, New York.

Nooe, R. M. 1977. A clinical model for rural practice. In R. K. Green and S. A. Webster (eds.), Social Work in Rural Areas. University of Tennessee School of Social Work, Knoxville, Tenn.

O'Leary, D. K., and Wilson, G. T. 1975. Behavior Therapy Applications and Outcome. Prentice-Hall, Englewood Cliffs, N.J.

Patterson, G. R. 1973. Reprogramming the families of aggressive boys. In C. E. Thoreson (ed.), Behavior Modification in Education. The University of Chicago Press, Chicago.

Patterson, G. R., Jones, R., Whitter, J., and Wright, M. A. 1965. A behavior modification technique for the hyperactive child. Behav. Res. Ther. 2:217–226.

Peters, L. H., and Rank, J. E. 1972. Techniques of Interviewing: A Programmed Text. Fort Sam Houston.

Perlman, H. H. 1957. Social Casework: A Problem-Solving Process. University of Chicago Press, Chicago.

Ramage, J. W. 1971. A basic philosophy in developing a rural mental health program. Public Welfare 29:475–479.

Reid, W. J. 1978. The Task Centered System. Columbia University Press, New York.

Research and Educational Association 1981. Handbook of Psychiatric Rating Scales. Research and Educational Association, New York.

Reul, M. 1972. A total community approach to rural development. In C. Moser (ed.), Manpower Planning for Jobs in Rural America. (Contract No. 82–26–71–44). Manpower Administration, U.S. Department of Labor, Washington, D.C.

Reul, M. R. 1974. Territorial Boundaries of Rural Poverty. Center for Rural Manpower and Public Affairs and the Cooperative Extension Service, Michigan State University, East Lansing, Mich.

Riggs, R. T., and Kugel, L. G. 1976. Transition from urban to rural mental health practice. Soc. Casework 57:562–567.

Rinn, R. C., and Vernon, J. C. 1975. Process evaluation of outpatient treatment in a community mental health center. J. Behav. Ther. Exper. Psychol. 6:5–11.

Tavormina, J. B. 1975. Relative effectiveness of behavioral and reflective group counseling with parents of mentally retarded children. J. Consult. Clin. Psychol. 43:22–31.

Tax, S. 1977. What do anthropologists do? In L. D. Holmes (ed.), Readings in General Anthropology. Ronald Press Co., New York.

Tranel, N. 1970. Rural program development. In H. Grunebaum (ed.), The Practice of Community Mental Health. Little Brown and Company, Boston.

Vitalo, R. L. 1975. Guidelines in the functioning of a helping service. Commun. Ment. Health J. 11:170–178.

Vittilow, D., Edwards, D., Pettit, J., and McCaffery, J. 1980. Approaching Living in a New Culture: A Workbook for Cross Cultural Learning.

Wells, R. A., and Miller, D. 1973. Developing relationship skills in social work students. Soc. Work Educ. Rep. 21:60–73.

Wodarski, J. S. 1979. Critical issues in social work education. J. Educ. Soc. Work 15:5–13.

Wodarski, J. S. 1980. Requisites for the establishment and implementation of competency based agency practice. Arete 6:17–28.

Wodarski, J. S., and Bagarozzi, D. A. 1979. A curriculum to train behavioral social workers. Behav. Ther. 2:19–21.

Wodarski, J. S., Feldman, R. A., and Pedi, S. J. 1976a. The comparison of anti-social and pro-social children on multi-criterion measures at summer camp. J. Abnorm. Child Psychol. 50:256–272.

Wodarski, J. S., Feldman, R. A., and Pedi, S. J. 1976b. The reduction of anti-social behavior in ten-, eleven-, and twelve-year-old boys participating in a recreational center. Small Group Behav. 7:183–196.

Wodarski, J. S., Filipczak, J., McCombs, D., Koustenis, G., and Rusilko, S. 1979. Follow-up on behavioral intervention with troublesome adolescents. J. Exp. Psych. Behav. Ther. 10:181–188.

Wodarski, J. S., and Pedi, S. J. 1977. The comparison of anti-social and pro-social children on multi-criterion measures at a community center: A three year study. Soc. Work 22:290–296.

Wolpe, J. 1973. The Practice of Behavior Therapy. Pergamon, New York.

Yates, A. J. 1970. Behavior Therapy. John Wiley, New York.

COURSE 1

Community Integration, Problem Identification, Assessment, and Planning of the Intervention

Course Description   Initially students complete the 3-weeks introduction to training segment. The remainder of the course centers on facilitating students in gaining information about the rural community in which they will practice. The course addresses what resources are available to solve a problem, such as other professionals; the role the student will take, including the integration process; and natural helping networks that will be employed in the intervention process. The course focuses also on helping the student isolate the power structure of the community, knowledge about the norms and folkways, the formal and informal communication patterns, organizational networks, social systems variables that influence the client, and how social work practice is perceived within the general community.

Course Objectives   Upon completion of this course, the student will be able to:

1. Understand the particular rural community in which the individual's practice endeavors will occur
2. Assess the folkways and the mores of the community and how they will influence practice endeavors
3. Isolate the social system components which play a major role in defining someone as needing help
4. Conceptualize the practitioner's role as change agent in terms of who should be the change agent
5. Make an initial assessment of client problems and plan interventions at the micro and macro levels

Outline of Topics

1. Getting to know the agency
2. Getting to know the community
3. Getting to know the community in terms of other services and professionals that are available
4. The feasible roles of social workers in the community
5. Integration procedures and activities
6. Assessment of client problems
7. Planning the intervention
8. Planning the evaluation of the intervention

Simulation Exercise   Students are required to do a community analysis in terms of the norms and the folkways of the community, isolation of natural helping networks, and the power structure of the community. They present their analysis to the field instructor and to other students. Additionally, students participate in an area event such as a picnic, church, or school activity and elucidate what they learned about the social style of the community.

Performance Criteria   By the end of this course the student should be able to:

1. Describe the attributes of the rural community and how they affect practice
2. Isolate significant problems in the community
3. Assess factors that are impinging upon these significant problems and the worker's ability to alter these problems in terms of energy and costs
4. Indicate what role they have in the change process
5. Plan requisite interventions based on the strongest theoretical and empirical rationale available
6. Plan adequate outcome criteria for said interventions

Texts

Collins, A. H., and Pancoast, D. L. 1978. Natural Helping Networks: A Strategy For Prevention. National Association of Social Workers, Washington.

Fischer, J. 1978. Effective Casework: An Eclectic Approach: McGraw Hill, New York.

Froland, C., Pancoast, D. L., Chapman, N. J., and Kimboko, P. J. 1981. Helping Networks and Human Services, Vol. 128. Sage Publications, Beverly Hills, Calif.

Green, R. K., and Webster, S. A. (eds.) 1982. Social Work in Rural Areas: Preparation and Practice. University of Tennessee School of Social Work, Knoxville, Tenn.

Reid, W. J. 1979. The Task Centered System. Columbia University Press, New York.

Wodarski, J. S. 1981. Role of Research in Clinical Practice. University Park Press, Baltimore.

Wodarski, J. S. 1983. Rural Community Mental Health Practice. University Park Press, Baltimore.

Articles

Gertz, B., Meider, J., and Pluckhan, M. L. 1975. Survey of rural community mental health needs and resources. Hosp. Commun. Psych. 26:816–818.

Winslow, W. W. 1982. Changing trends in CMHC's: Keys to survival in the eighties. Hosp. Commun. Psych. 33:273–277.

COURSE 2

Design and Implementation of Macro/Micro Intervention Programs

Course Description   The course centers on the implementation of an intervention for a problem that the student deems appropriate for alteration. Students first specify the variables, that is, biological, sociological, and psychological, controlling the phenomena of interest. Second, they isolate what variables can be altered and what energies and costs are involved in altering these variables. Third, they review criteria for choosing micro, macro, or a combination intervention to alter these variables. Fourth, they specify outcome an evluation may occur of the interventive attempt. Last, tenance procedures to ensure the continuance of the behavior is withdrawn.

Course Objectives   Upon completion of this course, students will be able to:

1. Assess a client problem situation in terms of micro and macro levels including psychological, sociological, and political factors impinging upon the client
2. Plan an intervention based on rational, theoretical knowledge
3. Conceptualize and implement the appropriate role of the change agent (This involves the role the worker will play in correspondence with significant others.)
4. Carry out the intervention in terms of beginning, intermediate, and advanced practice levels
5. Program strategies for the maintenance of the behavior
6. Collect data to evaluate how effective the intervention was.

Outline of Topics

1. Assessment of client problem
2. Delineation of micro/macro variables affecting the client's problem
3. Structuring of the intervention plan
4. Choosing the appropriate change agent
5. Developing adequate outcome criteria for the evaluation of the intervention plan
6. Executing the intervention plan
7. Programming for the maintenance of behavioral change
8. Collecting data which will help determine whether the plan was effectively carried out

Performance Criteria   The student should exhibit the ability to:

1. Specify a client problem
2. Specify variables impinging on the client's problem
3. Carry out requisite interventions
4. Evaluate those interventions

Texts

Cautela, J. R. (ed.) 1977. Behavior Analysis Forms for Clinical Intervention. Research Press, Champaign, Ill.

Feldman, R. A., and Wodarski, J. S. 1975. Contemporary Approaches to Group Treatment. Jossey-Bass, San Francisco.

Goldstein, A. P. 1973. Structured Learning Therapy: Toward a Psychotherapy for the Poor. Academic Press, New York.

Wodarski, J. S., and Bagarozzi, D. 1979. Behavioral Social Work. Human Sciences Press, New York.

Articles

Butcher, J. N., and Koss, M. P. 1978. Research on brief and crisis-oriented psychotherapies. In S. L. Garfield and A. E. Bergin (eds.), Handbook of Psychotherapy and Behavior Change: An Empirical Analysis. 2nd Ed. Wiley, New York.

Lorion, R. P. 1978. Research on psychotherapy and behavior change with the disadvantaged. In S. L. Garfield and A. E. Bergin (eds.), Handbook of Psychotherapy and Behavior Change: An Empirical Analysis. 2nd Ed. Wiley, New York.

COURSE 3

The Evaluation of Macro and Micro Programs

Course Description   The course centers on the student's evaluation of the programmed intervention and how to plan for the stabilization of new community programs that have been successful. During this part of the practicum the student continues to collect data, or data collection concludes. The student subsequently analyzes the data and comes to conclusions regarding whether or not said interventions were effective. If they were not effective, the student analyzes what factors were responsible for their ineffectiveness and plans a new intervention strategy with new outcome criteria.

Course Objectives   Upon completion of this course, the student will be able to:

1. Assess interventive attempts
2. Determine an appropriate time frame for conducting reliable and valid follow-up evaluations
3. Analyze data and relate it to the intervention
4. Make decisions on whether criteria used for the intervention evaluation are relevant and significant
5. Evaluate the intervention with the use of requisite statistical skills
6. Write up the intervention and subsequent data with appropriate conclusions
7. Plan another intervention if the one carried out was not successful and isolate variables that affected the unsuccessful evaluation
8. Understand the necessity for developing support structures in the community which will facilitate a program's maintenance
9. Understand the necessity of interpreting these findings to key individuals, groups, and officials in the community in order to offer them feedback and to ensure their support in the future
10. Understand the necessity for conducting periodic follow-up evaluations

Outline of Topics

1. Choice of outcome measures and means for assessment
2. Designs for daily practice evaluation
3. Application of statistical techniques in the evaluation of practice
4. Presentation of data in manuscript form
5. Interpretation of data
6. Deriving conclusions

Performance Criteria   The student should exhibit:

1. The ability to formulate outcome criteria
2. The ability to choose the strongest and most appropriate experimental design available
3. The ability to collect data
4. The ability to analyze the data

5. The ability to present the data in such a manner that specific conclusions can be supported
6. The ability to write up the study in manuscript form
7. The ability to derive conclusions about the intervention and subsequent interventions
8. The development of a professional attitude toward sharing one's findings with the community
9. The development of a professional attitude about receiving feedback from program recipients, community members, and other professionals
10. In cases in which the student's intervention attempts have been successful, the ability to carry out a component analysis of the program to discover precisely which aspects of the program contributed most to the program's overall effectiveness
11. The ability to plan for follow-ups and to prepare the community for such evaluation

Texts

Gottman, J. M., and Leiblum, S. R. 1974. How to Do Psychotherapy and How to Evaluate It. Holt, Rinehart & Winston, New York.

Hagedorn, H. J., Beck, K., Neubert, S., and Werlin, S. 1976. A Working Manual of Simple Program Evaluation Techniques for Community Mental Health Centers. Arthur D. Lettle, Inc., Cambridge, Mass.

Hersen, M., and Barlow, D. H. 1976. Single Case Experimental Designs: Strategies for Studying Behavior Change. Pergamon Press, New York.

Article

Jones, R. R. 1974. Design and analysis problems in program evaluation. In P. O. Davison, F. W. Clark, and L. A. Hamerlynck (eds.), Evaluation of Behavioral Programs in Community, Residential and School Settings: The Fifth Banff Research International Conference. Research Press, Champaign, Ill.

Chapter 9

Outcome Measures

Self and Behavioral

The term *competency* indicates an ability to demonstrate empirically that an individual possesses a certain skill. Depending upon the specified skill, evaluation can be conducted through means of: 1) videotapes of practitioner behavior; 2) inventories designed to measure specific academic and practice skills; 3) behavioral observations using time sampling procedures and critical incident reporting; and 4) structured and unstructured interviews with supervisors, clients, and seasoned agency practitioners. In all feasible instances, multicriterion measurement is utilized in order to provide for the assessment of the multidimensions of learning in the rural community mental health training program described here.

A COMPARISON OF COMPETENCY ASSESSMENT MECHANISMS

Videotaping student and worker interactions is the most rewarding evaluation mechanism in terms of capturing the richness of practice phenomena. Videotapes provide an excellent training medium through which beginning and established workers can learn competent practice behaviors through the observation of effective practitioners. Tapes provide a better medium through which client-worker interactions can be accurately recorded than do other means of evaluation. That is, they capture more verbal details, such as association and clustering of words, duration of utterances, number of interruptions, questions, summary and interpretative statements, and length of silent periods; and nonverbal details, such as posture, gestures, eye contact, and touching, than a worker can amass through traditional recording methods. Thus, with proper analysis, they can sharpen practice skills, can lead to an understanding of how behaviors exhibited by clients and workers influence their mutual interaction, and can illustrate how worker behaviors effect behavioral change in clients (Wodarski, 1976). Moreover, the recording of competent practitioners can reduce the length of time necessary to train inexperienced practitioners.

Behavioral observations are expensive in terms of cost of observers, energy involved in delineation of what behaviors should be observed and how, and the use of technical equipment necessary for accurate observation. However, they also capture the richness of clinical phenomena, and data they provide are highly reliable. Execution is facilitated when agencies have one-way mirrors and videotape equipment (Wodarski, 1975; Wodarski and Buckholdt, 1975).

Research has shown that interview schedules and self-inventories filled out by workers and/or clients are the least reliable of the evaluation methods. Therefore, they always should be checked with other measurement modes to ensure the data they are providing are consistent (reliable) (Wodarski, 1979).

SPECIFIC ASSESSMENT PROCEDURES
USED IN THE RURAL TRAINING PROJECT

In-Course Training Evaluation   Paper and pencil tests to assess the acquisition of academic knowledge were developed for each course in the educational curriculum relevant to the rural students. Pretesting of pre-entrance skills and posttesting of exit skills determine whether the curriculum materials have accomplished their objectives. For example, the trainees are asked to do a community analysis in terms of determining existing natural helping networks and how they can be used to enhance the mental health of community residents.

Practice Observation   As part of the training procedures, trainees are evaluated on relevant practice skills through audio and video tapes and by behavioral observations (protocols are contained within this chapter). Likewise, videotaping is used to provide reliability checks on the observational procedures and to provide feedback on implementation of practice training procedures.

Interviews and Attitude Testing   At designated times interviews are conducted with trainees, clients, supervisors, and agency executive personnel to assess the adequacy of the training experience. Such procedures facilitate any necessary modifications in the curriculum. Scales that measure interpersonal integration, concern for another's welfare, social values, self concept, self-disclosure, empathy, motivation to help others, critical personality attributes, anxiety, and need to help others are administered before the trainees commence their education, at the conclusion of training, and during follow-up to document the acquisition of competencies for practice in community mental health.

Follow-up   Several months after completion of training, trainees are contacted to determine what skills they are using that were acquired during their education. Also, observers are sent to their agencies to note which procedures are being used and how they are being used. These follow-up procedures provide data which are rarely available on the adequacy of training for professional careers but which nonetheless are necessary to ensure that relevant training experiences are provided in the future.

EDUCATIONAL OUTCOME MEASURES

Testing of any educational program must include adequate outcome measures. The measures used in this training program consist, basically, of self-inventories that purport to measure attributes necessary for effective practice, behavioral observation of student practice endeavors, and a content analysis, in terms of forms filled out by students and field work instructors and diaries kept by the students.

Self-Measures

After extensive review of the literature it was determined that the self measurement package should include the following fourteen scales as they measure the skills necessary for effective rural community mental health practice.

Internal-External Locus of Control This measure is a test of an individual's perception of the amount of control one believes one has over one's environment (Rotter, 1966). It measures the extent to which a person assigns responsibility for the occurences of favorable and unfavorable outcomes to the individual (that is, to internal causes) as compared to forces in the environment (that is, to external causes). The respondent is asked to endorse one of two paired alternatives, one of which is an "internal" and the other an "external" statement. Scores can range from zero (most internal) to 23 (most external). Statements indicative of internal control are: "Trusting to fate has never turned out as well for me as making a decision to take a definite course of action" and "In my case, getting what I want has little or nothing to do with luck." Statements indicative of external control are: "I have often found that what is going to happen will happen" and "Many times we might just as well decide what to do by flipping a coin." Test-retest reliability is reported by Rotter (1966), depending upon time interval and samples, from 0.49 to 0.83. Internal consistency estimates reported ranged from 0.65 to 0.79. Additional data suggest the inventory has sufficient convergent validity.

Rationale Student practitioners who work in rural settings in which there is little supervision, structure, or direction will need to exert more self-directed behavior in order to be effective in rural communities. Additionally, the practitioner needs to believe he or she can have an effect on the client and community and have the ability to communicate this expectation to the clients. Therefore, one might expect practitioners who are more internally controlled to perform more successfully in such settings.

Social Responsibility Scale The Social Responsibility Scale is composed of eight items scored according to a Likert scale format (Berkowitz and Lutterman, 1968). Four items are worded in the responsible direction, and the remaining four items are worded in the opposite direction. There are five response options, from strongly agree through strongly disagree. Typical items for which agreement would mean accepting social responsibility to help another individual are: "Every person should give some of his time for the good of his town or country'' and ''I feel bad when I have failed to finish a job I promised I would do.'' Agreement with the following statements, however, would indicate that a person feels little responsibility for others: ''Letting your friend down is not so bad because you can't do good all the time for everybody'' and ''People would be a lot better off if they would live far away from other people and never have to do anything with them'' (Berkowitz and Lutterman, 1968). This conclusion was based upon the data that high scores were more inclined not to deviate from the political traditions of their class and community.

Rationale   This measure is directly related to basic values of the profession, that is, concern for the person's welfare and the community.

Ascription of Responsibility for Another's Welfare   The Schwartz (1968) scale focuses on the differences in individuals' tendencies to take responsibility for the welfare of others. Respondents are asked to agree or disagree with a series of 20 stimulus statements. Half of the 20 statements are worded in such a way that agreement indicates ascription of responsibility to the self, whereas the other half are worded in such a way that agreement would mean that responsibility for others' welfare does not lie with oneself. Agreement with the following sample statement indicates acceptance of responsibility for another's welfare by the respondent: ''If a good friend of mine wanted to injure an enemy of his/hers, it would be my duty to try to stop him/her'' and ''Even if something you borrow is defective, you should still replace it if it gets broken.'' Agreement with the following sample items, however, would indicate the respondent's denial of responsibility for another: ''As long as a businessperson doesn't break laws, he/she should feel free to do his/her business as he/she sees fit'' and ''When you have a job to do it is impossible to look out for everybody's best interest.'' Schwartz (1973) reports internal consistency to range from 0.78 to 0.81.

Rationale   This measure, along with the two preceding, are related directly to social work values and ethics, and can measure the socialization process of students enrolled in a graduate social work program.

Social Values Test   This test consists of 40 items contained in a Social Attitudes Questionnaire. These items are intended to assess the positions of individuals on 10 relatively independent dimensions of social values. These values are believed to be of relevance throughout American society. They are of particular concern to those whose interests are directed toward general social welfare, such as social workers, teachers, clergy, and similar professions. Value positions, and quite often value conflicts, with regard to each of these dimensions are discussed throughout the ideological literature of such professions. In some instances a position is stated explicitly as part of the value premises of the profession.

In the following descriptions of the social value dimensions, drawn largely from McLeod and Meyer (1967, pp. 402–405), the first-named pole refers to a value position frequently set forth in the social work literature. The second-named pole is considered a contrasting position and, therefore, one unlikely to be accepted by professional social workers.

1. Public aid *versus* private effort
2. Personal freedom *versus* societal controls
3. Personal goals *versus* maintenance of group
4. Social causation *versus* individual autonomy
5. Pluralism *versus* homogeneity
6. Secularism *versus* religiosity
7. Self-determination *versus* fatalism
8. Positive satisfaction *versus* struggle denial
9. Social protection *versus* spiral redistribution
10. Innovation change *versus* traditionalism

The reliability of the test is indicated by the extent of adequate correlation within dimensions and by the stability of the clusters when the responses of two rather large samples of different respondents, such as social work majors versus business majors, on the same items are compared.

Rationale   This is the most extensively used inventory to assess social work values in the literature. These values are of direct concern to those professionals whose specific interests are directed toward social welfare professions such as teaching, social work, clergy, and so forth.

Index of Self-Esteem   The Index of Self Esteem (ISE) was designed as a 25-item category partition scale that purports to measure the evaluative components of self concept (Hudson and Proctor, 1977). Approximately half of the items were structured as positive statements, and the remainder were negatively worded in order to reduce or eliminate any response set by the client; scale items were ordered with the use of a table of random numbers. The ISE is self administered, contains minimal instructions, consists of a single page with items on each side, and can be completed in 3 to 5 minutes—rarely does the respondent need more than 7 minutes to complete the scale. The observed test-retest reliability was 0.92, which coincided with the mean corrected split-half reliability. Additional data indicate that the scale has high face, discriminant, and construct validity as a measure of self esteem.

Rationale   Moderate levels of self confidence are considered necessary for an individual to implement interpersonal helping skills (Corrigan et al., 1980; Wodarski, 1981).

Self-Disclosure Questionnaire   This is a 60-item questionnaire classified into six related groups: attitudes and opinions, tasks and interests, work (or studies), money, personality, and body (Jourard, 1971). It measures the amount and content of self-disclosure to target persons in the above areas. This is obtained by the use of a 4-point rating scale ranging from ''Have told the other person nothing about this aspect'' to ''Have hidden or misrepresented myself . . . ,'' for each of the five designated target persons for all the 60 questions. Thus, the questionnaire provides scores for self-disclosure for both target persons, such as mother, father, male friend, female friend, and spouse, and in certain areas, such as work and personality. A reliability test, using the odd-even method, produced a correlation of 0.94. Further examination of the instrument by Jourard (1971) showed that this method of assessment has validity.

Rationale   One indicator of a healthy personality is the ability to accurately portray oneself to others. Furthermore, the development and establishment of interpersonal skills of warmth, unconditional positive regard, empathy, and genuineness, necessary to build and maintain therapeutic relationships, are positively associated with self-disclosure. Research on psychotherapy has shown that client change will be facilitated by workers who use an appropriate number of self-disclosing statements (Johnson and Matross, 1977).

Recognition Assessment-Empathy (RA-E)   This measure is a pencil-and-paper inventory designed to measure a person's capacity for discrimminating the best empathic response from a given number of responses (*Administrator's Manual: RA-E,* 1975). This instrument is a forced-choice situational measure with four possible "helping" responses for each of 20 client statements. As such, it does not reflect or measure actual use of empathy in a helping relationship; rather, it reflects empathic sensitivity. Considering the previous research suggesting the utility of written measures for assessing change at an intitial level, the RA-E seemed an appropriate instrument (Gantt, Billingsley, and Giordano, 1980).

The RA-E is also an independent instrument that has been examined for reliability (test-retest correlation of 0.77 and 0.73) and for which national norm groups (based on testing of 1,000 persons) were available (*Administrator's Manual: RA-E,* 1975). Finally, it provides an economical standardized test for comparing different groups over extended periods of time.

Rationale   Accumulated research indicates that empathy is a necessary interpersonal skill for the successful implementation of social treatment models (Lambert, DeJulio, and Stein, 1978).

Hogan Empathy Scale   Empathy, the intellectual or imaginative apprehension of another's condition or state of mind, helps us understand moral development (Hogan, 1969). This 64-item self-report measure of empathy was constructed by comparing the responses of groups with high-and low-rated empathy. Of the 64 items on the test, 31 came from the California Psychological Inventory, 25 from the Minnesota Multi-Phasic Personality Inventory, and the remaining eight came from various experimental testing forms used in studies at the Institute of Personality Assessment and Research at Berkeley. By taking the moral point of view, a person is said to consider the consequences of his or her actions for the welfare of others.

The norms for the test are given for various groups from psychology majors rating high at 44.7, to young delinquents rating low at 29.1.

With a sample of 50 college undergraduates the reliability of the empathy scale, estimated by a test-retest correlation after a 2-month interval, was 0.84.

Rationale   The rationale is the same as for the Recognition Assessment-Empathy Scale.

Helping Skills Questionnaire   The scale consists of 16 excerpts that involve five responses to problems made by helpers (Carkhuff, 1980, 1981). Respondents are asked to formulate the most helpful or most effective responses that they would make to each of these expressions. They are asked to be as helpful as they can in communicating understanding and providing new direction for the helpees. Workers are asked to formulate responses directly, just as they would if they were talking with the helpee. The person presenting the problems is to be considered the helpee with whom one comes in contact in daily practice. Helpees are simply people who seek help at a time of need. In formulating responses, respondents are instructed to assume that they have been interacting with the helpees for some time before they presented the problems.

The instructions for administering the questionnaire are as follows: "The following 16 excerpts involve a number of responses that a helper might make to problems presented by persons with these concerns. In response to each excerpt there are five helper responses. Rate these responses from 1 to 5 as follows:

1 = Very ineffective—No understanding or direction.
2 = Ineffective—No understanding, some direction.
3 = Minimally effective—Understanding, no direction.
4 = Effective—Understanding and direction.
5 = Very effective—Understanding and specific direction."

Rationale   Accumulated research indicates skills of genuineness, nonpossessive warmth, and accurate empathic understanding are considered necessary for one to be an effective interpersonal helper (Wodarski, 1981).

Eysenck Personality Questionnaire (EPQ)   The EPQ measures three orthogonally independent dimensions of temperament: Extraversion-Introversion (E); Neuroticism-Stability (N); and Psychoticism or toughmindedness (P) (Eysenck and Eysenck, 1975). These dimensions are regarded as reflecting the major variance in the personality domain. The adult form of the EPQ consists of 90 items; 21 measuring E, 23 measuring N, 25 measuring P, and 21 providing data for the falsification scale. Individuals who score high on the E scale tend to be outgoing, impulsive, uninhibited, have many social contacts, and often take part in group activities. In contrast, the introvert tends to be quiet, retiring, and studious. High N scores indicate strong emotional stability and over-activity. High scorers may tend to develop neurotic disorders when under stress, which fall short of neurotic collapse. Persons with high P scores show a propensity toward making trouble for others, belittling, acting disruptively, and lacking in empathy. High scorers display tendencies toward developing psychotic disorders, while falling short of the actual psychotic conditions.

Reliability coefficients for the EPQ are determined both on test-retest investigations and on internal consistency studies, and have proved to be satisfactory in supporting the instrument as a reliable personality inventory with reliabilities lying in the 0.80 to 0.90 range.

Rationale   It has been posited that good emotional adjustment is necessary for a worker to be an effective interpersonal helper (Garfield, 1977).

Personality Scale of Manifest Anxiety   This 28-item questionnaire was based upon two assumptions: first, that variation in the level of internal anxiety of the individual is related to emotionality, and second, that the intensity of this anxiety could be ascertained by a paper-and-pencil test consisting of items describing what have been called overt or manifest symptoms of this state (Taylor, 1953). For example, items include such statements as "I am often sick to my stomach," "I wish I could be as happy as others," and "I am the kind of person who takes things hard."

A reliability test based on the test-retest scores showed a product-moment correlation of 0.88.

Rationale   A high level of anxiety does not facilitate the interpersonal helping process (Berzins, 1977).

The Gottesfeld Community Mental Health Critical Issues Test   The Gottesfeld Community Mental Health Critical Issues Test is an instrument to determine an individual's or group's standing on six major issues in the community mental health field. The categories are: 1) *Community Context,* these issues involve work directly in the community in which the community determines the needs and staff operate openly with community members; 2) *Radicalism,* rapid and drastic changes in mental health services should occur. Mental health services should be controlled by citizens and aimed at reaching the masses; 3) *Traditional Psychotherapy,* emphasis on psychotherapy and long-term treatment modeled after private practice; 4) *Prevention,* aimed at reducing the incidence of mental problems with emphasis on crisis intervention, identification of incipient problems, and consultations with human service agencies; 5) *Extending the Definition of Mental Health,* develop new areas for study from traditional diagnostic categories; and 6) *Role Diffusion,* professional roles are not restricted and new means of delivering service are employed (Gottesfeld, 1974).

The questionnaire consists of 12 questions in each of the six areas described above for a total of 72 questions.

When tested for reliability with 200 mental health workers in various mental health facilities, the instrument showed high internal consistency for all issues with a range of 0.86 to 0.95.

Rationale   This assessment scale is directly related to the major conceptual foci of the training program (Auerbach and Johnson, 1977).

Fundamental Interpersonal Relations Orientation-Feelings Scale (FIRO-F)   The FIRO-F is a self-report questionnaire designed to assess a person's need for inclusion, control, and affection in various aspects of interpersonal situations, such as feelings toward others (Schutz, 1978).

In the FIRO-F, separate subscales are constructed to assess each of the three needs (inclusion, control, and affection). The subscales assess each need separated for each of two modes of expression: expressed, what is done or felt toward others, and wanted, what is wanted of others. The subscales contain nine single-statement items, each of which is to be answered on a 6-point scale. Each item is keyed dichotomously and scoring results in high internal consistency of the keyed responses to the items in each subscale. There are no data on reliability.

Rationale The needs to show affection and to be close to individuals facilitate interpersonal helping; whereas, the desire to control others is detrimental to the interpersonal helping process (Parloff, Waskow, and Wolfe, 1978).

Rokeach Dogmatism Scale The primary purpose of this scale is to measure individual differences in openness or closedness of belief systems (Rokeach, 1960, 1980).

The Rokeach Dogmatism scale consists of 40 items to which the participant can respond in one of six ways from "I agree very much" to "I disagree very much." Sample items are: "A person who does not believe in some great cause has not really lived," and "Once I get wound up in a heated discussion I just can't stop." The Rokeach Dogmatism Scale was found to have a reliability of 0.81 for the English Colleges sample and 0.78 for the English worker sample.

Rationale This personality attribute is posited to relate to the ability to accept individual differences, a basic value premise of the profession (Friedlander and Apter, 1974).

Behavioral Measures

An extensive analysis of research literature occurred before choosing the behavioral measure profile for the training program. It is evident that research and the theoretical literature has centered at best on one of five worker attributes such as eye contact, number of questions, disclosures, number of interpretations, and summary statements. It was believed desirable to develop a general behavioral profile of interpersonal skills that are basic to the application of advanced micro and macro practice technologies (Larsen and Hepworth, 1978; Marshall, Charping, and Bell, 1979; Shulman, 1978). The data for these assessments were derived from two videotape interviews in which students were given a specific role to enact with another student. Student pairs were counterbalanced, that is, one initially played the role of client and subsequently switched to play the role of the worker. Typical roles included the alcoholic with a history of work problems, partners in marital breakup, and an individual losing a close relative. Measurement occurred before the student entered the field and at the conclusion of the 9-month field experience. Behavioral assessments were organized around five foci: verbal skills, nonverbal skills, verbal and nonverbal congruence, relationship-building skills, and higher order interpersonal helping skills.

Verbal Skills

Requisite to implementation of micro and macro practice technologies are adequate verbal skills, that is, the ability to communicate to the client the steps involved in the practice endeavor, to build the relationship, and to facilitate the influence attempt. The following basic verbal skills are measured:

1. Restatement
2. Open questions
3. Closed questions
4. Information giving
5. Minimal encouragement
6. Approval-reassurance
7. Directives
8. Reflection
9. Interpretation
10. Confrontation
11. Self-disclosure
12. Silence
13. Complex verbal responses

The Hill Counselor Verbal Response Category System (HCVRCS) was used to measure these verbal skills (Hill, 1978; Hill, Thames, and Rardin, 1979; Hill, Reed, and Charles, 1980): It consists of 14 nominal, muturally exclusive categories for judging worker verbal behavior: minimal encouragement, approval-reassurance, information, direct guidance, closed question, open question, restatement, reflection, nonverbal referent, interpretation, confrontation, self-disclosure, silence, and other. On a transcript of a session, each counselor response unit is judged by three persons as belonging in one of the 14 categories. In the two previous studies, agreement levels between judges were high (Kappas averaged 0.79 in Hill (1978), and 0.71 in Hill et al. (1979)). The system has acceptable face and content validity.

Speech Disfluencies   A significant variable seems to be the worker's ability to convey credibility regarding his or her abilities and treatment techniques. Studies indicate that workers can show credibility through being organized, providing structure in the client's and worker's role in therapy, suggesting appropriate topics for beginning discussions, and engaging in proper verbal and nonverbal communication; that is, being attentive, leaning toward the client, having responsive facial expressions and appropriate head nods, and maintaining an attentive posture (Corrigan et al., 1980; Schmidt and Strong, 1970). To measure verbal credibility the Mahl's Non-Ah Speech Disturbance Ratio (Mahl, 1956, 1963) was used, which seems to be the most reliable and widely used instrument for objectively measuring speech anxiety. Speech disturbances fall into seven categories:

1. Sentence change
2. Repetition
3. Stutter
4. Omission

5. Sentence incompletion
6. Tongue slip
7. Intruding incoherent sounds

Such things as "ah," sighs, silences, laughter, and figures of speech such as "you know" are not counted as anxiety. The ratio is a percentage of number of disturbances divided by the total number of words spoken by the counselor.

Higher Order Verbal Skills   Extensive research has been conducted that shows therapeutic attractiveness is increased if workers indicate to clients that verbal statements are being received and processed accordingly (Duehn and Proctor, 1977). The worker can signal that messages have been received through appropriate verbal statements and through nonverbal means, such as proper eye contact. These operations signify to the client that the worker has been listening, a rewarding process that should increase the probability of continuance in the relationship (Seabury, 1980). These component variables are conceptualized as *verbal congruence*. The foregoing would suggest again the efficacy of homogeneous grouping of clients and workers, especially in regard to language capacity and corresponding antecedents such as age and social class. Should a given treatment modality favor heterogeneous groupings, this postulate, at the minimum, would point to the desirability of pretherapy tutoring or coaching for selected clients and/or workers. (See Rosen and Lieberman (1972) for a discussion of the measurement process of verbal congruence.)

Content relevance refers to the extent to which the content of interactive response is perceived by participants as relevant and admissable to their own definition of the interactional situation. It can be postulated that the presentation of expected content in an interactional situation is likely to be highly reinforcing to all concerned and, consequently, the situation itself will be evaluated positively by the participants. This postulate has been supported by much social work literature concerning the compatibility between role expectations held by clients and therapists (Aronson and Overall, 1966; Mechanic, 1961; Oxley, 1966; Rosen and Lieberman, 1972; Rosenfeld, 1974; Sapolsky, 1970; Thomas, Polansky, and Kounin, 1967). (See Rosen and Lieberman (1972) for a discussion of the measurement process.)

Amount of speech was measured by obtaining a percentage of the number of words spoken by the trainee divided by the total number of words spoken in each client-worker session. The word count included the number of complete words, excluded incomplete words, distinct sounds caused by stuttering, incoherent sounds, and "ahs" (Hill, Charles, and Reed, 1981). Research indicates that the more active the worker is initially, the more successful is therapy (Goldstein, 1980).

Nonverbal Skills

Congruent nonverbal skills are considered essential to effective communication. A recurring theme throughout the research in nonverbal communication in counseling/psychotherapy is the degree of consistency between verbal and nonverbal channels of communication (Barrett-Lennard, 1962; Graves and Robinson,

1976; Tepper and Haase, 1978). Congruence is operationalized as consistency of response between verbal and nonverbal behavior. If some persons are more skilled than others in interpreting and communicating nonverbal messages, then this has implications for the selection of counselors for training and perhaps for the selection of clients for specified types of counseling. The following items were assessed through the use of the Profile of Nonverbal Sensitivity (PONS) (Hall et al., 1978; Rosenthal et al., 1974) Adequate reliability and validity have been demonstrated for this instrument.

1. Eye contact
2. Facial expressions
3. Body expression
   a. Body lean
   b. Legs
   c. Head nod
   d. Arms
   e. Hands
   f. Mouth
4. General body movement to indicate relaxed or anxiety level
5. Posture
6. Interpersonal space
7. Gestures and mannerisms
8. Total physical activity level
9. Voice
   a. Volume
   b. Rate

Verbal and Nonverbal Congruence

The definition of congruence used for this measure was Roger's (1957): "Congruence is a state in which feelings the counselor is experiencing are available to him/her, available to his/her awareness, that he/she is able to live these feelings, be them in the relationship, and be able to communicate them" (p. 90). For purposes of this study, it was assumed that this definition would hold for students. It was believed also that this definition would best be operationalized by allowing each student to rate his or her own experiences of congruence. Videotapes were made of student pairs described on page 228. Affect within the session was ascertained using a recall method, modeled after Kagan's (Kagan, Krathwohl, and Farquhar, 1965) Interpersonal Process Recall. A series of five standardized questions were asked for each 1-minute segment of replayed videotape. A 1-minute time period was used (based on a pilot experiment) so that the segment was long enough to judge congruence, yet not so long as to contain several affects. Student pairs were asked the following five questions: 1) What was your major feeling during this segment? 2) What feelings were you expressing through your words? 3) What feelings were you expressing through your voice tone? 4) What feelings were you expressing through your movements, facial expressions, and/or gestures? 5) What do you believe the other person was feeling in this segment? Each of these five questions was answered by recording 1 of the 13 categories on the Affect Adjective Checklist (Gazda, 1973; McNair, Lorr, and Droppleman, 1971; Zuckerman and Lubin, 1965). Adjectives were included on the checklist categorized as follows: calm-relaxed, happy-joyful, vigorous-active, competent-powerful, concerned-caring, respectful-loving, tense-anxious, sad-depressed, angry-hostile, tired-apathetic, confused-bewildered, criticized-ashamed, and inadequate-weak. Congruence was then operationalized as a consistency of response between two or more of the five questions; the same affect had to be recorded for congruence to be scored for any given minute. Five types of congruence were identified from the responses to the five questions: verbal congruence (consistency between Questions 1 and 2); paralinguistic congruence (consistency between Questions 1 and 3); kinesic congruence (consistency between Questions 1 and 4); intracongruence (consistency between Questions 1, 2, 3, and 4); intercongruence (consistency between Questions 1 and 5).

Relationship-Building Skills

Proponents of different therapeutic approaches disagree on many points. There is general consensus, however, that one potent treatment variable is the relationship formed between therapist and client (Goldstein et al., 1966). Many theorists have conceptualized this crucial treatment variable at a high level of abstraction but few have been able to conceptualize "relationship" in an operational and discrete manner. From a social learning perspective, however, Rosen (1971) has viewed the relationship between two or more individuals as an interactional situation that consists of a series of behavioral exchanges or, more specifically, of stimulus-response exchanges. At any point during their ongoing interaction either participant can draw upon a large pool of potential behaviors. Every behavior enacted by the worker or the client is considered to have certain cost and reward characteristics for each participant and, consequently, the interaction between any two behaviors results in its own unique cost and reward outcomes for each participant (Thibaut and Kelley, 1959). Likewise, any prolonged series of behavioral exchanges produces differing net cost and reward balances for the therapist or client(s). Although these outcomes, or differential results of social interaction, may vary for each individual, they influence crucial facets of treatment such as relationship formation, continuance, and involvement in the therapeutic process. The following skills were considered critical in the establishment, maintenance, and termination of therapeutic relationships.

1. Empathy
2. Warmth
3. Genuineness
4. Respect
5. Concreteness

6. Immediacy of the relationship
7. Activity level
8. Anxiety
9. Self composure and confidence
10. Trust
11. Expertness
12. Attractiveness

For measurement of these relationship-building skills see Byrne, 1961; Gazda et al., 1977; Ivy and Authier, 1978; Truax and Carkhuff, 1967.

Higher Order Skills

A substantial body of research indicates that a worker can influence a client's future verbal behavior, such as the number of utterances, pauses between verbal exchanges, rates of speech, number of interruptions, length of silence between verbal exchanges, and length of verbal statements. Hence, if a worker wishes to increase any of these behaviors, he or she should model them (Matarazzo and Saslow, 1968; Matarazzo and Wiens, 1977; Salzinger, 1969) and engage in other behavioral increasing activities, such as shaping and selective reinforcement, that is, reinforcing the client's closer approximation to the desired behaviors. For example, if a relevant treatment goal is to increase the client's rate of utterances the worker can reinforce the client's appropriate verbal responses to achieve this objective and model such behavior. However, virtually no investigators have looked at the pattern of an interview. Thus, the last focus of the assessment aspect of the training program consisted of the general category of skills called higher order communication skills. These are:

1. Timing of specific verbal communications
2. Appropriateness of the intervention
3. Managing course of treatment, that is, how and when to increase or decrease the intensity of treatment and appropriately planning for termination based on accurate assessment

The supervisor filled out a global scale weekly assessing these help qualities.

Other Data Sources

Students also kept diaries in which they indicated positive and negative events that influenced their educational experiences. Each day they were to briefly summarize the experiences. If no positive or negative experiences occurred, no entry was made. Traditional learning service plans and field instructors' evaluations also provided descriptive data on the activities in which they were engaged. Additionally, an attempt was made to implement on a pilot basis consumer assessment of practice endeavors. Inventories used are listed below.

  Barrett-Lennard Relationship Inventory (BLRI) The BLRI (Barrett-Lennard, 1962) measures perceptions of counselor-offered empathy, regard, congruence, and unconditionality of regard. There are 64 items (16 on each scale), each of which is rated on a 6-point scale (from −3 to +3). Split-half reliability of the scales ranges from 0.82 to 0.96. Content validation was established by counselor rating of the valence of the items; only those items were retained for which experienced counselors had full agreement as to the positive or negative valence.

Counseling Evaluation Inventory (CEI)   The CEI (Linden, Stone, and Schertzer, 1965) measures counseling climate, satisfaction with counseling, and counseling comfort. The measure consists of 19 randomly ordered items, each rated on a 5-point scale. Discriminative validity has been established for the three scales and the total score, using counselor trainees' practicum grades as a criterion. Total test-retest reliability ranges from 0.62 to 0.83.

Counselor Rating Form (CRF)   The CRF (Barak and LaCrosse, 1975) measures clients' perceptions of counselors' expertise, attractiveness, and trustworthiness. A total score combines the three scales. The total measure contains 36 randomly ordered 7-point bipolar items, with 12 items on each scale. Split-half reliability for the three dimensions, based on a normative group of undergraduates, ranges from 0.75 to 0.92.

SUMMARY

This chapter elucidates the various measurement techniques that were utilized to assess the training outcomes of the rural community mental health training program. Literature reviews led to the isolation of the chosen measurement processes. This chapter presents only a beginning in regard to the type of measurements that can be utilized to assess trainee acquisition of appropriate interpersonal skills. The future will probably witness the alteration and modification of this package to increase its strength in assessing competencies. As such alterations occur, the probability will be increased that educators can be more confident that students are acquiring the competencies necessary for effective practice.

REFERENCES

Administrator's Manual: RA-E 1975. Learning Designs, Toronto.

Aronson, H., and Overall, B. 1966. Treatment expectations of patients in two social classes. Soc. Work 11:35–41.

Auerbach, A. H., and Johnson, M. 1977. Research on the therapist's level of experience. In A. A. Gurman, and A. M. Razin (eds.), Effective Psychotherapy. Pergamon Press, New York.

Barak, A., and LaCrosse, M. B. 1975. Multidimensional reception of counselor behavior. J. Counsel. Psychol. 22:471–476.

Barrett-Lennard, G. T. 1962. Dimensions of therapist response as causal factors in therapeutic change. Psychol. Monogr. 43:No. 562.

Berkowitz, L., and Lutterman, K. 1968. The traditionally socially responsible personality. Public Opin. Q. 32:169–185.

Berzins, J. I. 1977. Therapist-patient matching. In A. A. Gurman and A. M. Razin (eds.), Effective Psychotherapy. Pergamon Press, New York.

Byrne, D. 1961. Interpersonal attraction and attitude similarity. J. Abnorm. Soc. Psychol. 62:713–715.

Carkhuff, R. R. 1980. Art of Helping IV. Human Resource Development Press, Amherst, Mass.

Carkhuff, R. R. 1981. Art of Helping. IV Student Workbook. Human Resource Development Press, Amherst, Mass.

Corrigan, J. P., Dell, D. M., Lewis, K. N., and Schmidt, L. E. 1980. Counseling as a social influence process: A review. J. Counsel. Psychol. 27:395–441.

Duehn, W. D., and Proctor, E. K. 1977. Initial clinical interaction and premature discontinuance in treatment. Am. J. Orthopsych. 47:284–290.

Eysenck, H. J., and Eysenck, S. B. 1975. Eysenck Personality Questionnaire, Test Manual. Educational and Industrial Testing Service, San Diego, Calif.

Friedlander, W., and Apter, R. Z. 1974. Introduction to Social Welfare. Prentice-Hall, Inc., Englewood Cliffs.

Gantt, S., Billingsley, D., and Giordano, J. 1980. Paraprofessional skills: Maintenance of empathic sensitivity after training. J. Counsel. Psychol. 4:27.

Garfield, S. L. 1977. Research on the training of professional psychotherapists. In A. A. Gurman and A. M. Razin (eds.), Effective Psychotherapy. Pergamon Press, New York.

Gazda, G. M. 1973. Vocabulary of Affective Adjectives in Human Relationship Development: A Manual for Educators. Allyn & Bacon, Boston, Mass.

Gazda, G. M., Asbury, F. R., Balzer, F. J., Childers, W. C., and Walters, R. P. 1977. Human Relations Development: A Manual for Educators. 2nd Ed. Allyn & Bacon, Boston.

Goldstein, A. P. 1980. Relationship-enhancement methods. In F. H. Kanfer and A. P. Goldstein (eds.), Helping People Change. Pergamon Press, New York.

Goldstein, A. P., Heller, K., and Sechrest, L. B. 1966. Psychotherapy and the Psychology of Behavior Change. John Wiley, New York.

Gottesfeld, H. 1974. The Gottesfeld Community Mental Health Critical Issues Test, Test Manual. Behavioral Publications, Inc., New York.

Graves, J. R., and Robinson, J. D. 1976. Proxemic behavior as a function of inconsistent verbal and nonverbal messages. J. Counsel. Psychol. 23:333–338.

Hall, J. A., Rosenthal, R., Archer, D., DiMatteo, M. R., and Rogers, P. L. 1978. Profile of nonverbal sensitivity. In P. McReynolds (ed.), Advances in Psychological Assessment, Vol. 4. Jossey-Bass, San Francisco.

Hill, C. E. 1978. Development of a counselor verbal response category system. J. Counsel. Psychol. 25:461–468.

Hill, C. E., Charles, D., and Reed, K. G. 1981. A longitudinal analysis of changes in counseling skills during doctoral training in counseling psychology. J. Counsel. Psychol. 28:428–436.

Hill. C. E., Reed, K., and Charles, D. 1980. Manual for Hill Counselor Verbal Response Category System. Unpublished manuscript. University of Maryland.

Hill, C. E., Thames, T. B., and Rardin, D. R. 1979. Comparison of Rogers, Perls, and Ellis on Hill Counselor Verbal Response Category System. J. Counsel. Psychol. 26:198–203.

Hogan, R. 1969. Development of an empathy scale. J. Consult. Clin. Psychol. 33:307–316.

Hudson, W. W., and Proctor, E. K. 1977. Assessment of depressive affect in clinical practice. J. Consult. Clin. Psychol. 45:1206–1207.

Ivy, A. E., and Authier, J. (eds.) 1978. Microcounseling. 2nd Ed. Charles C Thomas, Springfield, Ill.

Johnson, D. W., and Matross, R. 1977. Interpersonal influence in psychotherapy: A social psychological view. In A. A. Gurman, and A. M. Razin (eds.), Effective Psychotherapy. Pergamon Press, New York.

Jourard, S. 1971. The Transparent Self. D. Van Nostrand, New York.

Kagan, N., Krathwohl, D. R. and Farquhar, W. W. 1965. Interpersonal Process Recall: Simulated Recall by Videotape. Educational Research Series, No. 24. Bureau of Educational Research, Michigan State University, East Lansing, Mich.

Lambert, M. V., DeJulio, S. S., and Stein, D. M. 1978. Therapist interpersonal skills: Process, outcome, methodological considerations, and recommendations for future research. Psychol. Bull. 85:467–489.

Larsen, J., and Hepworth, D. H. 1978. Skill development through competency-based education. J. Educ. Soc. Work 14:73–81.

Linden, J. D., Stone, S. C., and Schertzer, B. 1965. Development and evaluation of an inventory for rating counselors. Personnel Guidance J. 43:267–276.

McLeod, D. L., and Meyer, H. J. 1967. The values of social workers. In E. J. Thomas, (ed.), Behavorial Science for Social Workers pp. 401–416. Free Press, New York.

McNair, D. M., Lorr, M., and Droppleman, L. F. 1971. Profile of Mood Manual. Educational and Industrial Testing Service, San Diego, Calif.

Mahl, G. F. 1956. Disturbances and silences in the patient's speech in psychotherapy. J. Abnorm. Soc. Psychol. 53:13.

Mahl, G. F. 1963. The lexical and linguistic levels in the expression of the emotions. In P. H. Knapp (ed.), Expression of the Emotion in Man. International University Press, New York.

Marshall, E. K., Charping, J. W., and Bell, W. J. 1979. Interpersonal skills training: A review of the research. Soc. Work Res. Abstr. 15:10–16.

Matarazzo, J. D., and Saslow, G. 1968. Speech and silent behavior in clinical psychology. In J. Shlien, H. Hunt, J. Matarazzo, and C. Savage (eds.), Research in Psychotherapy. American Psychology Association, Washington, D.C.

Matarazzo, J. D., and Wiens, A. N. 1977. Speech behavior as an objective correlate of empathy and outcome in interview and psychotherapy research: A review with implications for behavior modifications. Behav. Modif. 1:453–480.

Mechanic, D. 1961. Role expectations and communication in the therapist-patient relationship. J. Health Hum. Behav. 2:190–198.

Oxley, G. B. 1966. The caseworker's perceptions and client motivation. Soc. Casework 47:432–438.

Parloff, M. B., Waskow, I. E., and Wolfe, B. E. 1978. Research on therapists variables in relation to process and outcome. In S. L. Garfield and A. E. Bergin (eds.), Handbook of Psychotherapy and Behavior Change: An Empirical Analysis. 2nd Ed. John Wiley & Sons, New York.

Rogers, C. R. 1957. The necessary and sufficient conditions of therapeutic personality change. J. Consult. Psychol. 21:95–103.

Rokeach, M. 1960. The Open and the Closed Mind. Basic Books, New York.

Rokeach, M. 1980. Some unresolved issues in theories of beliefs, attitudes, and values. In M. Page (ed.), Nebraska Symposium on Motivation, pp. 261–304. University of Nebraska Press, Lincoln.

Rosen, A. 1971. Client-worker relationship: A conceptualization. J. Consult. Clin. Psychol. 38:329–337.

Rosen, A., and Lieberman, P. 1972. The experimental evaluation of interview performance of social workers. Soc. Sci. Rev. 46:395–412.

Rosenfeld, J. M. 1974. Strangeness between helper and client: A possible explanation of non-use of available professional help. Soc. Serv. Rev. 38:17–25.

Rosenthal, R., Archer, D., Koivumaki, J. H., DiMatteo, M. R., and Rogers, P. L. 1974.

Assessing sensitivity to nonverbal communications: The PONS test. Pers. Soc. Psychol. Bull (APA Division 8):1–3.

Rotter, J. B. 1966. Generalized expectancies for internal versus external control of reinforcement. Psychol. Monogr. 80:No. 609.

Salzinger, K. 1969. The place of operant conditioning of verbal behavior in psychotherapy. In C. Frank (ed.), Behavior Therapy: Appraisal and Status. McGraw-Hill, New York.

Sapolsky, A. 1970. Relationship between patient-doctor compatibility, mutual perception, and outcome of treatment. J. Abnor. Psychol. 17:115–118.

Schmidt, L. D., and Strong, S. R. 1970. Expertness and influence in counseling. J. Counsel. Psychol. 17:81–87.

Schutz, W. 1978. The Interpersonal Underworld. Consulting Psychologists Press, Inc., Palo Alto, Calif.

Schwartz, G. E. 1973. Biofeedback as therapy: Some theoretical and practical issues. Am. Psychol. 28:666–673.

Schwartz, S. H. 1968. Words, deeds and the perception of consequences and responsibility in action situations. J. Pers. Soc. Psychol. 10:232–243.

Seabury, B. A. 1980. Communication problems in social work practice. Soc. Work, 25:40–43.

Shulman, L. 1978. A study of practice skills. Soc. Work, July:274–280.

Taylor, R. A. 1953. A personality scale of manifest anxiety. J. Abnorm. Psychol. 48:285–290.

Tepper, D. T., and Haase, R. F. 1978. Verbal and nonverbal components of facilitative conditions. J. Counsel. Psychol. 25:35–44.

Thibaut, J. W., and Kelley, H. H. 1959. The Social Psychology of Groups. John Wiley, New York.

Thomas, E. J., Polansky, N. A., and Kounin, J. 1967. The expected behavior of a potentially helpful person. In E. J. Thomas (ed.), Behavioral Science for Social Workers. Free Press, New York.

Truax, C. B., and Carkhuff, R. R. 1967. Toward Effective Counseling and Psychotherapy Training and Practices. Aldine, Chicago.

Wodarski, J. S. 1975. Use of videotapes in social work. Clin. Soc. Work J. 3:120–127.

Wodarski, J. S. 1976. Procedural steps in the implementation of behavior modification programs in open settings. J. Exp. Psych. Behav. Ther. 7:133–136.

Wodarski, J. S. 1979. Requisites for the establishment, implementation, and evaluation of social work treatment programs. J. Sociol. Soc. Welfare 6:339–361.

Wodarski, J. S. 1981. Role of Research in Clinical Practice. University Park Press, Baltimore.

Wodarski, J. S., and Buckholdt, D. 1975. Behavioral instruction in college classrooms: A review of methodological procedures. In J. M. Johnson (ed.), Behavior Research and Technology in Higher Education. Charles C Thomas, Springfield, Ill.

Zuckerman, M., and Lubin, B. 1965. Multiple Affect Adjective Checklist Manual. Educational and Industrial Testing Service, San Diego, Calif.

Chapter 10

Competency-Based Education for Rural Community Mental Health Practice

Implications

Previous chapters elucidate the program for training social work students for practice in rural community mental health. The chapters center on conceptual foci of the curriculum, definition of practice competencies, and measurement of these competencies. In this chapter project findings are reviewed in terms of the implications for training social workers for rural community mental health practice and for competency-based education in general.

THE EVALUATION OF CONTENT AREAS FOR RURAL COMMUNITY MENTAL HEALTH PRACTICE

Primary data for the assessment of the adequacy of content areas are based on interviews with students and field instructors, and their evaluations of learning objectives are used to document the relevance of predetermined competencies. Student and field instructor interviews and evaluations were conducted at the end of each quarter during the program and thereafter during follow-up periods which occurred approximately 8 months after graduation.

The two data sources revealed information that confirmed posited competencies for effective preparation for rural practice, and provided more information on academic content and practice skills that are being incorporated in further development of the program. Information in three major categories emerged: professional acceptance and practice in rural areas; competencies that were predetermined to be relevant in the practice setting; and expansion and addition of competencies that would further professional practice in rural areas.

Acceptance

Acceptance in the rural setting is a prerequisite for effective practice. Many co-workers are para-professionals, and the degree of formal professional training is minimal. Students, therefore, were expected to show flexibility in accepting tasks and to "take it slow with no big words." Socialization and orientation were informal and unsystematic, that is, over coffee, at community social events such as picnics, and church suppers and so forth. As anticipated, students reported that clients and other community citizens were suspicious of mental health services. It was soon evident that acceptance for female practitioners was more difficult than for males. This is not surprising in light of the fact that professional roles in rural America traditionally are assigned to males. In general, findings are consistent with the characteristics of rural practice identified in Chapter 1. Toward the end of the project a substantial amount of time was spent preparing students for practice in rural communities.

Competencies

Previously specified knowledge and skills competencies initially deemed essential were confirmed by the investigators. The primary focus of most practicum experiences was direct practice and clinical services. Although administrative program planning and supervisory tasks were included, students were seen as less prepared for these macro-level tasks. This may be due to the inadequate delineation of tasks between bachelor's- and master's-level workers; that is, bachelor's-level personnel serving as primary providers of direct services and master's-level workers providing the supervision and consultation to ensure the quality of services provided. As rural agencies employ more bachelor's- and master's-level workers, differentiation of roles should be facilitated.

It was difficult for students to apply knowledge regarding labeling theory. Application of labeling theory may require a greater sophistication in how the power structure influences decision making regarding client groups, that is, who should be a candidate for service, type of behaviors and attributes that facilitate the labeling process, and the types of services clients will receive.

Although the area of deinstitutionalization received no direct ratings, related information emerged. The specific aspects related to deinstitutionalization that were expected of students are knowledge of psychotropic medication for community maintenance, knowledge concerning the assessment of attributes of the individual and his or her environment to ensure the probability of successful placement, and involvement with other community agencies in cooperative efforts to maintain the client in the community.

Regarding the implementation of change strategy, students could not differentiate their roles from those of associate-level or bachelor's-level workers. The idea that competencies should be on a continuum did facilitate the delineation of tasks for each level of worker. Students also could not provide a rationale for the duration of practice. Initially, they could not specify the criteria upon which termination of the treatment would be based. The process of specifying criteria in treatment termination was facilitated by having the student define concretely their practice objectives.

The prevention competency was not practiced to any extent that would allow for evaluation. Rural mental health practice in the prevention modes is virtually nonexistent. Furthermore, prevention activity outcome is typically difficult to document. The program did start the students thinking about preventive activities, and thus influenced practitioners in the agencies.

In the development of the training program, seven general practice skills were predetermined as being relevant to rural practice. The following conclusions were reached regarding the acquisition of these skills by trainees. Students' interpersonal skills were consistently rated as excellent. Skills in macro-level intervention, the ability to define the target of change, and the ability to determine the level on which change should be delivered were all rated as sufficient. Students were not typically provided the opportunity to choose the change agent, which usually was determined by the administration, location and availability of workers, as was the determining of where treatment should be provided. However, students did assess whether these attributes of the practice delivery system were adequate and how they affected their practice endeavors. Evaluation of treatment outcome initially received little attention. Field instructors' emphasis on this competency received increasing attention as the project progressed.

Expansion and Addition of Competencies

Additional competencies that became evident as necessary are as follows. There was an obvious need to increase short-term treatment knowledge and skills which would lay the foundation for the acquisition of knowledge of advanced treatment technologies. The majority of treatment expectations of clients focused on concrete solutions occurring within a limited time perspective, thus indicating the need for knowledge of task-centered casework (Reid, 1978). General interpersonal skills were expected as a base for all areas of practice and as a foundation for advanced practice. Students were involved in educational groups, therapeutic groups and maintenance groups, and requisite skills in conducting groups were expected. Students were inadequately prepared for such practice interventions as the appropriate applications of advanced interpersonal treatment technologies. Subsequently, practicums were altered to provide the necessary knowledge and intensive training experiences (see Chapter 8).

It had been anticipated that the modification of skills would be necessary to deliver services to specialized target groups. All students reported that half their caseloads were violence related, and alcohol abuse was present in the same number of cases. Two other target groups emerged, older adults, who were frequently served in nursing homes, and multi-problem families. Readings and clinical instruction were increased in all areas to alleviate these deficiencies.

Trainees needed additional preparation for the adequate management and treatment of chronic mental health clients, many of whom were deinstitutionalized and exhibited suicidal predilections. Knowledge of psychotropic medication and criteria for determination of reinstitutionalization were lacking.

A serious deficiency was the lack of medical backup for rural settings and a concurrent lack of medical knowledge. Students identified such macro-level skills as case coordination and public relations as necessary for effective practice.

Additional information was provided by field instructors in response to open-ended questions in the evaluations. Students were seen as having a firm base in human behavior but lacking in knowledge of a variety of treatment modalities. The apparent lack of formal preparation in group dynamics and group treatment was most frequently mentioned deficiency. Field instructors felt also that students should have been stronger in their knowledge of psychotropic medication, alcohol problems, and family dynamics. More preparation in administration, supervision, and program planning were seen as areas for curriculum emphasis in the future.

CRITICAL ISSUES IN COMPETENCY-BASED EDUCATION

Initial Levels of Competence

More concrete criteria must be developed as to when students are ready to practice in terms of knowledge, interpersonal skills, and practice skills levels. Levels of competence should be differentiated, such as the ability to initiate field work, readiness for graduation, and independent practice. The prepractice training experiences reviewed in Chapter 8 alleviated one of the major difficulties of practicum at the different agencies, that is, the variety of practice techniques in which trainees have to exhibit competency. Through the intensive training package which provided a basic level of knowledge and skills, students were adequately prepared to carry out requisite tasks. Differentiation of competencies will ensure that quality services are provided to clients by indicating what levels of supervision and consultation should be provided a worker.

Theoretical knowledge and acquisition of necessary practice skills should be assessed and demonstrated to be adequate through appropriate testing techniques before field practice. Before beginning an interventive process with a client, the worker should review a tape of a client or read a contrived case, make a diagnosis, design a corresponding intervention plan with specified outcomes and related means to measure said outcomes, and specify how the success of the plan will be evaluated. These should be accomplished to the satisfaction of the practicum instructor (Wodarski, 1980).

Securing Faculty and Student Agreement Regarding Evaluation

One of the most critical aspects of developing a competency-based education model is to secure professional agreement regarding the requisite competencies and their evaluation. Educators frequently will have concerns about stringent evaluation procedures that are deemed necessary. These concerns can be alleviated by providing rationale for the evaluation, by having faculty participate in the evaluation process, and in choosing items for evaluation, through indicating the types of procedures that will be evaluated, and through joint decisions regarding mechanisms for the evaluation. Professionals desiring to utilize evaluation may have to be prepared to provide rationale as to its benefits and to answer such questions as: Could evaluation be detrimental to the formation of the relationship between client and student? Will as much improvement take place in the client as would occur if evaluation procedures were omitted? And, finally, can the data be used to discredit my professional endeavors (Feldman and Wodarski, 1974; Wodarski and Feldman, 1974)?

Students, too, must be assured that the evaluation will not be used to criticize any one person or to portray anyone in a negative light, but will be implemented to provide him or her the necessary feedback on practice behavior to improve services provided to clients and to develop more adequate methods of education. One technique for reducing the amount of anxiety over being evaluated is to have all participants, including faculty and students, participate in the evaluation. Likewise, students should participate with faculty in the choice of criteria used in the evaluation of performances, for example, the amount of client improvement, and the means of evaluation, that is, video- and/or audiotaping, behavioral observation, interview schedules, and/or self-inventories. What will be evaluated, and how, must be clearly outlined before the initiation of evaluation procedures. It should be kept in mind, too, that evaluation procedures are most readily executed when they are unobtrusive and guarantee anonymity and/or confidentiality. To facilitate the acceptance of the evaluation procedures in the project described here, all of the foregoing procedures were employed (Wodarski, 1981).

Specific factors that may lead to the ready acceptance of evaluation in the educational environment include the administration's support of the use of evaluation to improve practice, the encouragement offered by individuals implementing the evaluation procedures, the professional manner employed by those executing the process, and the inclusion of the project's staff requisite job performance in the evaluation.

The review of competency must be handled in the most professional manner possible. Criticism offered in a positive manner can lead to improved practice; criticism offered in a degrading manner would not enable one to tap the potential in the use of these procedures to improve practice.

How the evaluation process is executed and how various professionals utilize the information for improving practice skills will depend upon developing mutual relationships among individuals using the data. These relationships should be characterized by mutual trust, sharing, respect, encouragement, and acceptance with the goal being the improvement of services provided to clients.

Use of Evaluation Data to Improve Practice

Adequate baseline data on practice competencies will provide the information needed to facilitate the development of a competency-based practice. After collection of baseline data, steps are taken to build or bolster initial competencies. Field supervision should be provided in such a manner that it will help the trainee alter dysfunctional practice behavior. Such a process should include:

1. Pinpointing the trainee's behaviors that need to be altered
2. Measuring the frequency of such behaviors
3. Developing a program to alter the behavior
4. Providing the trainee with feedback on targeted behaviors

Videotaping client and trainee interactions should facilitate isolation of those behaviors that need to be altered and likewise provide the opportunity for practicum instructors to reinforce the trainee's favorable practice behavior.

Cost

One cannot negate the cost involved in implementing a competency-based practice. Videotaping behavior, behavioral observation, and even administration of interview schedules and self-inventories are costly (Gamson, 1979; Wodarski, 1979b). The cost should be offset, however, by the benefits clients derive from effective practice and the increased ability of social work educators to document the relevance of the activities. Testing of theoretical knowledge is costly in terms of time and energy to construct inventories in a reliable and valid manner. Likewise, keeping the assessment current is a major investment. Pilot data indicate, however, the costs may well be worth it. Cummins and Arkava (1979), at the University of Montana, found a higher correlation between their competency exam and job performance ratings than with any other education aspect measured. Although this is encouraging, the authors are quick to point out that it is far from being a perfect predictor of later job success. The validity coefficient of 0.42 accounts for just under 18% of the variance of job performance scores. It is precisely more of this type of research design and data that are needed to relate competency-based education to job requisites.

Politics

One of the major issues in implementing a competency-based practice model is securing agreement on the criteria that will be used to assess educational outcome. These criteria are usually tied to theories of human behavior. Such theories and how they relate to practice effectiveness must be evaluated. Perhaps the one criteria that can be utilized universally concerning the effectiveness of a theory and the practice behaviors derived is whether it produced desired outcomes in client behaviors (Fischer, 1971, 1978; Wodarski, 1979a; Wodarski and Feldman, 1973).

A critical question involves the number of competencies necessary to ensure an adequate evaluation of a student's practice skills. Currently the number of competencies measured is massive. It is probable that future research will elucidate those competencies that are paramount to the preparation of social workers and will thus reduce the number and complexity of the measuring processes needed to ensure practice standards.

Research on the Instructional Process

There has been a minimal research effort to date to measure the effectiveness of the various instructional methodologies employed in social work practice. Briar (1973) called for the use of 20% of all social services budgets to conduct research on the effectiveness of social work practice. These funds could be used to seek answers to the following critical questions: What functions should social workers be educated to perform upon graduation? How are social work skills acquired? What are the qualities of the competent social work educator that facilitate student acquisition of knowledge? How are social work skills maintained? (Dwyer, 1976; Feldman, 1972; Grinnell and Kyte, 1976; Linnard and Greenwald, 1974; Miller, 1972; Radin, 1976; Seidl, 1973; Thomlison and Seidl, 1974). Another imminent question involves the parameters that affect the acquisition of new knowledge by social work educators and practitioners. Knowledge development is meaningless if only a few social workers utilize it. Answers to these questions will be difficult in terms of money, effort, time, and so forth but will provide a rationale for social work education (Wodarski, 1981).

SUMMARY

This text elucidates the conceptual, practice and methodological foci that guided the 5-year rural community mental health project. From the information received, considerable revision of the curriculum, with expansion and addition of competencies, is indicated. The exact roles of bachelor's- and master's-level social workers must be further delineated. Further conceptualizations and knowledge gains through research are needed in the areas of family violence, alcohol problems, problems of the elderly, group dynamics, multi-problem families, psychotropic medication, operation of criminal justice systems in rural areas, and rural culture. Regarding practice skills, more preparation seems necessary in individual and group advanced treatment techniques, administration, program planning, and community and public relations.

It is evident that the role of research in social work education will increase dramatically at all degree levels with initial training in the relevance of research in practice occurring at the baccalaureate level (Baer and Federico, 1978). An educational delivery system will include courses taught on the basis of the available empirical knowledge, the practice techniques derived from a verifiable empirical base, and the relevant practice issues that can be resolved through research. More faculty will engage in research relevant to practice and will move away from knowledge development without purpose. Moreover, students and beginning practitioners will begin to substantially integrate research findings into practice endeavors.

This prototype for the evaluation of a training program provides the opportunity to alter the program and thus ensure its future relevance in training practitioners for rural practice. Moreover, it illustrates how research can be used to provide students the education they need to prepare for effective practice.

REFERENCES

Baer, B. L., and Federico, R. 1978. Educating the Baccalaureat Social Worker: Report of the Undergraduate Social Work Curriculum Development Project. Ballinger Publishing Company, Cambridge, Mass.

Briar, S. 1973. The age of accountability. Soc. Work 18:114.

Cummins, D. E., and Arkava, M. L. 1979. Predicting posteducational job performance of BSW graduates. Soc. Work Res. Abstr. 15:33.

Dwyer, M. S. 1976. Mastering change in education: Involving others in educational change. Educ. Technol. 16:12.

Feldman, R. A. 1972. Towards the evaluation of teaching competence in social work. J. Educ. Soc. Work 8:5–15.

Feldman, R. A., and Wodarski, J. S. 1974. Bureaucratic constraints and methodological adaptations in community-based research. Am. J. Community Psychol. 2:211–224.

Fischer, J. 1971. A framework for the analysis and comparison of clinical theories of induced change. Soc. Serv. Rev. 45:110–130.

Fischer, J. 1978. Does anything work? J. Soc. Serv. Res. 1:215–243.

Gamson, Z. 1979. Understanding the difficulties of implementing a competence-based curriculum. In G. Grant et al. (eds.), On competence: A critical analysis of competency-based reforms in higher education. Jossey-Bass, San Franciso.

Grinnell, R. M., and Kyte, N. S. 1976. Measuring faculty competence: A model. J. Educ. Soc. Work 12:44–50.

Linnard, M. W., and Greenwald, S. R. 1974. Student attitudes, knowledge, and skill related to research training. J. Educ. Soc. Work 10:48–54.

Miller, R. I. 1972. Evaluating Faculty Performance. Jossey-Bass, San Francisco.

Radin, N. 1976. Follow-up of social work graduates. J. Educ. Soc. Work 12:103–107.

Reid, W. J. 1978. The Task-Centered System. Columbia University Press, New York.

Seidl, F. W. 1973. Teaching social work research: A study in teaching method. J. Educ. Soc. Work 9:71–77.

Thomlison, R. J., and Seidl, F. W. 1974. An experiment in curriculum innovation in graduate social work education. J. Educ. Soc. Work 10:93–98.

Wodarski, J. S. 1979a. Requisites for the establishment, implementation and evaluation of social work treatment programs. J. Sociol. Soc. Welfare 6:339–361.

Wodarski, J. S. 1979b. Critical issues in social work education. J. Educ. Soc. Work 15:5–13.

Wodarski, J. S. 1980. Requisites for the establishment and implementation of competency based agency practice. Arete 6:17–28.

Wodarski, J. S. 1981. Role of Research in Clinical Practice. University Park Press, Baltimore.

Wodarski, J. S., and Feldman, R. 1973. The research practicum: A beginning formulation of process and educational objectives. Int. Soc. Work 16:42–48.

Wodarski, J. S., and Feldman, R. 1974. Practical aspects of field research. Clin. Soc. Work J. 2:182–193.